ULTRASOUND OF THE PEDIATRIC ABDOMEN AND PELVIS

ULTRASOUND OF THE PEDIATRIC ABDOMEN AND PELVIS

A CORRELATIVE IMAGING APPROACH

HOOSHANG KANGARLOO, M.D.
Assistant Professor of Radiology
Chief, Section of Pediatric Radiology
University of California, Los Angeles, School of Medicine

W. FRED SAMPLE, M.D. (deceased)
Associate Professor of Radiology
Chief, Section of Ultrasound and CT Body Scanning
University of California, Los Angeles, School of Medicine

YEAR BOOK MEDICAL PUBLISHERS, INC.
CHICAGO•LONDON

Library of Congress Cataloging in Publication Data

Kangarloo, Hooshang.
　Ultrasound of the pediatric abdomen and pelvis.
　Includes index.
　1.　Pediatric gastroenterology – Diagnosis.
2.　Pediatric urology – Diagnosis.　3.　Diagnosis, Ultrasonic.　4.　Abdomen – Diseases – Diagnosis.
5.　Pelvis – Diseases – Diagnosis.　I.　Sample, William Frederick, 1939 – 1979 joint author.　II.　Title.
[DNLM: 1.　Abdomen.　2.　Pelvis.　3.　Diagnosis – In infancy and childhood.　4.　Ultrasonics – Diagnostic use.　WS310 K16u]
RJ449.U45K36　　　617'.55'0754　　　79 – 25906
ISBN 0 – 8151 – 4972 – 7

Dedicated to two great teachers,
W. Fred Sample
and
Leo G. Rigler

CONTRIBUTING AUTHORS

GARY M. AMUNDSON, M.D.
Assistant Professor of Pediatric Radiology
University of California, Los Angeles, School of Medicine
(Coauthor of Chapters 2–10)

DENNIS A. SARTI, M.D.
Assistant Professor of Radiology
Chief, Section of Ultrasound and CT Body Scanning
University of California, Los Angeles, School of Medicine
(Contributor to Chapter 1)

GAIL C. HANSEN, M.D.
Co-Director of Ultrasound Division
Los Angeles County Olive View Medical Center
(Contributor of text for Chapters 11–14)

DONALD A. ROSE, M.D.
Fellow in Nuclear Medicine
University of California, Los Angeles, School of Medicine
(Contributor of nuclear medicine studies)

Preface

EVALUATION OF DISEASE PROCESSES in the abdomen and pelvis requires a thorough understanding of the various imaging modalities available for assessment of pathological states. Recent advances in ultrasonography and computerized tomography have made it possible to establish a diagnosis faster and more accurately, but careful study of the application of these newer modalities is needed to prevent either excessive or inappropriate use.

The purpose of this text is to provide a correlative approach to the evaluation of abdominal and pelvic diseases in children as well as to assist in the selection of the best modality for establishing a diagnosis in the shortest period of time, at the lowest cost, and with the least harm to the patient.

Ultrasonography, because of its noninvasive and flexible nature, is one of the most acceptable modalities for the evaluation of disease processes in children and has received the main emphasis in this book. Ultrasonography has long passed the era of being limited to making the distinction between solid and cystic processes. It can frequently provide exact anatomical location and sometimes an accurate histological diagnosis. It is our intention to familiarize the reader with the detailed anatomy of the pediatric abdomen and pelvis and to review a spectrum of various disease processes in these areas. Since it is important to understand why we see what we see, each chapter begins with a description of particular pathological processes, which is then followed by appropriate illustrations. The illustrations are labeled in order to facilitate a grasp of the three-dimensional anatomy of the abdomen and pelvis.

We are thankful for the contributions of the following: Dr. Gary Amundson, who has been coauthor for chapters 2–10; Dr. Dennis Sarti, who contributed chapter 1; Dr. Gail Hansen, who provided the text for chapters 11–14; and Dr. Donald Rose, who provided the nuclear medicine studies and their interpretations.

We are indebted to many Residents and Staff of the UCLA School of Medicine for their strong support and stimulation during the preparation of this text. Anne Von, our secretary, in particular took a personal interest in this project and the final copy of the book emerged from her desk. She was assisted by three other secretaries who devoted time and energy to its preparation: Kathleen Ann Heitman, Marion M. Flowers, and Mary P. Frazier. We are in their debt. Georgia Keris, our very helpful librarian, provided all of the references and kept everything organized. We cannot thank her enough. We are especially grateful to Kimberly Willis, who produced all the illustrations, and any success this book may have will largely be because of her excellent job. We are also thankful to the supervisor of our photography lab, Paul E. Stout. For the quality of the images, we owe a special note of appreciation to the technologists in Ultrasound and Pediatric Radiology, and especially to Robert E. Clark and Rosemary Kozlowski. We also thank Jean Slater and Carol Mancel for their contributions. We are deeply grateful to our Chairman, Gabriel H. Wilson, M.D., and our Vice-Chairman for Education, Elias Theros, M.D., for their continuous encouragement and support of various projects. Last, but definitely not least, we are thankful to the Year Book Medical Publishers and their staff for their understanding and excellent advice. Without their personal interest, this project would have been impossible.

HOOSHANG KANGARLOO, M.D.

Acknowledgments

Acknowledgment is made to the following individuals and publishers for use of various illustrations in this text.

Figures 1–1, 1–2, 1–4 to 1–7, 1–9, 1–10, 1–13, and 1–15: Sarti, D. A., Kangarloo, H., and Sample, W. F.: Ultrasonic visualization of fetal anatomy, J. Perinatology-neonatology, 3(3):39, 1979.

Figure 1–14: Courtesy of Dr. Richard Hoffman, Torrance, California.

Figure 1–16: Courtesy of Dr. Roy Filly, San Francisco, California.

Figures 2–11 to 2–20: Kangarloo, H., Sukov, R., Sample, W. F., Lipson, M., and Smith, L.: Ultrasonographic evaluation of juxtadiaphragmatic masses in children, Radiology 125:785, 1977.

Figures 3–16, 3–20, 3–49, 4–3, 4–18, 4–21, 6–1, 6–2, 7–25, and 8–51: Sample, W. F., Gyepes, M. T., and Ehrlich, R. M.: Gray scale ultrasound in pediatric urology, J. Urol. 117:518, 1977.

Figures 4–52 and 4–55: Garris, J., Kangarloo, H., Sarti, D., Sample, W. F., and Smith, L. E.: The ultrasonic spectrum of prune-belly syndrome, J. Clin. Ultrasound, 8:117, 1980.

Figures 7–29 to 7–32: Kangarloo, H. and Sample, W. F.: Diagnostic oncology case study: Abdominal mass and cervical adenopathy in a child, A.J.R. 132:643, 1979.

Figures 7–40 to 7–43: Berger, P. E., Kuhn, J. P., and Munschauer, R. W.: Computed tomography and ultrasound in the diagnosis and management of neuroblastoma, Radiology 128:663, 1978.

Figures 9–19 and 10–41: Berk, J. E. (ed.): *Developments in Digestive Diseases: Clinical Relevance* (No. 1) (Philadelphia: Lea & Febiger, 1977).

Figures 9–59, 9–60, 9–67, 9–69, and 9–75: Kangarloo, H., Sarti, D. A., Sample, W. F., and Amundson, G.: Ultrasonographic spectrum of choledochal cysts in children, Pediatr. Radiol., in press.

Figures 9–87 and 9–90: Sample, W. F.: Techniques for improved delineation of normal anatomy of the upper abdomen and high retroperitoneum with gray-scale ultrasound, Radiology 124:197, 1977.

Figures 10–61 and 10–62: Courtesy of Dr. Ross Eto, Santa Monica Hospital, California.

Figure 11–25: Courtesy of Dr. Michael T. Gyepes, Long Beach Memorial Hospital, California.

Figures 11–40 to 11–42, 11–44, 11–46, and 11–47: Kangarloo, H., Sample, W. F., Hansen, G., Robinson, J. S., and Sarti, D.: Ultrasonic evaluation of abdominal gastrointestinal tract duplication in children, Radiology 131:191, 1979.

Figures 14–2, 14–7, 14–11, and 14–25: Sample, W. F. and Sarti, D. A.: Normal Anatomy of the Female Pelvis: Computed Tomography and Ultrasonography, in Rosenfield, A. T. and Taylor, K. J. W. (eds.): *Clinics in Diagnostic Ultrasound.* Volume 2: *Genitourinary Ultrasound* (New York: Churchill Livingstone & Longman, Inc., 1979).

Figures 14–4, 14–13, and 14–84: Lippe, B. M. and Sample, W. F.: Pelvic ultrasonography in pediatric and adolescent endocrine disorders, J. Pediatr. 92:897, 1978.

Contents

CONTENTS

1

Prenatal Anatomy and Anomalies

THE MOST DYNAMIC TIME of our lives occurs from conception to delivery; growth is rapid and future development is dramatically determined by those initial 9 months. Yet limited means are present that provide insight and information on this crucial time. The development of diagnostic ultrasound has provided a technique by which we can follow the progress of a developing fetus. This technique has improved in recent years, providing information and images during pregnancy that have helped us understand and monitor the growing fetus.

This chapter will deal with the fetus. Although the placenta, uterus and maternal anatomy are most important to pregnancy, they will not be discussed in this chapter. Instead we will concentrate on the normal and abnormal ultrasonic appearance of the developing fetus.

Diagnostic ultrasound was first used in examining the obstetrical patient in the late 1960s, with a "bistable" technique that recorded echoes from strong specular reflectors and yielded outlines of organ structures. The development of gray-scale echography has permitted recording of weaker reflectors arising from parenchymal tissue. This, along with improved transducer design and focusing, has produced images of markedly improved resolution and quality.

TECHNIQUE

Obstetrical studies are usually performed on a B-scan or real-time unit. A 3.5-MHz transducer, 13 or 19 mm in diameter, is used for most patients undergoing B-scan examination. Occasionally, a 2.25-MHz transducer will be necessary for increased penetration, especially on the obese, near-term patient.

Real-time examination is most often performed using a linear array, 2.25- or 3.5-MHz transducer. This provides an advantage over a "static" B-scan examination in that fetal activity can be assessed and monitored. This is of importance in ruling out fetal death or determining fetal extremity motion. Real-time examinations are also more quickly performed than B-scan studies. However, real-time images do not presently have the resolution of B-scan images. The patient is usually studied using the full-bladder technique, which serves 2 major purposes. First, it lifts the small-bowel loops out of the pelvis. This is extremely important in early pregnancy since air-filled bowel loops can completely obscure the uterus. Second, in later pregnancy a filled urinary bladder will provide better visualization of the lower uterine segment as it elevates the uterus out of the pelvis.

GESTATIONAL AGE

Accurate determination of gestational age is extremely helpful to the obstetrician in monitoring pregnancy. Ultrasound provides a means of assessing gestational age by measuring 3 rapidly growing anatomical structures: (1) mean diameter of gestational sac, (2) crown-rump length (CRL) and (3) biparietal diameter (BPD).

From the 5th to 11th menstrual week of pregnancy, gestational age can be determined by measuring the mean diameter of the gestational sac. The sac is first visualized in the uterus at the 4th–5th menstrual week as a circular to oval, highly echogenic region with central sonolucency. This undergoes rapid growth, with an increase in diameter of approximately 7–10 mm per week. By the 10th menstrual week it is 5–6 cm in diameter. The surrounding high-amplitude echoes of the gestational sac are formed by the lace-like vascular network of the chorionic villi and decidual reaction. The gestational sac eventually disappears around the 11th menstrual week as the chorionic villi, which are opposite the placental implantation site, atrophy. However, the rapid growth of the gestational sac from the 5th to the 11th menstrual week provides an excellent measurable anatomical structure for assessing gestational age.

From the 6th to 15th menstrual week, the CRL can be measured by ultrasound to estimate gestational age. Its rapid growth from 7 mm to approximately 8 cm during this time provides an excellent means for dating the pregnancy. A major difficulty in obtaining a CRL is the marked activity of the fetus during early pregnancy. It is easier to obtain a CRL using real-time ultrasound since fetal activity can be dynamically monitored and a quick scan parallel to the long axis of the fetus obtained.

After the 15th week of pregnancy, gestational age is determined by measuring the BPD, which is the widest distance between the parietal bones. The BPD should be visualized in 100% of pregnancies by the 15th menstrual week. It can occasionally be obtained as early as the 11th or 12th week. The BPD grows approximately 3 mm per week in the 2d trimester. Therefore, the earlier in pregnancy that one obtains the BPD, the more accurate the assessment of gestational age.

Several sources of error can arise in obtaining a BPD. Variation in technique among ultrasonographers leads to a large source of error. It is important to use a reproducible technique, such as that described by Campbell (1968, 1969), in obtaining the BPD. Fetal activity and position are also sources of error.

Since the 3 anatomical structures just discussed are easily identified by ultrasound, they can be measured at various appropriate times during pregnancy to give an estimate of gestational age.

NORMAL FETAL ANATOMY

The embryo is first visualized by present-day ultrasound equipment at approximately the 7th menstrual week. As the fetus enlarges, numerous anatomical structures can be seen in the 2d and 3d trimesters. Besides the skull and falx cerebri, numerous other structures of the fetal head can be identified, such as lateral ventricles, thalamus, 3d ventricle, corpus callosum, foramen magnum, middle fossa and bony orbits. Structures of the normal fetal thorax and abdomen that can be visualized include ribs, heart, lungs, aorta, inferior vena cava, spine, kidneys, spleen, stomach, urinary bladder, umbilical vessels, bowel, scrotum and penis. The various bones of the upper and lower extremities can also be identified. It becomes extremely important to recognize normal fetal anatomy in order to detect abnormal fetal detail during a routine obstetrical study.

AMNIOCENTESIS

Ultrasound has proved of assistance in patients undergoing amniocentesis for fetal karyotyping, sexing, α-fetoprotein (AFP) levels, lung maturity and serial evaluation of Rh-sensitized pregnancies.

The primary use of ultrasound in these instances is to locate a readily accessible pool of amniotic fluid. However, it also provides other important information, such as (1) gestational age, which aids in AFP determination, (2) the presence of twins and tap sites for sacs, (3) fetal death, which can elevate AFP and (4) gross fetal abnormalities. When chemical studies from amniocentesis are found to be abnormal, it is advisable to reexamine the patient and perform a thorough fetal study.

ABNORMALITIES OF THE FETAL HEAD

The fetal head is easily recognizable during routine ultrasound examination in 100% of normal pregnancies after 15 weeks' gestation. Anencephaly, microcephaly, hydrocephalus, encephaloceles, posterior fossa cysts and cystic hygromas have all been detected by ultrasound. The AFP levels in amniotic fluid decline from 2 mg/dl at 12 weeks to less than 0.5 mg/dl at 20 weeks. An elevated AFP level may be caused by neural tube defects. This should lead to close scrutiny of the fetal head. Anencephaly yields a markedly elevated AFP level and can be easily recognized by ultrasound. A cluster of echoes is found in the region of the suspected fetal skull. Very often the fetus is quite active and hydramnios is present secondary to interruption of the fetal swallowing mechanism. Microcephaly is more difficult to detect. Comparison of the relative size of the fetal head to fetal body can assist in the early detection of microcephaly.

Ultrasonic visualization of an enlarged or abnormally sonolucent fetal head has been noted in hydrocephalus and posterior fossa cysts. Sonolucent masses adjacent to the fetal skull can be seen in encephaloceles, meningoceles and cystic hygromas. Such abnormalities within and about the fetal skull are usually detected when one is attempting to obtain a BPD for gestational age. Real-time examination is often quite helpful in detecting such an abnormality since a three-dimensional concept of the fetus can be derived quite quickly.

SPINAL ABNORMALITIES

Since an elevated AFP level is often secondary to a neural tube defect, close examination of the fetal spine is also necessary. Spinal abnormalities, such as meningoceles, meningomyeloceles, spina bifida and sacrococcygeal teratomas, have been reported. The fetal spine can be easily identified with present-day equipment in both longitudinal and transverse sections. A longitudinal scan slightly anterior will display the tubular aorta. Transverse scans of the fetal spine demonstrate a highly echogenic area surrounding a central sonolucent region situated in the posterior aspect of the thorax or abdomen. When the AFP level is elevated, close scrutiny of the region posterior to the cervical and sacral spine is undertaken to rule out the presence of any masses secondary to meningoceles and meningomyeloceles. The fetal spine is also examined in the transverse plane in an effort to detect any posterior defects suggesting spina bifida. Finally, real-time examination of the lower extremities is performed to detect normal motion.

ABNORMALITIES OF THE FETAL ABDOMEN

As mentioned earlier, some sonolucent areas are normally present in the fetal abdomen. When they are too numerous or large, closer examination is necessary to rule out a pathological state. High gastrointestinal tract obstruction involving the stomach, duodenum or proximal part of the jejunum will produce large sonolucent masses in the upper part of the abdomen, accompanied by hydramnios. Interruption of the normal fetal swallowing and absorption mechanism will lead to hydramnios, as is the situation in proximal gastrointestinal tract obstruction. Mesenteric cysts have been visualized by ultrasound in utero and appear as sonolucent abdominal masses. When fluid-filled abdominal masses are noted in the presence of oligohydramnios, a genitourinary tract abnormality should be considered. Hydronephrosis, megaureter, obstructed upperpole calix secondary to ectopic ureterocele and fetal polycystic kidney disease have been reported. If multiple abdominal fluid masses are present, the fetal renal beds should be examined closely in an effort to identify the fetal kidneys. This is especially necessary in the presence of oligohydramnios. Abdominal fluid present within the peritoneal cavity and not within bowel loops has also been identified. Fetal ascites is most often seen in Rh sensitization and has an ultrasonic appearance similar to that seen in the adult. The fluid is not contained within bowel loops. It is located peripherally, with bowel loops and liver displaced centrally.

THORACIC AND SKELETAL ABNORMALITIES

Examination of the fetal thorax is most often concerned with fetal cardiac activity to document fetal viability. However, fetal echocardiography is being performed in an effort to detect cardiac anomalies. Pleural effusions appear as fluid within the pleural space similar to that seen in the adult. A collapsed or "empty" thorax is manifested in fetal death as a relatively lucent thorax with distortion of the normal architecture.

Evaluation of proximal to distal extremity length and the relative size of the extremities in relation to the fetal head and body have been undertaken. This has raised the possibility of intrauterine diagnosis of skeletal abnormalities. Thanatophoric dwarfism and chondroectodermal dysplasia (Ellis-van Creveld syndrome) have been reported.

INTRAUTERINE GROWTH RETARDATION

The early diagnosis of intrauterine growth retardation (IUGR) is of importance since the fetus will be delivered as soon as lung maturity is present. The fetus will do better outside the uterus once lung maturation is present. Since IUGR results in higher perinatal mortality and morbidity, early diagnosis is critical. Leveling growth rate of the BPD has been used to detect IUGR. However, this will detect only 50% of affected fetuses. The reason is that 2 patterns of growth retardation have been noted. In the first, or diffuse, type, the entire fetus is small and the BPD will not grow at the usual rate. In the second, the fetal head is spared at the expense of the body and the BPD may appear normal throughout pregnancy. Because of this finding, total intrauterine volume (TIUV) is more useful in detecting IUGR. The TIUV takes into account the fetus, placenta and amniotic fluid in detecting IUGR and has proved more sensitive than the BPD alone.

FETAL DEATH

Numerous ultrasonic findings should alert the ultrasonographer of fetal distress or death. A "double ring" sign about the fetal head or body is indicative of fetal edema. It can be seen in Rh sensitization, congestive heart failure and 24–48 hours after fetal death. Ultrasonic visualization of overlapping skull bones indicates fetal death and degeneration. Marked tortuosity and angulation of the fetal spine can occasionally be demonstrated by ultrasound and roentgenograms when fetal death occurs. Since ultrasound detects acoustical interfaces, separation of the amnion from the chorion can be easily demonstrated and can suggest fetal death. Lack of fetal activity during the course of a routine B-scan examination should alert one to the possibility of fetal difficulty.

When any of the above findings are present, examination for fetal viability by either real-time or Doppler is necessary. Fetal viability can be quickly determined by locating the fetal thorax and documenting cardiac activity.

REFERENCES

Campbell, S.: An improved method of fetal cephalometry by ultrasound, J. Obstet. Gynecol. Br. Comm. 75:568, 1968.

Campbell, S.: The prediction of fetal maturity by ultrasonic measurement of the biparietal diameter, J. Obstet. Gynecol. Br. Comm. 76:603, 1969.

Cecuk, A. K., and Breyer, B.: Prediction of maturity in the first trimester of pregnancy by ultrasonic measurement of fetal crown-rump length, J. Clin. Ultrasound 4:83, 1976.

Cederqvist, L. L., Williams, L. R., Symchych, P. S., and Saary, Z. I.: Prenatal diagnosis of fetal ascites by ultrasound, Am. J. Obstet. Gynecol. 128:229, 1977.

Crandall, B. F., Lebherz, T. B., and Freihube, R.: Neural tube defects: Maternal serum screening and prenatal diagnosis, Pediatr. Clin. North Am. 25:619, 1978.

Cremin, B. J., and Sheff, M. I.: Ultrasonic diagnosis of thanatophoric dwarfism in utero, Radiology 124:479, 1977.

Cunningham, M. E., and Walls, W. J.: Ultrasound in the evaluation of anencephaly, Radiology 118:165, 1976.

Donald, I.: Diagnostic uses of sonar in obstetrics and gynecology, J. Obstet. Gynecol. Br. Comm. 72:907, 1955.

Donald, I.: Ultrasonic echo sounding in obstetrical and gynecological diagnosis, Am. J. Gynecol. 93:935, 1965.

Duenhoelter, J. H., Santos-Ramos, R., Rosenfeld, C. R., and Coln, C. D.: Prenatal diagnosis of gastrointestinal tract obstruction, Obstet. Gynecol. 47:618, 1970.

Field, B., Mitchell, G., Garrett, W., and Kerr, C.: Prenatal diagnoses and selective abortion for anencephaly and spina bifida, Med. J. Aust. 1:608, 1974.

Freeman, R. K., McQuown, D. S., Secrist, L. J., and Larson, E. J.: The diagnosis of fetal hydrocephalus before viability, Obstet. Gynecol. 49:109, 1977.

Garrett, W. J., Greenwald, G., and Robinson, D. E.: Prenatal diagnosis of fetal polycystic kidney by ultrasound, Aust. N.Z.J. Obstet. Gynecol. 10:7, 1970.

Garrett, W. J., Kossoff, G., and Osborn, R. A.: The diagnosis of fetal hydronephrosis, megaureter and urethral obstruction by ultrasonic echography, Br. J. Obstet. Gynecol. 82:115, 1975.

Garrett, W. J., Pil, D., Fisher, C. C., and Kossoff, G.: Hydrocephaly, microcephaly and anencephaly diagnosed in pregnancy by ultrasonic echography, Med. J. Aust. 2:587, 1975.

Ghorashi, B., and Gottesfeld, K.: The gray-scale appearance of the normal pregnancy from 4–16 weeks of gestation, J. Clin. Ultrasound 5:195, 1977.

Gohari, P., Berkowitz, R. L., and Hobbins, J. C.: Prediction of intrauterine growth retardation by determination of total intrauterine volume, Am. J. Obstet. Gynecol. 127:255, 1977.

Gottesfeld, K. R.: The ultrasonic diagnosis of intrauterine fetal death, Am. J. Obstet. Gynecol. 108:623, 1970.

Gottesfeld, K. R.: Ultrasound in obstetrics and gynecology, Semin. Roentgenol. 10:305, 1975.

Hellman, L. M., Kobayashi, M., Fillisti, L., et al.: Growth and development of the human fetus prior to the 20th week of gestation, Am. J. Obstet. Gynecol. 103:789, 1969.

Kassner, E. G., and Cromb, E.: Sonographic diagnosis of fetal hydrops, Radiology 116:399, 1975.

Kobayashi, M., Hellman, L. M., and Bromb, I.: *Atlas of Ultrasonography in Obstetrics and Gynecology* (New York: Appleton-Century-Crofts, 1972).

Kossoff, G., and Garrett, W. J.: Intracranial detail in fetal echograms, Invest. Radiol. 7:159, 1972.

Kossoff, G., Garrett, W. J., and Radovanovich, G.: Grey-scale echography in obstetrics and gynecology, Aust. Radiol. 18:62, 1974.

Lee, T. G., and Blake, S.: Prenatal fetal abdominal ultrasonography and diagnosis, Radiology 124:275, 1977.

Lee, T. G., and Newton, B. W.: Posterior fossa cyst: Prenatal diagnosis by ultrasound, J. Clin. Ultrasound 4:29, 1976.

Lee, T. G., and Warren, B. H.: Antenatal ultrasonic demonstration of fetal bowel, Radiology 124:471, 1977.

Mahoney, M. J., and Hobbins, J. C.: Prenatal diagnosis of chondroectodermal dysplasia (Ellis-van Creveld syndrome) with fetoscopy and ultrasound, N. Engl. J. Med. 297:258, 1977.

Morgan, C. L., Haney, A., Christakos, A., et al.: Neonatal detection of fetal structural defects with ultrasound, J. Clin. Ultrasound 3:287, 1975.

Platt, L. D., Manning, F. A., and Lemay, M.: Real-time B-scan directed amniocentesis, Am. J. Obstet. Gynecol. 130:700, 1978.

Queenan, J. T., Kubarych, S. F., Cook, L. N., et al.: Diagnostic ultrasound for detection of intrauterine growth and retardation, Am. J. Obstet. Gynecol. 124:871, 1976.

Robinson, H. P.: Sonar measurements of fetal crown-rump length as a means of assessing maturity in the first trimester of pregnancy, Br. J. Med. 4:28, 1973.

Sabbagha, R. E., Depp, R., Grasse, D., and Kippler, I.: Ultrasound diagnosis of occipitothoracic meningocele at 22 weeks gestation, Am. J. Obstet. Gynecol. 131:113, 1978.

Sanders, R. C., and Conrad, M. R.: Sonography in obstetrics, Radiol. Clin. North Am. 13:435, 1975.

Santos-Ramos, R., and Duenhoelter, J. H.: Diagnosis of congenital fetal abnormalities by sonography, Obstet. Gynecol. 45:279, 1975.

Shapiro, L. J., Kaback, M. M., Toomey, K. E., Sarti, D., et al.: Prenatal diagnosis of the Meckel syndrome: Use of serial ultrasound and alpha-fetoprotein measurements, Birth Defects 13:267, 1977.

Shaub, M., and Wilson, R.: Erythroblastosis fetalis: Ultrasonic diagnosis, J. Clin. Ultrasound 4:19, 1976.

Shaub, M., Wilson, R., and Collea, J.: Fetal cystic lymphangioma (cystic hygroma): Prepartum ultrasonic findings, Radiology 121:449, 1976.

Wladimiroff, J. W., Barentsen, R., Henk, C. S., et al.: Fetal urine production in a case of diabetes associated with polyhydramnios, Obstet. Gynecol. 46:100, 1975.

Zimmerman, H. B.: Prenatal demonstration of gastric and duodenal obstruction by ultrasound, J. Can. Assoc. Radiol. 29:138, 1978.

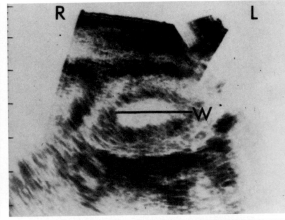

Fig 1—1.

Fig 1—2.

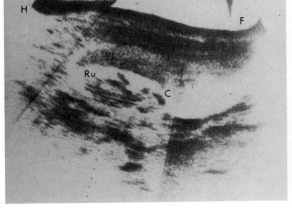

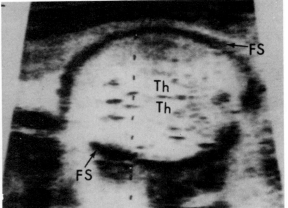

Fig 1—3.

Fig 1—4.

Figs 1—1 to 1—4. — Gestational age. Ultrasonic determination of gestational age is obtained by measuring 3 easily recognizable structures at different times of pregnancy. In early pregnancy, from 5th to 10th week, determination of mean diameter of gestational sac gives estimate of gestational age. In Figures 1—1 and 1—2, length (L), height (H) and width (W) of gestational sac are added and then divided by 3. Mean diameter of gestational sac grows from 1 cm at 5 postmenstrual weeks to approximately 5 cm at 10—11 weeks. P = symphysis pubis; B = urinary bladder; R = toward right of patient; L = toward left of patient.

Crown-rump length (CRL) is 2d measurement used to determine gestational age. This is most often used from 7th to 14th week of pregnancy. Figure 1—3 is an example of CRL determination that measures distance from fetal crown (C) to fetal rump (Ru). This measurement can often be difficult to obtain on B-scan unit secondary to fetal activity. This problem is overcome with real-time ultrasound, which

enables more rapid determination of long axis of fetus. H = toward head of patient; F = toward foot of patient; Pl = placenta.

From the 15th week until term, gestational age is determined by measurement of fetal biparietal diameter (BPD). The BPD should be identifiable in 100% of cases by 15 weeks and can often be seen as early as 11 or 12 weeks. The measurement in Figure 1—4 is obtained from near fetal skull (FS) to far fetal skull echoes once appropriate midline structures are identified. It is necessary not only to identify linear midline echoes of falx cerebri and 3d ventricle but also the relatively lucent thalamic regions (Th) in order to be certain you are at correct level. The BPD grows 3 mm/week up to 30—32 weeks and then decreases its growth rate to 1—2 mm/week until term. Therefore, a more accurate determination of gestational age from BPD is obtained earlier in pregnancy.

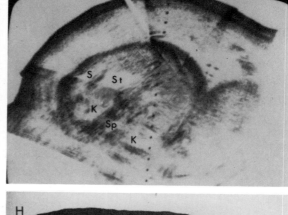

Fig 1–5.

Fig 1–6.

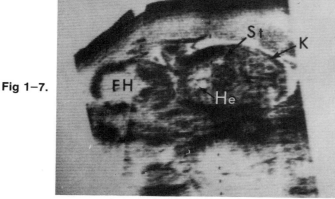

Fig 1–7.

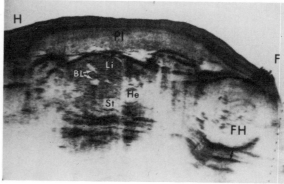

Fig 1–8.

Figs 1–5 to 1–8. — Normal fetal anatomy. During obstetrical ultrasound study, numerous normal anatomical structures can be identified within fetus. Fetal head is routinely examined for biparietal diameter with midline echoes arising from falx cerebri, 3d ventricle, pineal gland, etc. Examination of fetal body yields numerous normal structures that can be easily identified. Figure 1–5 demonstrates highly echogenic steplike echoes *(arrows)* arising from fetal ribs. Acoustical shadowing is present deep to fetal ribs, which denote location of the fetal thorax. This can be of assistance when trying to locate fetal heart (see Figs 1–7 and 1–8). H = toward head of fetus; F = toward foot of fetus; A = aorta. Fetal viability is documented by demonstrating fetal cardiac activity by B-scan, M or A mode, and Doppler. Ultrasonic localization of fetal thorax makes documentation of fetal cardiac activity quite easy. Figure 1–6 is an example of numerous abdominal structures that can be identified. Fetal spine (Sp) is circular cluster of high echoes in posterior aspect of fetus. On either side of fetal spine, one can identify both kidneys (K), which have an ultrasonic appearance similar to that seen in adult. These are located on transverse scans of fetus just below heart and diaphragm. St = stomach; S = spleen. Figure 1–7 is a coronal scan of fetus in which we see kidney (K) in coronal section. Spleen can occasionally be identified lateral to left kidney in left upper quadrant (LUQ). Often one will identify oval-shaped, fluid-filled mass in LUQ anterior to left kidney that represents normal stomach (St). It is important to recognize this as a normal structure so that mistaken diagnosis of gastrointestinal or genitourinary obstruction or mesenteric cyst is not made. FH = fetal head; He = heart. Occasionally, other fluid-filled bowel loops (BL in Fig 1–8) may be identified. In these instances, obstruction must be ruled out. Real-time studies of such bowel loops should show normal peristaltic activity with emptying. If there is any question, another examination will confirm that these bowel loops have disappeared or changed position. If they remain constant in position and contour, possibility of gastrointestinal or genitourinary obstruction should be considered. H = toward head of fetus; F = toward foot of fetus; FH = fetal head; Li = liver; St = stomach; He = heart; Pl = placenta.

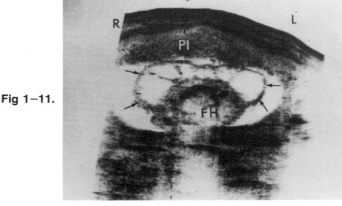

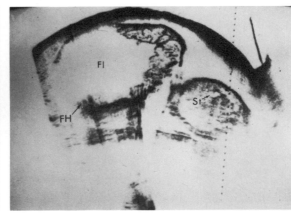

Fig 1–9.

Fig 1–10.

Fig 1–11.

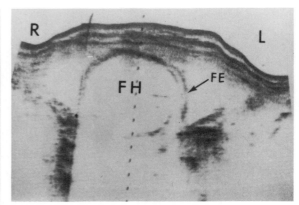

Fig 1–12.

Figs 1–9 to 1–12.—Abnormal fetal head. Abnormalities of fetal head may involve structures within or adjacent to fetal skull. When α-fetoprotein determinations are elevated, close scrutiny of fetal skull is necessary to rule out anencephaly. Anencephaly appears as cluster of echoes in region of fetal head (Fig 1–9). Notice disparity in size between anencephalic head (An) and fetal body (FB). These structures should normally be approximately equal in size. When marked discrepancy is present, possibility of anencephaly or microcephaly should be raised. Fetus must be carefully scanned since fetal head may be off to the side of individual scan. On thorough examination of fetus, one will not be able to identify biparietal diameter (BPD) and normal fetal skull in anencephaly. Instead, cluster of high-level echoes much smaller in diameter than fetal body will be identified. Very often these fetuses are active and difficult to examine and hydramnios may be present.

Large fluid collections within or about fetal skull may be identified. Hydrocephalus displays relatively lucent fetal head secondary to large, dilated, fluid-filled ventricles. These are more easily recognized under real-time examina-

tion. Unfortunately, hydrocephalus has usually been detected in later pregnancy. Figure 1–10 is an example of large cystic mass (Fl) within fetal head (FH). This large fluid-filled area was found to be secondary to obstruction and dilatation of 4th ventricle in Dandy-Walker syndrome. Fluid and solid masses may also be visualized adjacent to fetal head in encephaloceles, myeloceles, meningomyeloceles and cystic hygromas. St = stomach. In Figure 1–11, we see septated fluid-filled mass *(arrows)* surrounding fetal head (FH) that might represent one of the above entities. However, this is a case of fetal death in which amnion has separated and collapsed away from chorion but has appearance of fluid mass adjacent to fetal head. R = toward right of patient; L = toward left of patient. Figure 1–12 is classic-appearing "halo" or "double ring" sign of fetal edema that is often seen in fetal death or Rh sensitization. Strong outer ring arises from skin interface, which is displaced away from fetal head (FH) by edema (FE). Other signs of fetal death include overlapping of skull echoes and inability to obtain BPD secondary to degeneration. R = toward right of patient; L = toward left of patient.

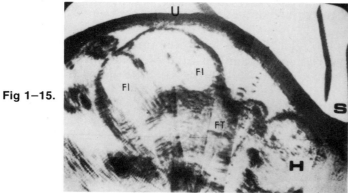

Fig 1–13.

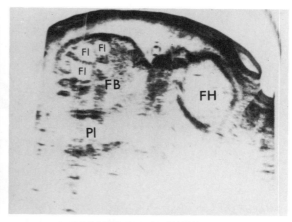

Fig 1–14.

Fig 1–15.

Fig 1–16.

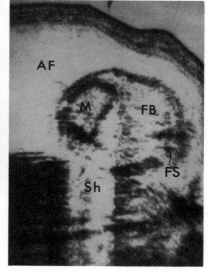

Figs 1–13 to 1–16.—Abnormalities of fetal body. Numerous fluid-filled structures that can normally be visualized within fetal abdomen include stomach, bowel loops, umbilical vein, urinary bladder, aorta and inferior vena cava. It is important to recognize this routinely so that abnormal masses can be more easily identified. An abnormal fluid collection within peritoneal cavity of fetus gives ultrasonic appearance similar to that seen in adult. Liver and bowel loops can be seen floating freely within sonolucent fluid-filled abdomen. Figure 1–13 is an example of fetal ascites secondary to Rh sensitization. The sonolucent ascitic fluid (As) is seen to completely surround liver (Li), indicating its intraperitoneal location. Pl = placenta; AF = amniotic fluid; FH = fetal head; FL = fetal limbs.

Occasionally, fluid-filled bowel must first be ruled out. This may be done by real-time or repeated examination. Figure 1–14 is an example of high gastrointestinal tract obstruction in which numerous loops of fluid-filled bowel (Fl) may be identified. These were persistent in configuration and location, suggesting the diagnosis. FB = fetal body; Pl = placenta; FH = fetal head.

Figure 1–15 is an example of large abdominal fluid (Fl) collections secondary to dilated ureters. Notice size of fetal abdomen in relation to thorax (FT) and head (H). When persistent fluid-filled loops are noted, one should examine fetal renal area in an effort to identify fetal kidneys. Rarely, one may be able to identify solid mass within fetal abdomen. S = level of symphysis; U = umbilical level. Figure 1–16 is solid mass (M) with highly echogenic borders. Acoustical shadowing (Sh) present deep to mass indicates calcification. This was a case of calcified meconium peritonitis visualized in utero. AF = amniotic fluid; FB = fetal body; FS = fetal spine.

9

2

Diaphragm

THE DIAPHRAGM (of Greek origin: *phragma,* partition; *dia,* across) is a musculotendinous structure that separates the thoracic and abdominal cavities. The heart depresses the middle portion of the diaphragm, allowing the lateral portions to form domes (hemidiaphragms). This concept of hemidiaphragms is of importance since each responds independently in most pathological conditions.

The diaphragm develops mainly from 4 structures: (1) the septum transversum, (2) the dorsal mesentery of the esophagus, (3) the pleuroperitoneal membranes and (4) the body walls. The septum transversum becomes the central tendon of the diaphragm. The dorsal mesentery of the esophagus forms the medial portion of each hemidiaphragm. The crura of the diaphragm develop from the extension of muscle fibers into the dorsal mesentery of the esophagus. The pleuroperitoneal membranes fuse with the dorsal mesentery of the esophagus and the dorsal portion of the septum transversum to complete the partition between the thoracic and abdominal cavities.

DIAPHRAGMATIC LESIONS

Lesions of the diaphragm include congenital lesions, such as diaphragmatic hernias or diaphragmatic eventration; traumatic lesions, such as hematomas or acquired diaphragmatic hernias; and diaphragmatic tumors.

Defective fusion of the costal and vertebral origins (pleuroperitoneal canal) results in a congenital dia-phragmatic (Bochdalek) hernia. Since the left pleuroperitoneal opening fuses later than the right, congenital diaphragmatic hernias are more common on the left side (80–90%). In most instances of Bochdalek's hernia, there is free communication between the thoracic and abdominal cavities; rarely, there may be a thin peritoneal sac covering the abdominal viscera in the chest. The small intestine, left colon, stomach and spleen may be found in the thorax with left-sided hernias. There is usually an associated malrotation with nonfixation of the intestine. On the right side, the hernia usually contains the liver but may also contain bowel or the right kidney. The ipsilateral lung is usually collapsed and may be hypoplastic. The mediastinal structures are shifted to the opposite side of the chest. The contralateral lung is partially compressed and may be hypoplastic.

Similarly, defective fusion of the xiphoid and costal origins of the diaphragm will result in an anterior diaphragmatic hernia (Morgagni). This is an uncommon abnormality and seen only rarely in children. Morgagni hernias usually have a peritoneal sac that limits the cephalad herniation of the abdominal viscera.

EVENTRATION

Eventration is less common than diaphragmatic hernias and is due to abnormal thinness of the diaphragmatic muscle; in some instances, there is complete absence of the muscle layer in a part of the diaphragm. This muscular defect results in stretching of

10

the diaphragm, allowing abdominal viscera to ascend into the hemithorax. In severe cases, the diaphragm is markedly elevated and compresses the ipsilateral lung; there is acute respiratory embarrassment in the newborn; and it may be difficult to distinguish this lesion from true diaphragmatic hernia. In less severe cases, there may be a combination of respiratory and gastrointestinal symptoms in later life and the diagnosis is usually established without any difficulty. An acquired form of diaphragmatic eventration is the result of phrenic nerve injury. In the newborn, there usually is a history of difficult breech delivery. Diaphragmatic paralysis and eventration may also occur as a rare complication of pneumonia or following cardiac surgery. The diagnosis is usually established by ultrasonography or fluoroscopy without any difficulty.

TUMORS

Primary tumors of the diaphragm are rare, particularly in children; most reported cases are of patients 40–50 years of age. However, primary tumors can occur at any age; the youngest patient described was a 26-day-old girl with a hemangioendothelioma. The incidence of primary diaphragmatic tumors is almost equal in males and females. Benign lesions are more common than malignant ones at any age, particularly in children. The most common benign lesions include lipomas, hemangioendotheliomas, cystic lymphangiomas and neurilemomas. Most malignant tumors are sarcomas, rhabdomyosarcomas or fibrosarcomas.

JUXTADIAPHRAGMATIC LESIONS

The differential diagnosis of juxtadiaphragmatic lesions is extensive and includes (1) hepatic lesions (abnormal size or position, neoplasms, cysts), (2) pulmonary or mediastinal lesions (inflammatory, neoplastic, cystic), (3) cardiac lesions (pericardial cysts, fluid), (4) gastric lesions (tumors), (5) splenic lesions (hematomas, cysts), (6) retroperitoneal lesions (lipomas, liposarcomas) and (7) inflammatory lesions (abscesses, effusions above or below the diaphragm).

DIAGNOSTIC MODALITIES

Visualization of the diaphragm by conventional methods such as plain x-ray films, fluoroscopy, double-exposure technique and pneumoperitonography are well known. However, visualization of the diaphragm using ultrasonography can be achieved without difficulty, particularly on the right side. Ultrasonography, using B-mode with gray-scale in conjunction with A-mode, M-mode or real-time, will accurately demonstrate abnormalities of the diaphragm.

Patients are examined in the supine or decubitus position. A 3.5- or 5.0-MHz transducer is placed on the patient's abdomen immediately inferior to the anterior costal margin or in an intercostal space. With the transducer initially angled cephalad, a longitudinal sweep caudally at various points along the transverse axis allows sagittal visualization of a hemidiaphragm. The hemidiaphragm appears as a convex-domed band of dense echoes.

If scans are performed in inspiration and expiration, diaphragmatic movement, or the lack of it, can easily be ascertained. M-mode and, more recently, real-time ultrasound are of particular value in the evaluation of diaphragmatic movement in very young children who cannot cooperate for the previously described technique. A-mode ultrasound may be used initially and the gain reduced until only the diaphragmatic echo remains. Subsequently, an M-mode tracing of diaphragmatic movement is obtained. This technique is the method of choice in patients with rapid respiratory rates or diaphragmatic flutter. Normally, there is 1–2 cm of diaphragmatic excursion with quiet breathing. This may increase to 4 or 5 cm depending on the respiratory effort and the patient's age. Real-time ultrasound allows a continuous in vivo visualization of the diaphragm.

The juxtadiaphragmatic areas are also easily evaluated using ultrasonography. If a juxtadiaphragmatic abnormality is suspected on an abdominal or chest roentgenogram, ultrasonography is helpful in either making the proper diagnosis and obviating the need for further, more invasive studies or in indicating what specific test or procedure is necessary to make the diagnosis. It will also aid in differentiating the origin of the juxtadiaphragmatic lesion, e.g., liver, heart, lungs or diaphragm, and may suggest a histological diagnosis by visualization of the internal architecture of the lesion. Further diagnostic studies can then be performed depending on the sonographic findings.

The examination is individually tailored to the specific clinical problem. In general, perpendicular views of the region of interest are obtained using the liver or spleen as a sonographic window. Prone, supine, decubitus or oblique positioning may be necessary, depending on the patient's habitus and the location of the lesion.

The distinction between subpulmonic and subphrenic fluid can be made by using the liver or spleen as ultrasonic windows. This technique is of particular assistance in the delineation of subphrenic abscesses that might be associated with subpulmonic effusions.

REFERENCES

Callen, P. W., et al.: Computed tomographic evaluation of the diaphragmatic crura, Radiology 126:413, 1978.

Callen, P. W., et al.: Ultrasonography of the diaphragmatic crura, Radiology 130:721, 1979.

Doust, B. D., et al.: Ultrasonic evaluation of pleural opacities, Radiology 114:135, 1975.

Feigin, D. S., et al.: Pericardial cysts: A radiologic-pathologic correlation and review, Radiology 125:15, 1977.

Ferguson, D. D., et al.: Lipoma of the diaphragm, Radiology 118:527, 1976.

Gold, R. P., et al.: Efficacy of combined liver-lung scintillation imaging, Radiology 117:105, 1975.

Goldberg, B. B.: *Abdominal Gray-Scale Ultrasonography* (New York: John Wiley & Sons, Inc., 1977).

Haber, K., et al.: Echographic evaluation of diaphragmatic motion in intra-abdominal diseases, Radiology 114:141, 1975.

Hesselink, J. R., et al.: Congenital partial eventration of the left diaphragm, A. J. R. 131:417, 1978.

Hirsch, J. H., et al.: Ultrasonic evaluation of radiographic opacities of the chest, A. J. R. 130:1153, 1978.

Kangarloo, H., et al.: Ultrasonographic evaluation of juxta-diaphragmatic masses in children, Radiology 125:785, 1977.

Laing, F. C., et al.: Problems in the application of ultrasonography for the evaluation of pleural opacities, Radiology 126:211, 1978.

Landay, M., et al.: Ultrasonic differentiation of right pleural effusion from subphrenic fluid on longitudinal scans of the right upper quadrant: Importance of recognizing the diaphragm, Radiology 123:155, 1977.

Moore, K. L.: *The Developing Human: Clinically Oriented Embryology* (Philadelphia: W. B. Saunders Co., 1974).

Olafsson, G., et al.: Primary tumors of the diaphragm, Chest 59:568, 1971.

Rashad, F. A., et al.: Arteriovenous malformation of the right leaf of the diaphragm communicating with vascular malformation of the right lung, A. J. R. 131:507, 1978.

Satyanath, S., et al.: Infra pulmonary effusion, J. Asso. Physicians India 24:77, 1976.

Stadler, H.E.: paroxysmal diaphragmatic flutter in a young infant, J. Ind. State Med. Assoc. 69:151, 1976.

Wiener, M. F., et al.: Primary tumors of the diaphragm, Arch. Surg. 90:143, 1965.

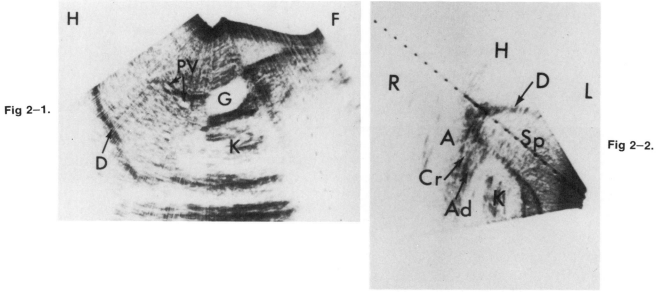

Figs 2–1 and 2–2.—Normal diaphragm. Diaphragm and adjacent areas can easily be identified with ultrasonography. Since liver acts as ultrasonic window, it is easier to identify right hemidiaphragm accurately. H = head; F = feet; R = right; L = left; D = diaphragm; Sp = spleen; A = aorta; Cr = crus of diaphragm; Ad = adrenal gland; K = kidney; G = gallbladder; PV = portal veins.

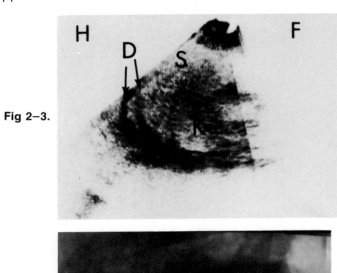

Fig 2–3.

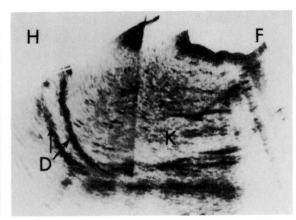

Fig 2–4.

Fig 2–5.

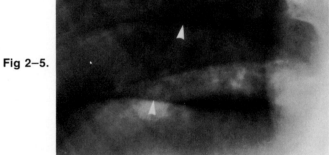

Figs 2–3 to 2–5. — Diaphragmatic motion. Diaphragmatic motion can be evaluated by scanning in inspiration and expiration. This can be done with ultrasonography (Figs 2–3 and 2–4, *arrows*) as well as roentgenographically (Fig 2–5, *arrowheads*). H = head; F = feet; D = diaphragm; S = spleen; K = kidney.

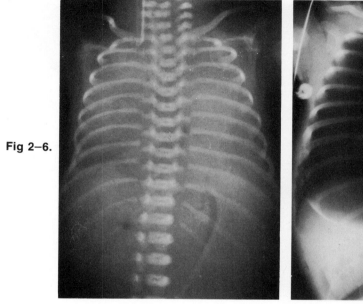

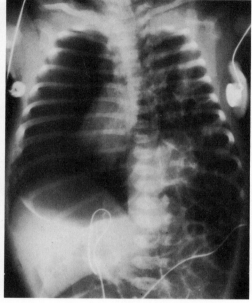

Fig 2–6.

Fig 2–7.

Figs 2–6 and 2–7.—Bochdalek's hernia. Diagnosis of Bochdalek's hernia is usually established without difficulty on plain chest and abdomen films, even when loops of bowel are not filled with gas (Fig 2–6). Figure 2–6 demonstrates opaque chest, displacement of umbilical venous line toward left side which is due to herniation of abdominal organs into chest on left side. Figure 2–7 shows more typical form of Bochdalek's hernia, with gas-filled bowel loops.

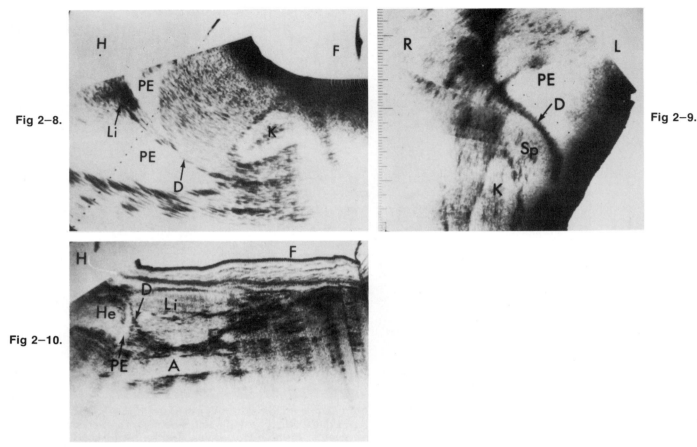

Fig 2–8.

Fig 2–9.

Fig 2–10.

Figs 2–8 to 2–10.—Fluid accumulation adjacent to dia-phragm can be identified ultrasonographically, and distinction between pleural effusion and subpulmonic effusion can be made without difficulty (Figs 2–8 and 2–9). Peri--cardial effusion also can be identified ultrasonographically (Fig 2–10). H = head; F = feet; PE = pleural effusion (Figs 2–8 and 2–9) and pericardial effusion (Fig 2–10); Li = lung (Fig 2–8), liver (Fig 2–10); D = diaphragm; K = kidney; Sp = spleen; He = heart; A = aorta; R = toward right of patient; L = toward left of patient.

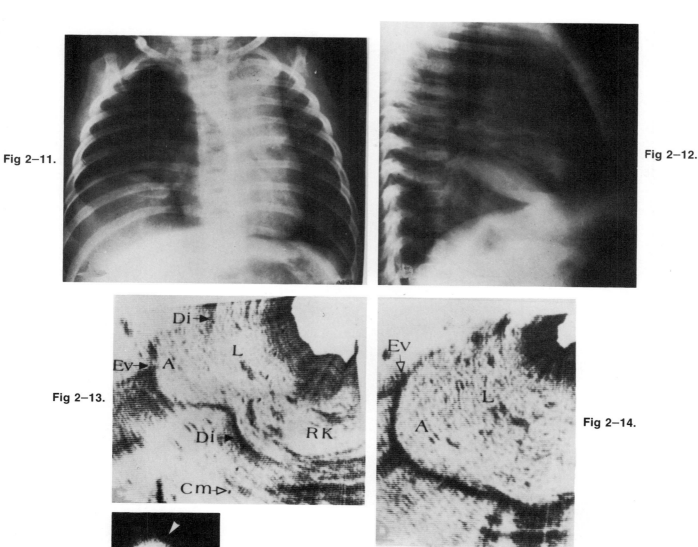

Fig 2–11.

Fig 2–12.

Fig 2–13.

Fig 2–14.

Fig 2–15.

Figs 2–11 to 2–15.—Eventration of diaphragm. Frontal (Fig 2–11) and lateral (Fig 2–12) views of chest demonstrate soft tissue mass inseparable from right hemidiaphragm. There is also evidence of right upper lobe emphysema. Longitudinal scan (Fig 2–13) demonstrates that this mass is result of eventration of diaphragm. Limited longitudinal scan (Fig 2–14) with gain setting adjusted to best visualize internal architecture of this mass clearly demonstrates that this lesion represents normal liver. Ev = eventration; Di = diaphragm; L = liver; RK = right kidney; A = part of normal liver; cm = centimeter marker. Depending on ultrasonographic findings, further diagnostic studies, such as 99mTc-sulfur colloid scans (Fig 2–15), may be performed that can further confirm the diagnosis of eventration *(arrowhead).*

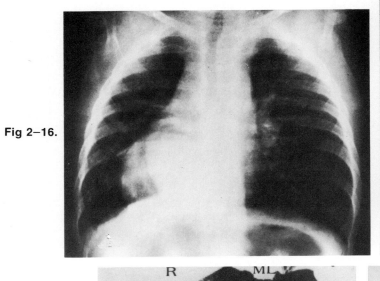

Fig 2–16.

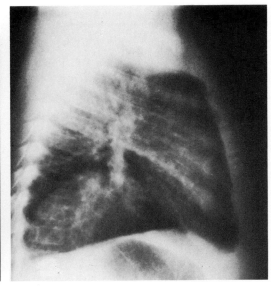

Fig 2–17.

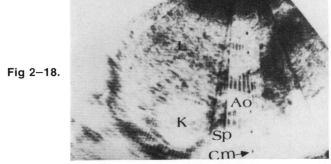

Fig 2–18.

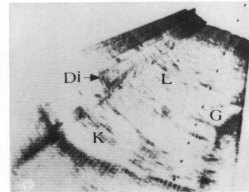

Fig 2–19.

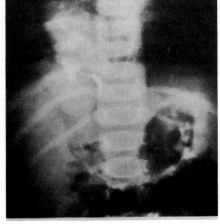

Fig 2–20.

Figs 2–16 to 2–20.—Intrathoracic kidney. Frontal (Fig 2–16) and lateral (Fig 2–17) views of chest demonstrate a soft tissue mass adjacent to right hemidiaphragm. There is also evidence of cardiac mesoversion. Transverse scan (Fig 2–18) performed for topography with transducer angled 30° cephalad demonstrates a mass that probably represents normal kidney. Limited longitudinal scan, using liver as sonic window and oriented along axis of intrathoracic kidney, clearly demonstrates internal architecture of malpositioned kidney (Fig 2–19). R = right; ML = midline; L = liver; K = kidney; Ao = aorta; Sp = spine; cm = centimeter marker; Di = diaphragm; G = gallbladder. Excretory urogram (Fig 2–20) further demonstrates intrathoracic position of right kidney.

3

Congenital Anomalies of the Urinary Tract

ANOMALIES OF THE URINARY TRACT are the most common congenital malformations found in children. Various authors have reported the overall incidence in the general population as just under 10%. Many anomalies are of minor or no importance; however, if 1 anomaly is present, about 20% of patients will have a 2d anomaly.

A knowledge of the embryologic development and normal anatomy of the genitourinary system is essential to understanding anomalies involving the urinary tract. The final formation of a structurally intact and functional kidney requires the intimate union between the endodermal elements forming the collecting system and the mesodermal elements forming the parenchyma. The urinary system develops in an orderly progression, beginning with the pronephros, blending into the mesonephros and ending in the metanephros. At about the 4th week of intrauterine life, the earliest nephric stage consists of 6–10 paired tubules, the pronephros, that drain into the pronephric duct. This in turn empties into the terminal portion of the hindgut, termed the cloaca. At about the 5th week of life, the pronephric tubules begin to degenerate and a 2d set of tubules, the mesonephros, develop. As these tubules join the pronephric duct, the name is changed to the mesonephric (wolffian) duct. The ureteral bud and specific portions of the genital tract will arise from the wolffian duct. At about 6–8 weeks, the metanephros, definitive kidney, begins to develop from the mesonephros by induction from the ureteric bud. The

actively growing portion of the ureteric bud (ampulla) undergoes several divisions and ultimately forms the ureter, pelvis, calyces and other portions of the collecting system. The nephrogenic blastema, under the influence of the ampulla, develops into functioning nephrons and supporting stromal elements. The kidneys show apparent ascent from their fetal position to the normal position at birth. During this time the vascular supply to the kidneys continuously changes, with the initial supply from the iliac vessels and the later supply from the renal arteries.

The lower part of the urinary and genital tract also develops in an orderly sequence and is, in part, dependent on the development of a normal upper tract. The major structure that forms the lower tract is the terminal, blind-ending portion of the hindgut, the cloaca. Its primary function is to serve as the primitive receptacle into which the reproductive and excretory tracts empty. At about the 6th week of gestation, the urorectal septum forms and divides the cloaca into the rectum dorsally and the urogenital sinus ventrally. At this time the wolffian duct is still present and drains into the urogenital sinus. As a result of differential growth of the sinus, the distal wolffian duct, as well as the point of origin of the ureter, is incorporated into the urogenital sinus and forms the area that will become the bladder trigone. The urogenital sinus then divides into a distal pars phallica, into which the wolffian duct opens, and a proximal pars pelvina, into which the ureters open. These 2 parts of the sinus then mature to form the urethra and bladder, respectively.

Additional embryologic structures of direct importance are the urachus, wolffian duct and müllerian duct. The urachus is a narrow, epithelial-lined tube that in embryonic life connects the primitive bladder to the allantoic duct. Normally, as the bladder "descends" into the pelvis, this tube becomes obliterated and remains as a fibromuscular remnant.

In males, most of the müllerian duct degenerates but the caudal end forms the prostatic utricle. In females, the müllerian duct forms the uterus, proximal vagina and fallopian tubes.

The wolffian ducts, in addition to giving origin to the ureters, form the efferent tubules, duct of the epididymis, vas deferens, seminal vesicles and ejaculatory ducts in males, and the epoophoron, para-oophoron and Gartner's duct in females.

The kidneys of infants and children are relatively large with fetal lobulations. The renal sinus is much smaller during infancy and most of the renal pelvis lies within the renal sinus. The ureters of infants are relatively shorter and wider, and the bladder is an abdominal organ that attains its pelvic position later in childhood. A physiologic sphincteric mechanism exists at the junction of the minor and major calyces, the major calyces and the renal pelvis, and the pelviureteric junction.

ANOMALIES OF THE KIDNEYS

Anomalies of Number

Supernumerary kidneys are one of the rarest urinary anomalies. To be considered truly supernumerary, the additional tissue must have its own vascular supply and renal capsule and must not be fused with adjacent renal tissue by fibrous or parenchymal bands. It is a separate, ectopic, functioning unit located either above or below the normally positioned kidneys. The ureter usually inserts ectopically into the bladder.

A much more common anomaly is that of a decreased quantity of renal tissue in the form of agenesis (no vestige of renal tissue present), dysgenesis (nodules of tissue present without pathological or histological resemblance to or organization of renal tissue and having no renal function; some authors would term this condition aplasia or dysplasia) or hypoplasia (small but otherwise normal kidney, morphologically and functionally).

Renal agenesis may be unilateral or bilateral. The bilateral form is extremely rare and incompatible with life. The abnormality is believed to be a failure of the wolffian ducts to generate the ureteric bud. Therefore, the ureters are absent and the bladder is hypoplastic secondary to lack of the stimulus of urine volume. Associated oligohydramnios will cause "Potter's facies" and pulmonary hypoplasia. Death usually occurs in a few hours or days from the pulmonary hypoplasia.

Unilateral renal agenesis is caused by failure of the development of the nephrogenic blastema, the ureteric bud or the vascular supply. The ipsilateral ureter is rudimentary or absent. The ureterovesical orifice and adjacent portion of the trigone are absent in the majority of cases. Associated genital anomalies are the most frequently encountered structural defects and, in females, may range from an ipsilateral absence of the oviduct to a unicornuate uterus with an absent ovary and atretic vagina. In males, associated anomalies, such as absence of the vas deferens, seminal vesicles or ipsilateral testicle, may be present. The overall incidence of unilateral agenesis is slightly higher in men, but this condition is more frequently discovered in women because of the associated gynecological problems. Some degree of compensatory hypertrophy of the contralateral kidney is generally seen. The problem of a dysgenetic (or aplastic) kidney presents a similar picture. In this instance, renal tissue may be demonstrated but there is essentially no function. The ureter may be present or partially or completely atretic.

The hypoplastic kidney is best considered as an abnormality of structure and will be discussed below.

Anomalies of Structure

In general, anomalies of structure may be divided into 2 major categories: (1) small kidney: (a) with normal structure (hypoplastic kidney) or (b) with abnormal structure (small multicystic kidney disease, Potter's type IIB) and (2) large kidney: (a) with normal structure (compensatory hypertrophy or duplicated collecting system) or (b) with abnormal structure (Potter's type I polycystic disease or Potter's type IIA multicystic kidney disease).

A hypoplastic kidney is abnormally small, positioned more medially than normal, and is supplied by one or more arteries of diminished size. Clinical symptomatology is secondary to infection or hypertension. On an excretory urogram, renal function is usually normal or slightly diminished. The calyces are frequently clubbed, probably the result of maldevelopment of the papillae. The incidence of associated genital anomalies is not increased.

The Ask-Upmark kidney, which is a small kidney with an indentation in its marginal contour and a subjacent dilated, elongated calyx, may be considered a segmental hypoplasia or a sequel of chronic atrophic pyelonephritis.

Anomalies of Position

Abnormal position of 1 or both kidneys can be divided into 3 main categories: malrotation, ectopia and ptosis. Malrotation is common and can usually be classified as 1 of 4 basic types depending on the position of the renal pelvis: (1) nonrotation (the pelvis is in an anterior position), (2) incomplete rotation (the pelvis is in an anteromedial position), (3) reverse rotation (the pelvis is in a lateral position) and (4) hyperrotation (the pelvis is in a posteromedial position). Malrotation, either unilateral or bilateral, may be encountered as an isolated entity. More commonly, however, malrotation is associated with ptotic or ectopic kidney.

An ectopic kidney, by definition, never attains a normal retroperitoneal position. Its ureter is abnormally short but appropriate for the kidney's position. Its vascular supply is aberrant, the specific origin of the vessel(s) again determined by its position.

Renal ectopia can be subdivided into crossed and uncrossed types. Crossed ectopia is usually (90–95%), but not necessarily, associated with fusion. Most ectopic kidneys are located in the pelvis or lower part of the abdomen inferior to their normal position in the renal fossa. Rarely, the kidney will be located above the renal fossae and may even be in the thorax. If the left kidney is ectopically located, plain x-ray films of the abdomen show a characteristic medial displacement of the anatomical splenic flexure of the colon. The same appearance of the colon may be seen in left renal agenesis. Similarly, a characteristic position of hepatic flexure can be seen with right renal agenesis or ectopia.

The mechanism of crossed ectopia is theorized to be a failure of the ureteric bud to invaginate into the ipsilateral nephrogenic ridge. Instead, it migrates to the contralateral ridge because of the close proximity of the ureteric buds and nephrogenic ridges during this phase of development. At this site, the usual nephron induction begins, usually partially fusing the 2 renal masses. The most common pattern of fusion is for the superior pole of the ectopic kidney to fuse with the inferior pole of the normally positioned kidney. The ureterovesical orifices are always in a normal position.

All forms of renal fusion are associated with ectopia, since at least one kidney is in an abnormal position. Contralateral fusion may cause any number of bizarre-appearing abnormalities, depending on the site of fusion. The resulting anomalies have been given descriptive names, including horseshoe, sigmoid, disc, doughnut or lump kidney.

A horseshoe kidney is the most common type of fusion anomaly. The lower poles are fused by a band of either functioning renal parenchyma or fibrous tissue. This fixation of the lower poles abnormally orients the kidney's axis, the lower poles positioned more medial than the upper poles. The fusion is thought to represent an impediment to renal "ascent" and therefore these kidneys are usually found at the level of the 4th or 5th lumbar vertebra. Malrotation (either nonrotation or incomplete rotation) is almost always associated, the ureter and pelvis located anteriorly and overlying the isthmus. This may impair urine flow, with resultant obstruction and calculus formation.

A ptotic kidney, by definition, reaches a normal position but does not maintain it. The ureter has a normal length but becomes redundant secondary to the low position of the kidney. The vascular supply, however, is normal.

Extrarenal Anomalies

Extrarenal anomalies include (1) an extrarenal pelvis, which is commonly associated with ectopia and fusion abnormalities, and (2) vascular anomalies, such as aneurysms and multiple renal arteries.

ANOMALIES OF THE RENAL PELVIS AND URETER

Anomalies of Number

Duplication of the renal pelvis and ureter, partial or complete, is a frequent anomaly of the genitourinary tract. It is estimated to occur in 0.5% of the general population and is bilateral in 10% of the cases. The malformation occurs if 2 ureteric buds arise from the wolffian duct, or if the single bud bifurcates during its development. Thus, there may be either complete duplication with both ureters entering the bladder at separate orifices, or, more commonly, incomplete duplication with the 2 ureters uniting anywhere proximal to their entry into the bladder. Associated abnormalities are common, such as an ectopic insertion of the ureter, ureteroceles or structural renal anomalies.

A rare form of incomplete duplication is a blind-ending ureteral stump with or without an associated normal ureter connected to it. This resembles a large diverticulum 1–2 cm in length. These can be located anywhere along the ureter, but are most common at either the ureterovesical junction or pelviureteric junction.

Anomalies of Structure

Calyceal diverticula will be described in chapter 5.

True ureteral valves are rare anomalies. According to Busch (1963), a true valve must meet 3 criteria: (1) transverse folds containing bands of smooth muscle must be anatomically demonstrable, (2) proximal obstruction must be present and (3) no other cause for the obstruction can be identified. The counterpart of ureteral valves, ureteral stenosis, has no sound pathologic basis for its existence. In most cases, what was thought to be a ureteral valve or stenosis has been shown pathologically to be an inflammatory stricture or an aberrant vessel.

The prune-belly syndrome is another example of a ureteral anomaly. This entity is described in chapter 4.

Primary megaureter is another infrequently encountered entity that roentgenographically resembles the dilated ureter seen in the prune-belly syndrome. In this disorder, there is atonic dilatation of the entire ureter except at its most distal end. Here, there is a smooth, concentric, rapid tapering as it enters the vesical wall. The important roentgenographic features that separate this entity from other causes of a dilated ureter are as follows: there is no ureterovesical junction obstruction, there is no evidence of vesicoureteral reflux and there is no evidence of ureteral peristalsis at fluoroscopy.

The intrarenal counterpart of megaureter is megacalyces. The calyces are enlarged without distal obstruction and are associated with underdevelopment of the renal pyramids. The defect probably occurs as the ureteric bud and nephrogenic blastema unite. Most reported cases have been bilateral. Roentgenographically, an increased number of calyces are seen that are dilated and "clubbed." The renal medulla assumes a semilunar appearance with a normal renal cortical thickness. The pelvis and ureters are normal. Patients are usually asymptomatic.

Anomalies of Position

Pelviureteric junction obstruction and ureteroceles will be discussed in chapter 4.

Ureteral orifices located in other than their normal trigonal position are termed ectopic ureters. Approximately 90% of ectopic ureters are associated with duplicated collecting systems, the upper moiety being the ectopic component. This anomaly may clinically present as incontinence or enuresis in females.

Although most children with enuresis have no underlying structural abnormality, excretory urography should be performed on selected patients depending on clinical findings. The anatomical causes of enuresis may be divided into 4 categories: (1) An ectopic ureter associated with a duplicated collecting system. This is a well-recognized cause of enuresis in females; however, in males, insertion of the ureter is proximal to the external sphincter and will not cause incontinence. The duplicated upper pole is often small and functions poorly. Contralateral duplication aids in the diagnosis. (2) An ectopic ureter with a single collecting system. In this type, the kidney is often small and functions very poorly. Although the renal tissue is often dysplastic, it produces enough urine to cause wetting. (3) Vaginal reflux. Vaginal reflux during micturition is common but normally drains promptly. If there is delay in vaginal drainage, it can produce prolonged seepage and "incontinence." (4) Sacral anomalies. Spinal dysraphia and caudal regression are among the most common causes of incontinence secondary to the associated neurological abnormalities.

The final anomaly that can be classified in this section is that of a retrocaval ureter. This occurs almost exclusively on the right side at the level of L3–4, but has been reported on the left side if there is a left-sided inferior vena cava. The embryological defect is a persistence of the subcardinal vein rather than the supracardinal vein as it forms the infrarenal portion of the inferior vena cava. Patients may be symptomatic if the inferior vena cava produces an obstructive uropathy.

ANOMALIES OF THE BLADDER

Anomalies of Number

Agenesis of the bladder and an accessory bladder are extremely uncommon anomalies. Duplication of the bladder is also very rare. In this entity, each ureter drains into its respective orifice but the bladder is divided by a complete sagittal septum. Duplication of the urethra is often associated.

Anomalies of Structure

Anomalies of structure are far more common than anomalies of number. "Bladder ears" represent extraperitoneal herniation of the bladder through the internal inguinal ring under 6 months of age. Inguinal hernias are clinically evident in a high percentage of these children.

Bladder diverticula are produced by mucosal herniation through defects in the muscular wall. A frequent form is the paraureteral (Hutch) diverticulum. These are generally associated with either a low urinary tract obstruction or, more commonly, neurogenic bladder from any cause. The explanation for these diverticula, as proposed by Hutch et al. (1965), is that the ureteral insertion is an inherent weak point in the bladder wall. A saccule is formed in the region of the ureteral orifice, usually laterally and superiorly. As the saccule enlarges, it incorporates the ureteral orifice on its inframedial aspect. Therefore, the intramural course of the distal ureter is lost allowing vesicoureteral reflux.

Another entity sometimes associated with Hutch diverticula is the megacystis syndrome. In this disorder of unknown cause, the bladder is large and thin-walled, with the trigone 2–3 times its normal size. The ureteral orifices are large with associated vesicoureteral reflux. This entity is more commonly seen in young girls. The megacystis may be a part of the megacystis-microcolon-intestinal hypoperistalsis syndrome described by Berdon (1976).

Exstrophy of the bladder is one of the common structural anomalies of the bladder and is more common in males. In this disorder, abnormal persistence of the cloacal membrane acts as a mechanical barrier to mesodermal movement during the first 6 weeks of embryonic life. Since this membrane extends from the hindgut to the allantoic duct, the associated anomalies may involve portions of the urinary, genital, musculoskeletal and gastrointestinal systems. Depending on the degree of involvement, various types of the anomaly have been described. (1) Classically, exstrophy of the bladder represents eversion of the bladder through a defect in the anterior abdominal wall associated with separation of the pubic symphysis. The upper urinary tract is frequently normal. (2) Cloacal exstrophy occurs when the cloacal membrane prematurely dehisces prior to the development of the urorectal septum. The bladder, urethra and intestine are everted through the diastasis of the anterior abdominal wall. Gonadal agenesis and spina bifida are frequently associated. (3) Duplicated exstrophy is rare. There is a normal urinary tract, but remnants of the primitive bladder are externalized and associated with defects in the abdominal musculature. (4) A superior vesical fissure may be present and represents a relatively mild form. The vesical opening is just inferior to the umbilicus. The remaining urinary tract is frequently normal. (5) An inferior vesical fissure is a type of epispadias in which the urethral meatus may be located anywhere from the pubic symphysis to the glans penis.

Abnormality of Position

An abnormal position of the bladder is rare but, if present, is usually associated with urachal abnormalities. In the fetus, the bladder is located at the umbilicus and communicates with the allantoic canal. The urachus is formed as the bladder begins its descent into the true pelvis. As this occurs, the vertex of the bladder elongates, forming a fibromuscular appendage approximately 5 cm long and surrounding the allantoic canal. This canal is normally obliterated by the time of birth; however, several anomalies of the urachus may develop.

A patent urachus is the result of persistence of the allantoic canal between the bladder and the umbilicus. It may be associated with persistence of the fetal position of the bladder without descent, with partial bladder descent or with a normal descent of the bladder.

A partially patent urachus means that the urachus either communicates with the umbilicus but not the bladder (urachal sinus), or communicates with the bladder but not the umbilicus. If the allantoic canal is obliterated at both ends but patent in between, a urachal cyst will form. An excretory urogram should be obtained in all instances of urachal anomalies as there is increased association with other anomalies of the urinary tract.

ANOMALIES OF THE URETHRA

A duplicate or accessory urethra is an uncommon malformation occurring almost exclusively in males. True duplication is associated with duplication of the bladder and, usually, duplication of the genitalia. One urethra drains each bladder and the diagnosis is generally obvious.

Hypospadias, epispadias and meatal stenosis are best diagnosed clinically. Fistulous communication with the vagina and rectum (in rectal atresia) may occur.

Congenital megaurethra is the result of a deficiency of erectile tissue and may be associated with the prune-belly syndrome.

OTHER ANOMALIES OF THE LOWER URINARY TRACT

Other abnormal cystic structures in males are derived from the müllerian duct. Normally, the structure forms the appendix testis and prostatic utricle. Abnormal remnants of this structure can be found anywhere from the scrotum, along the vas deferens, to the region of the utricle. The usual location is in the midline between the bladder and the rectum. Initial symptoms depend on the size and the presence or absence of infection. A müllerian duct cyst will be demonstrated roentgenographically as a mass between the bladder and the rectum. Cysts of the seminal vesicles may be confused with müllerian duct cysts but are generally not in the midline and contain spermatozoa.

REFERENCES

Abeshouse, B. S., et al.: Crossed renal ectopia with and without fusion, Urology 9:63, 1959.

Abowitz, J.: Obstructive hydronephrosis, Radiology 48:33, 1947.

Allen, R. P., et al.: Transitory extraperitoneal hernia of the bladder in infants (bladder ears), Radiology 77:979, 1961.

Amar, A. D.: Reflux in duplicated ureters, Br. J. Urol. 40:385, 1968.

Ambos, M. A., et al.: The pear-shaped bladder, Radiology 122:85, 1977.

Anderson, K. N., et al.: Congenital valves of the posterior urethra, J. Urol. 95:783, 1966.

Arduina, L. J.: Crossed ectopy without fusion, J. Urol. 93:125, 1965.

Arey, L. B.: *Developmental Anatomy* (7th ed; Philadelphia: W. B. Saunders Co., 1974).

Ashley, D. J. B., et al.: Renal agenesis and dysgenesis, J. Urol. 83:211, 1960.

Aurora, A. L., et al.: Bladder stone disease of childhood, Acta Paediatr. Scand. 59:177, 1970.

Barnes, J. C., et al.: The VATER Association, Radiology 126:445, 1978.

Berdon, W. E., et al.: Megacystis–microcolon–intestinal hypoperistalsis syndrome, A.J.R. 126:957, 1976.

Bernstein, J.: Developmental abnormalities of the renal parenchyma: Renal hypoplasia and dysplasia, Pathol. Annu. 3:213, 1968.

Bischkoff, P.: Megaureter, Br. J. Urol. 29:411, 1957.

Blackard, C. E., and Mellinger, G. T.: Cancer in horseshoe kidneys, Arch. Surg. 97:616, 1968.

Bodian, M.: Some observations on the pathology of congenital "idiopathic bladder neck obstruction" – Marion's disease, Br. J. Urol. 29:393, 1957.

Burkland, C. E.: Clinical considerations in aplasia, hypoplasia and atrophy of the kidney, J. Urol. 71:1, 1954.

Busch, F. M., et al.: Congenital ureteral valve, J. Urol. 90:43, 1963.

Carlson, H. E.: Supernumerary kidney: A summary of 51 cases, J. Urol. 4:224, 1950.

Chang, C. V.: Anterior urethral valves: A case report, J. Urol. 100:29, 1968.

Chem, D., et al.: Ectopic ureter with congenital absence of the urethral sphincter, Br. J. Urol. 37:320, 1968.

Cook, J. H., et al.: Ultrasonic demonstration of intrarenal anatomy, A.J.R. 129:831, 1977.

Currarino, G., et al.: Anal agenesis with rectobulbar fistula, Radiology 126:457, 1978.

Curtis, J. A., et al.: Malposition of the colon in right renal agenesis, ectopia, and anterior nephrectomy, A.J.R. 129:845, 1977.

Danforth, D. N.: *Textbook of Obstetrics and Gynecology* (2d ed.; New York: Harper & Row, 1971).

Daniel, J., et al.: Congenital anterior urethral valve: Diagnosis and treatment, Br. J. Urol. 40:589, 1968.

Dees, J. E.: Clinical importance of congenital anomalies of the upper urinary tract, J. Urol. 46:659, 1941.

Drummond, K. N.: Renal anatomy, in Nelson, W. E. (ed.): *Textbook of Pediatrics* (Philadelphia: W. B. Saunders Co., 1975).

Drummond, K. N.: Renal physiology, in Nelson, W. E. (ed.): *Textbook of Pediatrics* (Philadelphia: W. B. Saunders Co., 1975).

Drummond, K. N.: Developmental abnormalities, in Nelson, W. E. (ed.): *Textbook of Pediatrics* (Philadelphia: W. B. Saunders Co., 1975).

Drummond, K. N.: Congenital malformation of the urinary collecting system, bladder and urethra, in Nelson, W. E. (ed.): *Textbook of Pediatrics* (Philadelphia: W. B. Saunders Co., 1975).

Effman, E. L., et al.: Renal growth, Radiol. Clin. North Am. 15:3, 1977.

Ellis, D. G.: Duplicate exstrophy of the bladder, J. Urol. 106:295, 1971.

Ellis, D. G., et al.: Congenital posterior urethral valves, J. Urol. 95:549, 1966.

Emmett, J. L., et al.: *Clinical Urography* (Philadelphia: W. B. Saunders Co., 1971).

Engel, R. M., et al.: Bladder exstrophy, J. Urol. 104:699, 1970.

Exley, M., et al.: Supernumerary kidney with clear-cell carcinoma, J. Urol. 51:569, 1944.

Forgoard, D. M., et al.: Trifurcation of the anterior urethra: A case report, J. Urol. 95:785, 1966.

Gayanna, R., et al.: The pathologic and anomalous conditions associated with duplication of the renal pelvis and ureter, J. Urol. 54:1, 1945.

Greenwald, P.: Relation of müllerian and wolffian ducts and its genesis in malformations, Anat. Rec. 26:33, 1937.

Harcke, H. T., et al.: Bladder diverticula and Menkes' syndrome, Radiology 124:459, 1977.

Hutch, J. A., et al.: Etiology of non-occlusive ureteral dilatation, J. Urol. 93:177, 1965.

Kittredge, R. D., et al.: Urethral diverticula in women, J. Urol. 98:200, 1966.

Laughlin, V. C.: Retrocaval ureter associated with solitary kidney, J. Urol. 71:195, 1954.

Leadbetter, G. W., et al.: Urethral stricture in male children, J. Urol. 87:409, 1962.

Lich, R.: The obstructed ureteropelvic junction, Radiology 68:337, 1957.

Lich, R.: A clinical-pathologic study of ureteropelvic junction obstruction, J.Urol. 77:382, 1957.

Mandler, J. I., et al.: Polyps of the posterior urethra in children, J. Urol. 100:317, 1968.

Marshall, V. F., et al.: Variations in exstrophy, J. Urol. 88:766, 1962.

Mascatello, V., et al.: Malposition of the colon in left renal agenesis and ectopia, Radiology 120:371, 1976.

McDonald, D. G.: Ultrasound of the urinary tract, Curr. Probl. Diag. Radiol. 7:1, 1977.

Meyers, M. A., et al.: Malposition and displacement of the bowel in renal agenesis and ectopia: New observations, A.J.R. 117:323, 1973.

Mindell, H. J., et al.: Horseshoe kidney: Ultrasonic demonstration, A.J.R. 129:526, 1977.

Moore, K. L.: *The Developing Human: Clinically Oriented Embryology* (Philadelphia: W. B. Saunders Co., 1973).

Moore, T.: Hydrocalicosis, Br. J. Urol. 22:304, 1950.

Morin, M. E., et al.: Urachal cyst in the adult: Ultrasound diagnosis, A.J.R. 132:831, 1979.

Ney, C.: *Radiographic Atlas of the Genito-urinary System.* (Philadelphia: J. B. Lippincott Co., 1966).

Palubinskas, A. J.: Medullary sponge kidney, Radiology 76:911, 1961.

Paquin, A. J., et al.: The megaceptis syndrome, J. Urol. 83:634, 1960.

Pinckney, L. E., et al.: Renal malposition associated with omphalocele, Radiology 129:677, 1978.

Potter, E. L.: *Normal and Abnormal Development of the Kidney* (Chicago: Year Book Medical Publishers, Inc., 1972).

Purpon, I.: Crossed renal ectopy with solitary kidney: A review of the literature, J. Urol. 90:13, 1963.

Rank, W. B., et al.: Ureteral diverticula etiologic considerations, J. Urol. 83:566, 1960.

Reilly, B. J., et al.: Renal tubular ectasia in cystic disease of the kidneys and liver, A. J. R. 84:546, 1960.

Schumaker, H. B.: Congenital anomalies of the genitalia associated with unilateral renal agenesis, Arch. Surg. 37:586, 1938.

Shopfner, C. E.: Ureteropelvic junction obstruction, A.J.R. 98:148, 1966.

Smith, D. W.: Recognizable patterns of human malformations, Major Probl. Clin. Pediatr., no. 7, 1976.

Smith, R. C., et al.: A clinical and statistical study of 471 congenital anomalies of the kidney and ureter, J. Urol. 53:11, 1945.

Stannard, M. W., et al.: Urography in the child who wets, A.J.R. 130:959, 1978.

Stephens, F. D.: *Congenital Malformations of the Rectum, Anus, and Genitourinary Tracts* (Edinburgh: E. & S. Livingstone Ltd., 1963).

Sussman, M. L., et al.: *Urologic Roentgenology* (Baltimore: Williams & Wilkins Co., 1967).

Swenson, O., et al.: A new concept of the etiology of megaloureters, N. Engl. J. Med. 246:41, 1952.

Talner, L. B., et al.: Megacalyces, Clin. Radiol. 23:355, 1972.

Tanagho, E. A., et al.: Trigonal hypertrophy: A cause of ureteral obstruction, J. Urol. 93:678, 1965.

Teele, R. L.: Ultrasonography of the genitourinary tract in children, Radiol. Clin. North Am. 15:109, 1977.

Teele, R. L., et al.: The anatomic splenic flexure: An ultrasonic renal impostor, A.J.R. 128:115, 1977.

Teichmann-Duplessis, H., et al.: *Illustrated Human Embryology*, vol. 1 (New York: Springer-Verlag New York, Inc., 1972).

Thompson, G. J., et al.: Ureterocele: A clinical study and a report of 37 cases, J. Urol. 47:800, 1942.

Thompson, G. J., et al.: Congenital solitary kidney, J. Urol. 68:63, 1952.

Vezina, W. C. et al.: Megacystis-microcolon-intestinal hypoperistalsis syndrome: Antenatal ultrasound appearance, A. J. R. 133:749, 1979.

Waterhouse, K., et al.: The importance of urethral valves as a cause of vesical neck obstruction in children, J. Urol. 87:404, 1962.

Wepfer, J. F., et al.: Mesonephric duct remnants (Gartner's duct), A.J.R. 131:499, 1978.

White, P., et al.: Exstrophy of the bladder, Radiol. Clin. North Am. 15:93, 1977.

Williams, D. I.: Renal Anomalies, in *Urology in Childhood*, vol. 15 (suppl.), *Encyclopedia of Urology* (New York: Springer-Verlag New York, Inc., 1974).

Williams, D. I., et al.: The prune-belly syndrome, J. Urol. 98:244, 1967.

Williams, D. I., et al.: Further progress with reconstruction of the exstrophied bladder, Br. J. Surg. 60:203, 1973.

Williams, J. L., et al.: Congenital multiple diverticula of the ureter, Br. J. Urol. 37:299, 1965.

Zatz, L. M.: Combined physiologic and radiologic studies of bladder function in female children with recurrent urinary tract infections, Invest. Urol. 3:278, 1965.

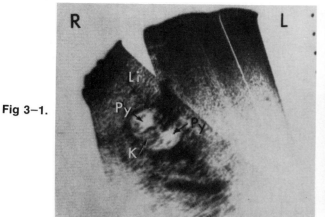

Fig 3–1.

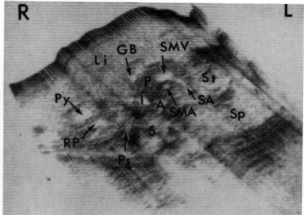

Fig 3–2.

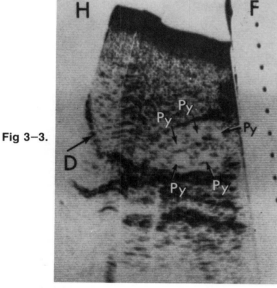

Fig 3–3.

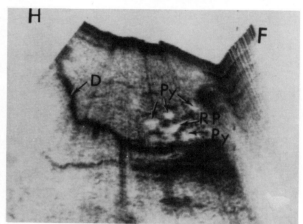

Fig 3–4.

Figs 3–1 to 3–4.—Normal neonatal kidneys. In the neonatal period the right kidney can be examined both transversely (Figs 3–1 and 3–2) and longitudinally (Figs 3–3 and 3–4) with the patient in the supine position. The liver acts as acoustic window, and in this age group 5-MHz transducers usually provide excellent renal architectural detail. Differentiation of renal pyramids from cortical portions of renal parenchyma is frequently possible. In fact, sonolucent nature of renal pyramids may be so striking that they may be mistaken for cysts within kidney. Careful attention should be paid to lack of through transmission as well as absence of sharp specular reflection from deep wall, which are distinguishing characteristics. Frequently relationship of kidneys to psoas muscle, inferior vena cava, gallbladder and head of pancreas· can be delineated. In this age group, very little renal sinus fat is present and therefore renal sinus echoes that are seen so frequently in adult are not as prominent. However, with higher-frequency transducers, it is not uncommon to see a small amount of fluid normally in renal pelvis. This should not be mistaken for mild hydronephrosis.

Left kidney is rarely well visualized transversely or longitudinally with the patient in supine position. Usually overlying gas prevents penetration of sound beam and sonographer must place the patient in either prone or lateral decubitus position to image the left kidney. R = right; L = left; H = head; F = feet; Li = liver; Py = pyramid; K = kidney; RP = renal pelvis; GB = gallbladder; Ps = psoas muscle; S = spine; I = inferior vena cava; A = aorta; P = pancreas; SMV = superior mesenteric vein; SA = splenic artery; SMA = superior mesenteric artery; St = stomach; Sp = spleen; D = diaphragm.

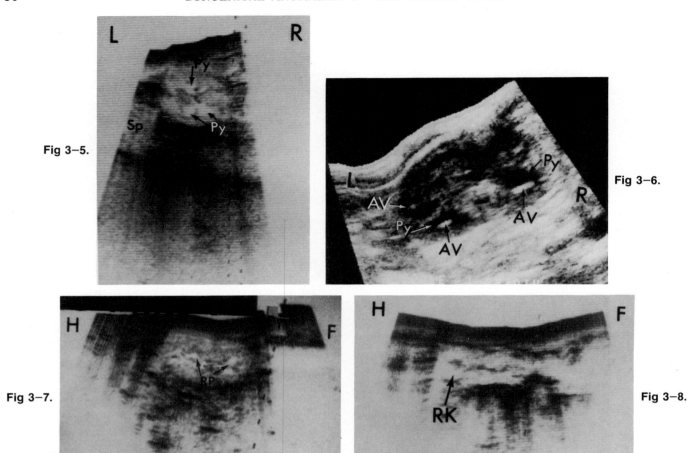

Figs 3–5 to 3–8. — Normal neonatal kidneys. Either kidney may be satisfactorily visualized with the patient in prone position. Both transverse (Figs 3–5 and 3–6) and longitudinal (Figs 3–7 and 3–8) scans are necessary to obtain 3-dimensional picture of kidney. Sonolucent nature of renal pyramids can frequently be appreciated. In addition, strong reflection at central portion of corticomedullary junction is occasionally seen and represents arcuate vasculature. Although these are small vessels, they are specular reflectors and beam-width artifact produces large echo complex. Absence of prominent renal sinus echo in neonate should be emphasized since this is normal. In addition, small amount of fluid in renal pelvis that is frequently seen with patient in prone position should not be mistaken for mild hydronephrosis. Upper pole of either kidney may be difficult to define accurately due to air in the lung in the overlying costophrenic angle. In these situations, decubitus scan of kidney is frequently more satisfactory. L = left; R = right; Sp = spleen; Py = pyramid; AV = arcuate vessels; H = head; F = feet; RP = renal pelvis; RK = right kidney.

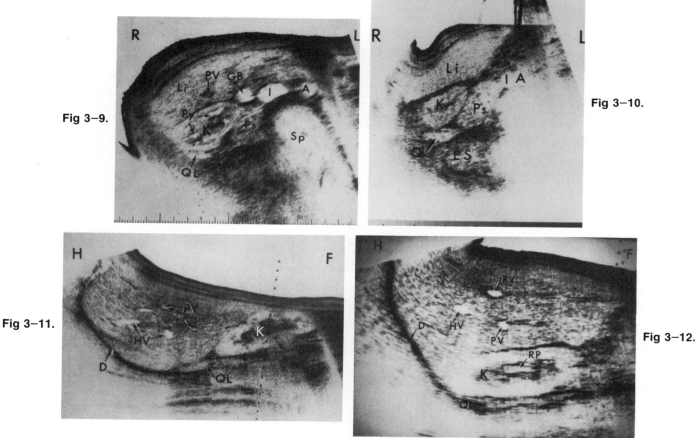

Fig 3–9.

Fig 3–10.

Fig 3–11.

Fig 3–12.

Figs 3–9 to 3–12.—Normal kidneys in older child. Right kidney can be well visualized in older child in supine position. Transverse (Figs 3–9 and 3–10) and longitudinal (Figs 3–11 and 3–12) scans will give 3-dimensional picture of intimate relationships of kidney and surrounding musculature. In addition, positional relationship of kidney to liver is frequently best appreciated on longitudinal scans. Excellent renal architecture can usually be obtained in thinner patients, including differentiation of pyramids from renal cortex. Although perirenal fascia usually cannot be separately distinguished, echogenic perinephric and paranephric fat is evident.

In older child renal sinus fat is more abundant and stands out as separate echogenic region in central portion of kidney. Small fluid areas within this renal sinus complex may be appreciated with high-resolution transducers representing the normal renal pelvis. Because of this finding, it may be difficult to differentiate this from early hydronephrosis. R = right; L = left; H = head; F = feet; Li = liver; PV = portal vein; GB = gallbladder; Py = pyramid; K = kidney; Ps = psoas muscle; QL = quadratus lumborum; I = inferior vena cava; A = aorta; Sp = spine; ES = erector spinae muscle; HV = hepatic vein; D = diaphragm; RP = renal pelvis.

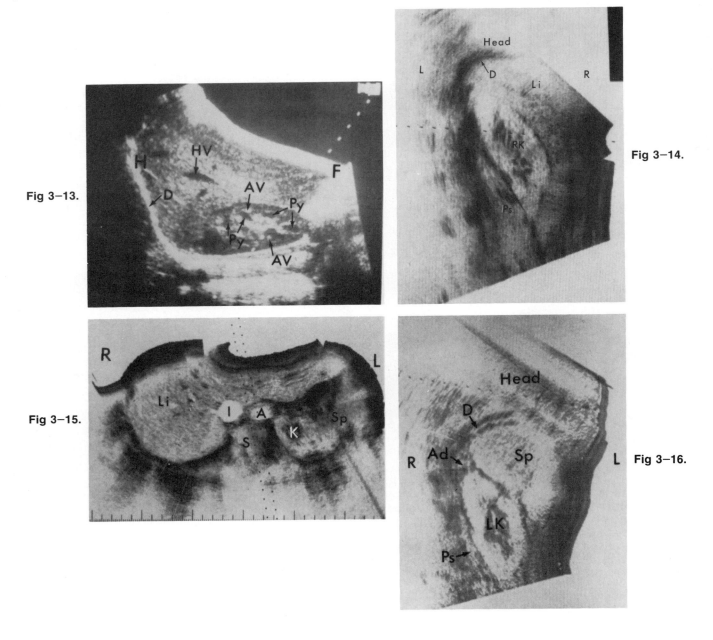

Fig 3-13.

Fig 3-14.

Fig 3-15.

Fig 3-16.

Figs 3–13 to 3–16.—Normal kidneys in older child. Although frequently the best intrarenal architecture of right kidney can be obtained in longitudinal scans performed with patient in supine position (Fig 3–13), medial and upper-pole relationships are often best demonstrated utilizing coronal scan with patient in a decubitus position (Fig 3–14). In addition, the relationship of the kidney to the psoas muscle and abnormalities in the renal axis are also maximally displayed.

Left kidney is only rarely well delineated with the patient in supine position (Fig 3–15). In addition to prone scans, coronal scan performed with the patient in decubitus position is frequently optimal (Fig 3–16). Intimate relationships of left kidney to psoas muscle, spleen and adrenal gland can be demonstrated in this view.

Decubitus positions are also preferable for suspected lesions along lateral or medial aspect of kidney. In addition, evaluation for suspected hydronephrosis is often best performed in this position so that communication between dilated calyces and renal pelvis can best be appreciated. Therefore, decubitus position should be standard view in all renal studies. H = head; F = feet; L = left; R = right; D = diaphragm; HV = hepatic vein; Py = pyramid; AV = arcuate vasculature; RK = right kidney; Ps = psoas muscle; Li = liver; I = inferior vena cava; A = aorta; S = spine; K = kidney; Sp = spleen; LK = left kidney; Ad = adrenal gland.

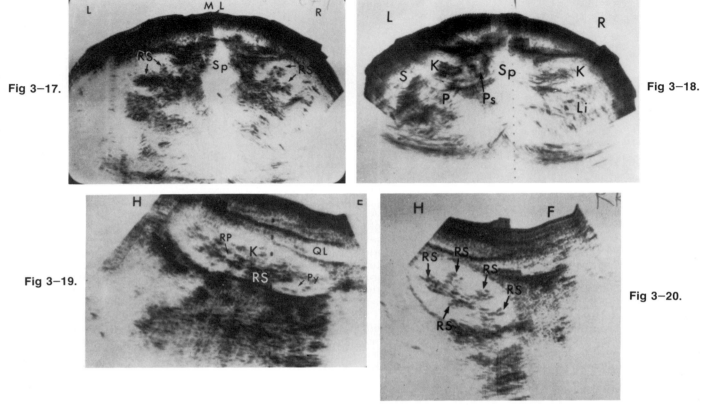

Figs 3–17 to 3–20. — Normal kidneys in older child. Transverse (Figs 3–17 and 3–18) and longitudinal (Figs 3–19 and 3–20) scans performed with the patient in prone position frequently give excellent 3-dimensional view of either kidney in older child. Corticomedullary junction is not seen as often in these views as in supine views of right or decubitus views of either kidney. Nevertheless, considerable renal sinus branching detail frequently can be visualized in these views. Considerable variation occurs in renal sinus branching pattern for each individual and normal variations must be learned. Small fluid areas in middle of renal sinus representing normal renal pelvis may also be visualized. Relationship of left kidney to pancreas is usually best appreciated in these views. L = left; R = right; ML = midline; RS = renal sinus; Sp = spine; S = spleen; K = kidney; P = pancreas; Ps = psoas muscle; Li = liver; RP = renal pelvis; Py = pyramid; QL = quadratus lumborum muscle; H = head; F = feet.

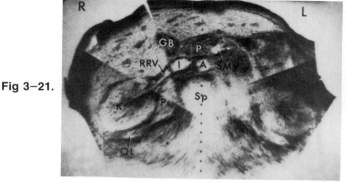

Fig 3–21.

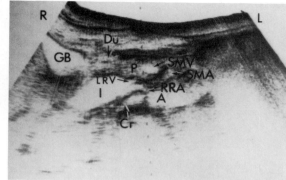

Fig 3–22.

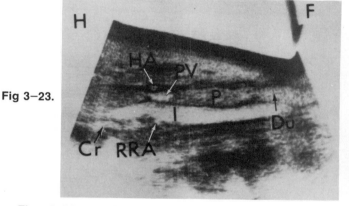

Fig 3–23.

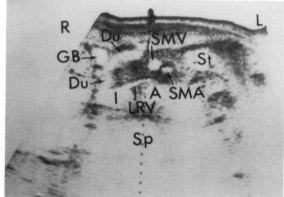

Fig 3–24.

Figs 3–21 to 3–24.—Normal renal vasculature. In most children, portions of normal renal vasculature can be visualized in either transverse or longitudinal scans. Right renal vein is frequently best visualized in transverse scans performed with the patient in supine position (Fig 3–21). Right renal vein arises from right lateral aspect of inferior vena cava (IVC) and courses directly into right renal sinus. Right renal artery is frequently confused with right crus of diaphragm (Fig 3–22). Right renal artery, however, arises from right anterolateral aspect of aorta and passes between thickened right crus of diaphragm and IVC. This vessel may be traceable all the way into renal sinus. Right renal artery is best visualized in longitudinal scans (Fig 3–23) performed with the patient in supine position. Vessel can be seen to notch dorsal aspect of IVC as it passes anterior to right crus of diaphragm.

Left renal vein arises from left lateral aspect of IVC and passes anterior to aorta but posterior to superior mesenteric vessels (Fig 3–24). Vessel is intimately related to posterior aspect of head and uncinate process of pancreas. R = right; L = left; GB = gallbladder; RRV = right renal vein; K = kidney; QL = quadratus lumborum muscle; Ps = psoas muscle; Sp = spine; I = inferior vena cava; P = pancreas; A = aorta; SMV = superior mesenteric vein; Du = duodenum; LRV = left renal vein; SMA = superior mesenteric artery; RRA = right renal artery; Cr = crus of diaphragm; HA = hepatic artery; PV = portal vein; St = stomach; H = head; F = feet.

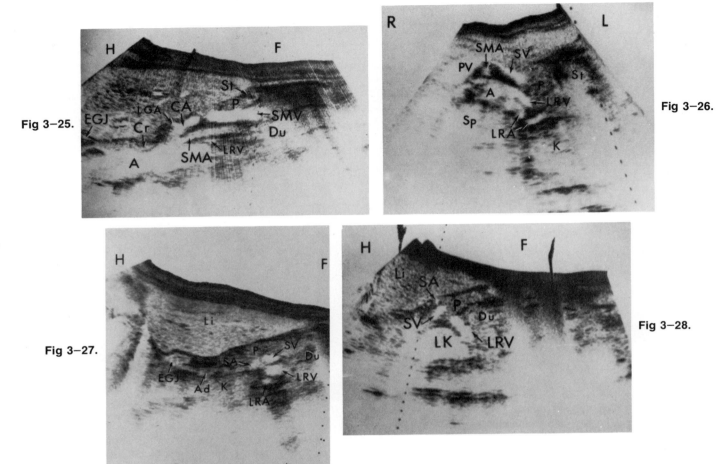

Figs 3–25 to 3–28.—Normal renal vasculature. Left renal vein can frequently be identified in the midline of longitudinal scans performed with patient in supine position (Fig 3–25). Vessel will be seen to lie posterior to superior mesenteric artery and anterior to aorta. After passing over the aorta, left renal vein courses into left kidney. In this region, it may be separable from left renal artery on either transverse (Fig 3–26) or longitudinal (Fig 3–27) scans. Frequently, however, vessels cannot be individually distinguished and are seen as 1 prominent left renal vascular bundle (Fig 3–28). Longitudinal scans performed with patient in supine position but inclined laterally to left are often best means of distinguishing left renal vascular bundle from splenic vessels (Figs 3–27 and 3–28). Furthermore, relationship of left renal vessels to adrenal gland and 4th portion of duodenum are often best demonstrated in these views. H = head; F = feet; R = right; L = left; EGJ = esophagogastric junction; A = aorta; Cr = crus of diaphragm; LGA = left gastric artery; CA = celiac artery; SMA = superior mesenteric artery; LRV = left renal vein; St = stomach; P = pancreas; SMV = superior mesenteric vein; Du = duodenum; PV = portal vein; SV = splenic vein; LRA = left renal artery; Sp = spine; K = kidney; Ad = adrenal gland; SA = splenic artery; Li = liver; LK = left kidney.

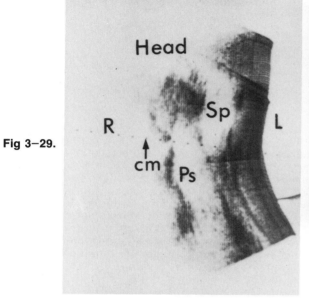

Fig 3–29.

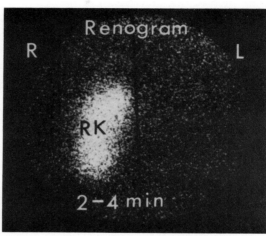

Fig 3–30.

Figs 3–29 and 3–30.—Renal agenesis. Longitudinal scan of the left renal fossa with patient in decubitus position (Fig 3–29) fails to demonstrate left kidney here. Isotope studies on same patient (Fig 3–30) demonstrate normal functioning right kidney and no evidence of function on left side. R = patient's right; L = patient's left; Sp = spleen; cm = centimeter marker; Ps = psoas muscle; RK = right kidney.

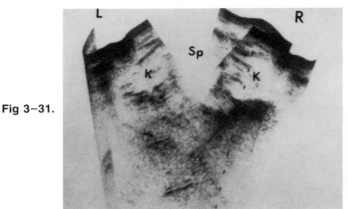

Fig 3–31.

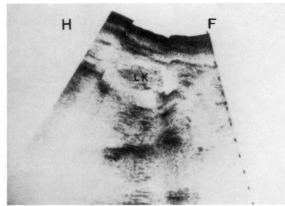

Fig 3–32.

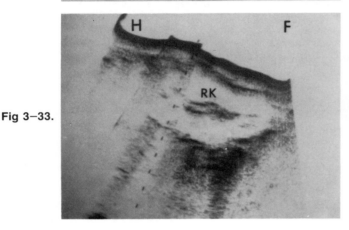

Fig 3–33.

Figs 3–31 to 3–33.—Hypoplastic kidney. A hypoplastic kidney may be only minimally smaller than contralateral normal kidney (Figs 3–31 to 3–33). In many of these cases reniform nature of mass with acoustic texture differentiation of renal sinus and renal parenchyma is possible. However, considerable irregularity in thickness of renal parenchyma will usually be evident on hypoplastic side. This type of irregularity is difficult to distinguish from asymmetrical chronic pyelonephritis. Clinical and laboratory correlation is usually necessary to make this differentiation. L = left; R = right; Sp = spine; K = kidney; LK = left kidney; RK = right kidney; H = head; F = feet.

Figs 3–34 to 3–39.—Hypoplastic right kidney. One of the more challenging diagnoses may be hypoplasia of the kidney. Sonograms should be performed with patient in all positions in an attempt to identify reniform mass in renal fossa (Figs 3–34 to 3–36). In some views, mass may be difficult to define; in other views, it may be more readily apparent. In addition, usually compensatory enlargement of normal kidney may be appreciated. It is also important to evaluate the pelvis (Fig 3–37) for presence of pelvic kidney. As hypoplastic kidneys become less reniform in nature, they become more difficult to delineate ultrasonographically. Furthermore, loops of bowel and other intra-abdominal organs may occupy partially empty fossa, mimicking renal hypoplasia. At present, a number of correlative imaging techniques can be utilized to aid in diagnosis. Computerized tomography is an excellent way to differentiate interposed bowel as well as other abdominal organs. Renal scintigraphy may help identify hypoplastic but functioning renal tissue; however, absence of renal function does not completely rule out presence of small hypoplastic kidney. Similarly, an excretory urogram, particularly with nephrotomography (Fig 3–38), may demonstrate minimally functioning reniform mass. If all noninvasive imaging modalities fail, a retrograde pyelogram (Fig 3–39) can then be performed to demonstrate hypoplastic kidney. L = left; R = right; K = kidney; S = spine; LK = left kidney; H = head; F = feet; Li = liver; HK = hypoplastic kidney; B = bladder; Ut = uterus.

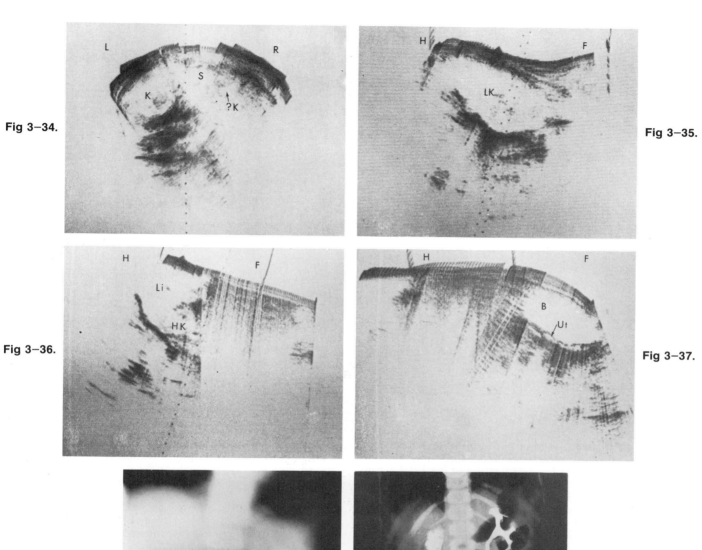

Fig 3–34.

Fig 3–35.

Fig 3–36.

Fig 3–37.

Fig 3–38.

←See legend on facing page.

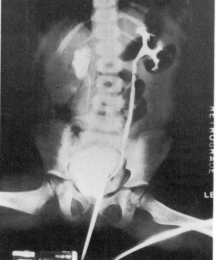

Fig 3–39.

Fig 3—40.

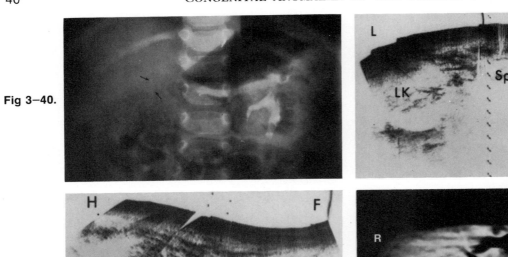

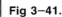
Fig 3—41.

Fig 3—42.

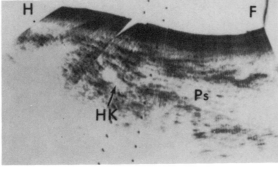

Fig 3—43.

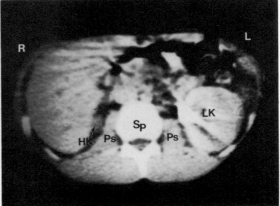

Figs 3—40 to 3—43.—Renal dysgenesis (aplasia or dysplasia). An excretory urogram (Fig 3–40) demonstrates a normal left kidney with no visualization of the right kidney. Delayed films failed to demonstrate any function on this side. On plain film and excretory urogram there were faint calcifications adjacent to 2d lumbar vertebra *(arrows)* that were suggestive of intrauterine renal vein thrombosis. However, the calcifications were pathologically proved to be in renal arteries. Transverse scan on same patient (Fig 3–41) shows normal left kidney and small "nubbin" of tissue on right side that does not have reniform appearance. Longitudinal scan (Fig 3–42) on same patient again fails to demonstrate normal reniform appearance on right side. Computerized tomography (Fig 3–43) shows normal left kidney and a "nubbin" of tissue in the area of the right kidney. L = patient's left; R = patient's right; LK = normal left kidney; HK = aplastic (dysgenetic) right kidney; Sp = spine; Ps = psoas muscle; H = toward patient's head; F = toward patient's feet.

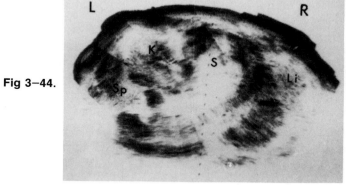

Fig 3–44.

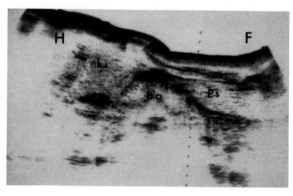

Fig 3–45.

Figs 3–44 and 3–45.—Renal agenesis. One of the most difficult diagnoses to make on ultrasound is agenesis of the kidney (Figs 3–44 and 3–45). Scans of renal fossa should be performed in all available positions as well as throughout midabdomen and pelvis. Latter scans should help rule out abnormal position of kidney, and former scans will document empty renal fossa. It should be noted that bowel or other organs may fall into empty renal fossa and mimic small hypoplastic kidney. As a result, if ultrasonography is nondiagnostic and/or nonspecific, additional studies, such as computerized axial tomography, renal scintiscan or excretory urogram, are needed to determine if there is any functioning renal tissue in the apparently empty renal fossa. H = head; F = feet; K = kidney; Sp = spleen; S = spine; Li = liver; Ps = psoas muscle; Bo = bowel; L = patient's left; R = patient's right.

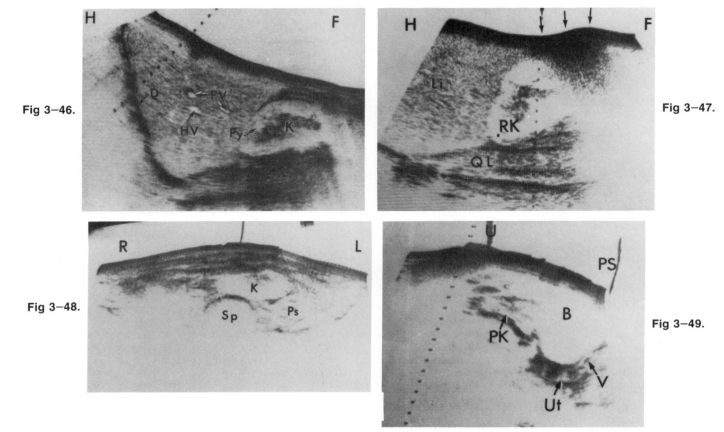

Fig 3—46.

Fig 3—47.

Fig 3—48.

Fig 3—49.

Figs 3—46 to 3—49. — Anomalies of renal position. Since kidney undergoes "migration" as well as rotation during embryogenesis, variable degrees of ectopia and malrotation can be seen. Normal relationship of kidney to liver or spleen can be demonstrated on ultrasonograms (Fig 3—46). When malrotation presents as palpable abdominal mass (Fig 3—47), normal renal origin of this palpatory finding usually can be demonstrated by ultrasound. Furthermore, the normal renal architecture, as opposed to a pathological renal mass, can usually be imaged and no additional studies are required.

Variable degrees of renal ectopia can be seen, including midabdominal kidney (Fig 3—48) and pelvic kidney (Fig 3—49). It should be emphasized that pelvic kidneys may have bizarre reniform configuration that is difficult to distinguish from true pathological pelvic mass. When equivocal, one should proceed to excretory urogram or renal scintiscan for confirmation. Many times, however, reniform nature of mass can be appreciated on sonogram and correct diagnosis made. H = head; F = feet; D = diaphragm; PV = portal vein; HV = hepatic vein; Py = pyramid; K = kidney; Li = liver; QL = quadratus lumborum muscle; RK = right kidney; Sp = spine; Ps = psoas muscle; U = umbilicus; PS = pubic symphysis; B = bladder; V = vagina; Ut = uterus; PK = pelvic kidney; L = patient's left; R = patient's right.

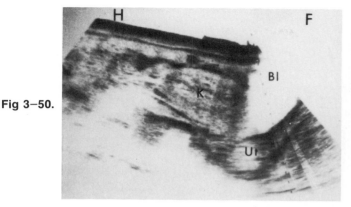

Fig 3–50.

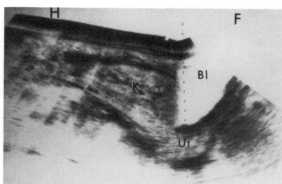

Fig 3–51.

Fig 3–52.

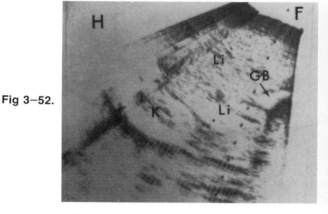

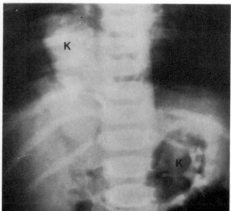

Fig 3–53.

Figs 3–50 to 3–53.—Anomalies of renal position. A pelvic kidney may mimic slightly enlarged uterus (Figs 3–50 and 3–51). With newer instrumentation, renal and uterine acoustical texture is somewhat similar. Confusion may exist if tissue plane between pelvic kidney and uterus is not demonstrated. Furthermore, since reniform configuration of pelvic kidney may not be apparent, careful scanning to try to image a renal pelvis-type echogenic pattern is necessary. Again, if possibility of a pelvic kidney is considered but the acoustical pattern is not definitive, excretory urography may be performed for confirmation.

Rarely, anomalous position of kidney may be demonstrated as intrathoracic kidney. This anomaly may be detected on chest x-ray as a mass adjacent to the diaphragm. Longitudinal scans using liver as sonic window will clearly demonstrate intrathoracic position of kidney (Fig 3–52). If necessary, this may be confirmed by performing excretory urography (Fig 3–53). H = head; F = feet; K = kidney; Bl = bladder; Ut = uterus; Li = liver; GB = gallbladder.

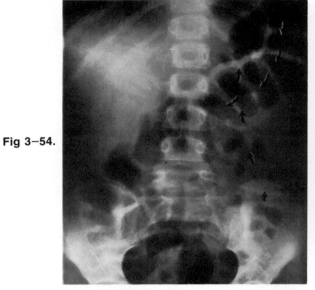

Fig 3–54.

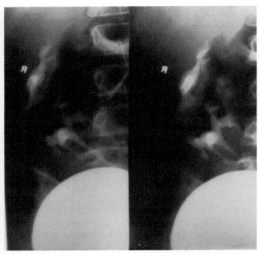

Fig 3–55.

Figs 3–54 and 3–55.—Cross-fused renal ectopia. Plain film of abdomen (Fig 3–54) demonstrates medial displacement of the anatomical splenic flexure of colon. Arrows point to location of descending colon, anatomical splenic flexure, roentgenographic splenic flexure and transverse colon. Notice anatomical splenic flexure is displaced medi- al to roentgenographic splenic flexure. This may also be seen in left renal agenesis (see Figs 3–44 and 3–45) as well as renal ectopia, as in this patient. Voiding cystourethrogram on same patient (Fig 3–55) shows vesicoureteral reflux and cross-fused renal ectopia with left kidney abnormally positioned on right side inferior to right kidney.

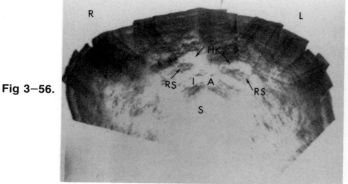

Fig 3–56.

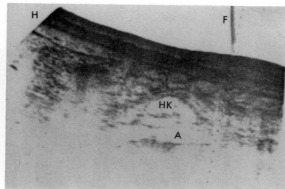

Fig 3–57.

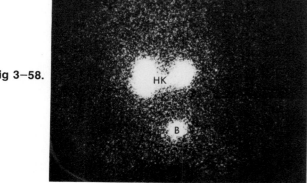

Fig 3–58.

Figs 3–56 to 3–58. — Horseshoe kidney. A variety of renal fusion anomalies may occur; the most common is horseshoe kidney. This anomaly is usually asymptomatic; however, it may present as palpable midabdominal mass or be mistaken for aortic aneurysm. On ultrasound, the mass will be found anterior to prevertebral vessels (Figs 3–56 and 3–57), which may mimic a mass in head of the pancreas, retroperitoneal adenopathy or primary retroperitoneal tumor. Careful scanning should help to bring out reniform nature of the mass with differentiation of renal sinus from renal parenchyma. In addition, usually renal sinus opens anterolaterally rather than medially, since there is rotational abnormality as well as fusion across midline. If reniform nature of mass cannot be delineated by sonography, an intravenous urogram or renal scintiscan (Fig 3–58) can be performed for confirmation. H = head; F = feet; R = right; L = left; RS = renal sinus; I = inferior vena cava; A = aorta; S = spine; HK = horseshoe kidney; B = bladder.

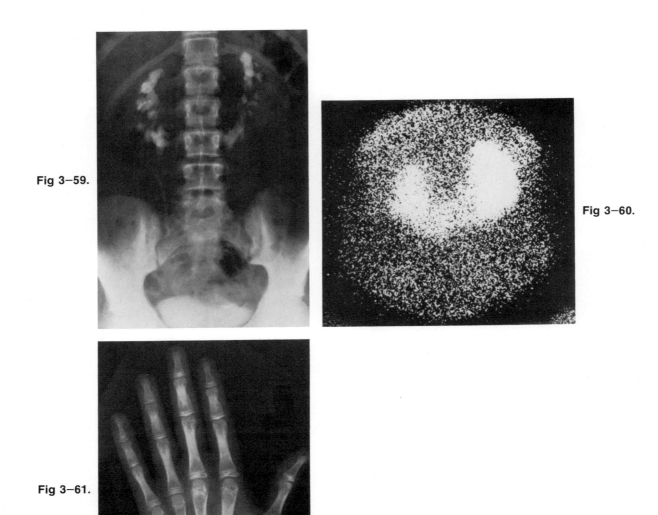

Fig 3–59.

Fig 3–60.

Fig 3–61.

Figs 3–59 to 3–61.—Horseshoe kidney in patient with Turner's syndrome. Excretory urogram (Fig 3–59) demonstrates medial displacement of lower poles and malrotation of both kidneys. This is typical appearance of horseshoe kidney. A functioning renal isthmus can be demonstrated in the renal isotope scan (Fig 3–60). Hand x-ray film demonstrates short 4th metacarpal, which is characteristic of Turner's syndrome (Fig 3–61).

46

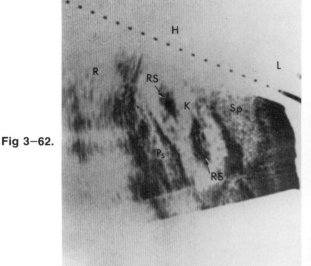

Fig 3—62.

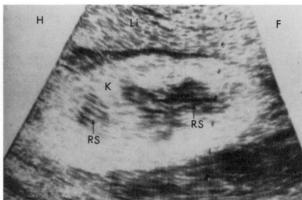

Fig 3—63.

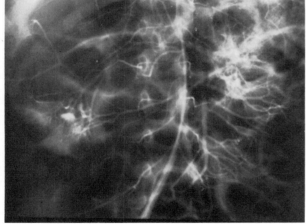

Fig 3—64.

Figs 3—62 to 3—64.—Duplication of kidney. One of the most common congenital anomalies of the urinary tract is partial or complete duplication of kidney. If no associated abnormality exists, such as hydronephrosis of the upper moiety and/or an ectopic ureterocele, then kidney will have normal reniform ultrasonic texture with differentiation of echogenic renal sinus and more sonolucent renal parenchyma. However, renal sinus will be symmetrically or asymmetrically divided by a band of sonolucent tissue (Figs 3–62 and 3–63). Key ultrasonic feature that distinguishes this anomaly from centrally located renal mass is normal acoustical texture of this band of tissue, which is similar to the rest of renal parenchyma. Although diagnosis of obstructed duplex system may be made by a variety of roentgenographic modalities including arteriograms (Fig 3–64), easiest method for diagnosis of hydronephrosis is ultrasound. H = head; F = feet; Li = liver; K = kidney; RS = renal sinus; Ps = psoas muscle; Sp = spleen; R = right; L = left.

Fig 3-65.

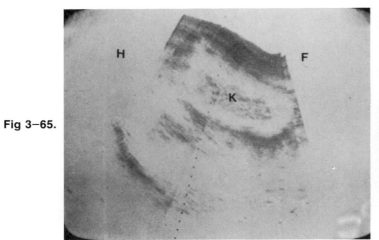

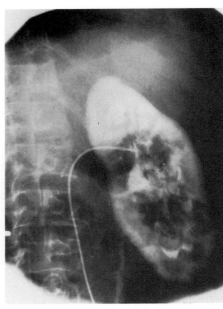

Fig 3-66.

Fig 3-67.

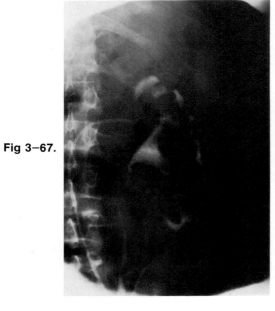

Figs 3-65 to 3-67. — Megacalyces. This anomaly is intrarenal counterpart of megaloureter. The kidney may appear enlarged sonographically (Fig 3-65) but there is no evidence of hydronephrosis. Calyces appear clubbed and are increased in number. Thickness of renal cortex and caliber of ureter are normal (Figs 3-66 and 3-67). H = head; F = feet; K = kidney.

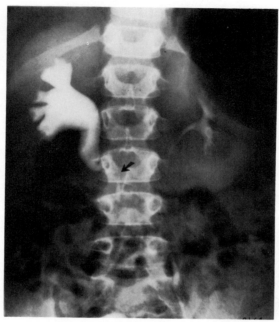

Fig 3–68.—Retrocaval ureter. Excretory urogram demonstrates medial displacement of right ureter (medial to vertebral pedicle), which is marked with arrow. Mild hydronephrosis is seen proximal to this point of partial obstruction. This anomaly is result of persistent subcardinal vein rather than supracardinal vein. Ureter is posterior to inferior vena cava.

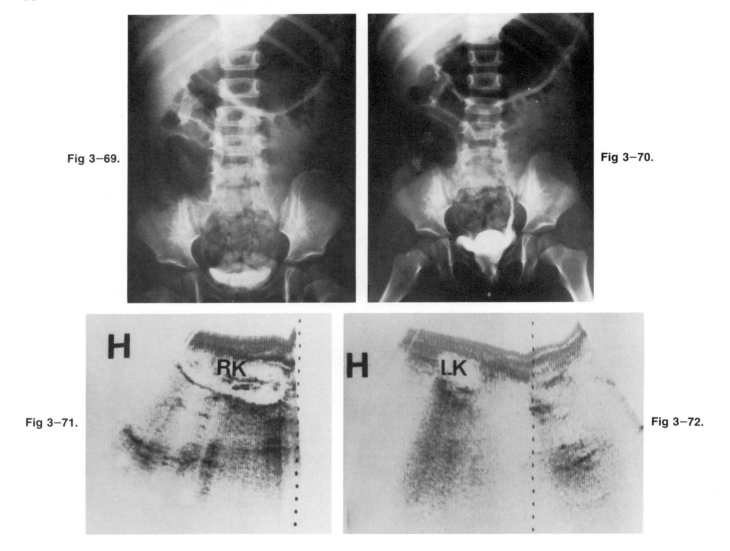

Fig 3–69.

Fig 3–70.

Fig 3–71.

Fig 3–72.

Fig 3–73.

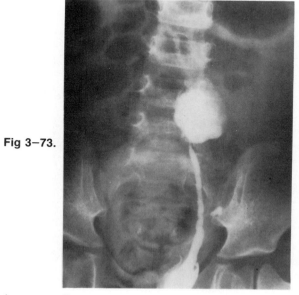

Figs 3–69 to 3–73.—Ectopic ureter. Excretory urogram (Fig 3–69) shows normal functioning right kidney and no visualization of the left kidney. This finding in association with clinical history of enuresis should suggest ectopic insertion of left ureter with abnormal function of left kidney. During micturition, there is reflux of contrast material from vagina into ectopic left ureter (Fig 3–70). Ultrasonographi-cally, normal right kidney (Fig 3–71) and small hypoplastic or dysplastic left kidney (Fig 3–72) is demonstrated. Retrograde studies show ectopic insertion of left ureter into vagina and small dysplastic left kidney (Fig 3–73). Although this kidney is dysplastic, it does have enough function to cause enuresis. H = head; RK = right kidney; LK = left kidney.

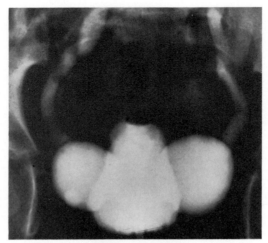

Fig 3–74.—Bilateral Hutch diverticula. Bladder diverticula are formed by mucosal herniation through defects in muscular wall. Bladder diverticula have been described in prune-belly syndrome, Menkes' kinky-hair syndrome, Eh-lers-Danlos syndrome, William's syndrome and cutis laxa. Hutch diverticula can be associated either with lower urinary tract obstruction or with neurogenic bladder.

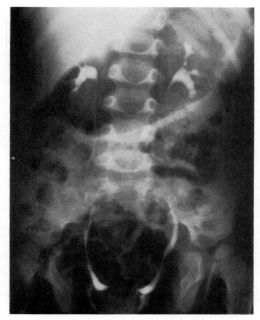

Fig 3–75.—Exstrophy of bladder. Excretory urogram in this patient shows the typical appearance of exstrophy of the bladder with diastasis of the symphysis pubis. Notice normal renal function and appearance of the collecting system. Upper urinary tracts are frequently normal in patients with classic exstrophy of bladder.

Fig 3–76.

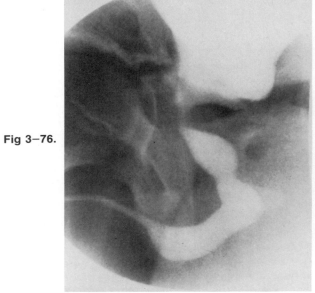

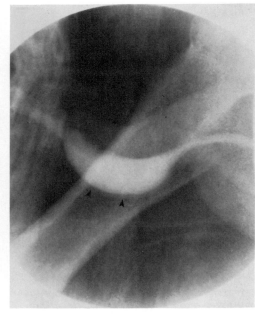

Fig 3–77.

Figs 3–76 and 3–77. — Megalourethra. Two films of voiding cystourethrogram demonstrate megalourethra. This anomaly may be associated with prune-belly syndrome.

However, in this patient it was an isolated finding. Notice close proximity of urethra to skin on the ventral aspect of the penis due to absence of erectile tissue.

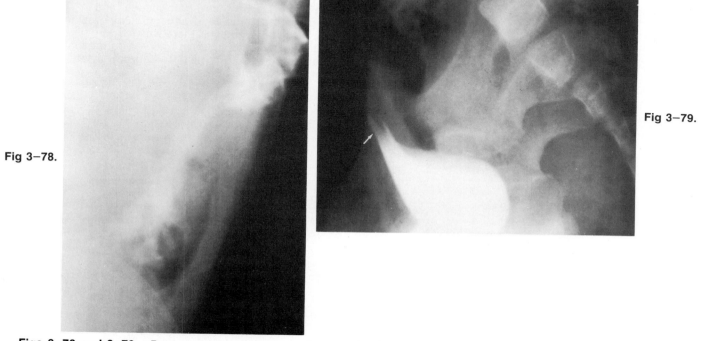

Fig 3–78.

Fig 3–79.

Figs 3–78 and 3–79.—Patent urachus. Injection of contrast material into umbilicus demonstrates connection of urachal sinus to umbilicus (Fig 3–78). Lateral view of bladder following excretory urogram (Fig 3–79), demonstrates that apex of bladder is pointing toward patent urachus *(arrow).*

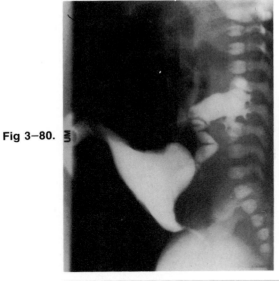

Fig 3–80.

Figs 3–80 to 3–82.—Patent urachus. Figure 3–80 shows persistent urachus that is connected to both bladder and umbilicus (UM). Figures 3–81 and 3–82 show urachal cysts in a different patient. In the latter patient, there was no connection to bladder or umbilicus but an intervening urachal remnant has formed cystic structure (US). R = right; L = left; H = head; F = feet; Bl = bladder; Sp = spine.

Fig 3–81.

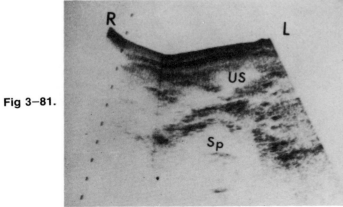

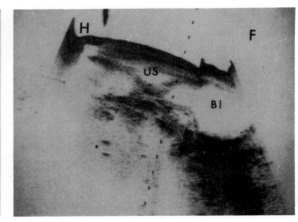

Fig 3–82.

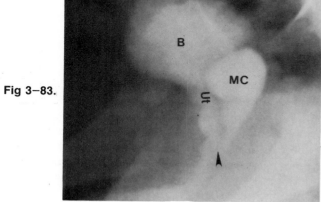

Fig 3–83.

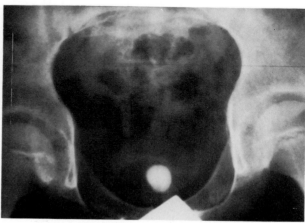

Fig 3–84.

Figs 3–83 and 3–84.—Müllerian duct cysts. Oblique film during micturition (Fig 3–83) demonstrates filling of utricle, which is somewhat dilated (müllerian duct cyst) from posterior urethra *(arrowhead)*. B = bladder; Ut = posterior urethra; MC = müllerian duct cysts. Figure 3–84 shows residual contrast material in utricle in another patient following complete voiding.

4

Hydronephrosis

THE TERM "HYDRONEPHROSIS" (of Greek origin: *hydro*, water; *nephros*, kidney; *osis*, state of) is technically a misnomer but it is used radiologically to indicate abnormal dilatation of the renal pelvis and calyces. Similarly, "hydroureter" indicates abnormal dilatation of the ureter. The compound term, "hydroureteronephrosis," defines the combination of the two conditions.

Although the most common cause of dilatation of the renal calyces, pelvis or ureter is some type of obstruction, dilatation can occur without obstruction. Therefore, it is important to distinguish between obstructive and nonobstructive dilatation. Surgery can potentially correct the former condition; however, it has only limited usefulness, if indicated at all, in the latter condition.

Since obstructive or nonobstructive urinary tract dilatation may appear identical on the excretory urogram, two tests are now being used to determine whether or not an obstruction is present. These replace the older method of measuring the drainage time following retrograde pyelography. The first, the Whitaker test, is a measurement of the urine flow rate through a suspected obstruction, and the measurement of the hydrostatic pressure in the pelvis or ureter proximal to the obstruction at that particular flow rate. This requires a percutaneous antegrade puncture of the renal pelvis and equipment capable of quantitating the desired measurements. The second, the Lasix test, is the much simpler method and gives useful qualitative results. A diuretic (Lasix) is injected intravenously (2 mg/kg) immediately following the excretory urogram. If there is an obstruction, the proximal collecting system becomes progressively more dilated. If there is no obstruction, the proximal collecting system does not become dilated, and the contrast is cleared rapidly from the collecting system.

Urinary tract obstruction has a number of renal as well as extrarenal complications. These include renal parenchymal atrophy (back-pressure atrophy), which is the most common long-term effect of postnatal obstruction; renal cystic dysplasia, which is a direct result of long-standing intrauterine obstruction; pulmonary hypoplasia, which occurs indirectly as a result of the oligohydramnios secondary to decreased fetal urine excretion (most commonly a posterior urethral valve) and its resultant therapeutic respiratory complications of interstitial emphysema, pneumothorax or pneumomediastinum. Anemia, polycythemia and hypertension may also result from the obstructive uropathy.

ROENTGENOGRAPHIC TECHNIQUE

In performing an excretory urogram, it is essential to inject a sufficient amount of contrast material. Dosages using a mixture of diatrizoate sodium and diatrizoate meglumine (Renografin-60) or an equivalent contrast agent vary with the body weight. Neonates and infants weighing less than 5.5 kg require a dose of 4 ml/kg; infants weighing 5.5 – 11 kg may receive a total dose of 25 ml; and children weighing over 11 kg require a dose of 2 ml/kg.

It is also essential to optimally visualize the entire cortical surface of the kidney. If needed, placing the patient in a prone position, insufflating the stomach with air or inflating a balloon paddle over the renal areas aids in displacing the overlying bowel gas and stool. Oblique views, and occasionally lateral views, may be necessary for accurate evaluation of the kidneys.

Routinely, following the intravenous injection of the bolus of contrast material, a coned film of the kidneys is taken at 1 minute. This is followed by a 4-minute full abdominal film, which normally shows the pyelographic phase and may be helpful in identifying lesions such as an ectopic ureterocele before the bladder becomes distended with contrast material. Immediately thereafter, coned oblique views of the kidneys may be obtained. Following the initial routine views, the urogram should be tailored as dictated by the early roentgenographic findings and the clinical suspicions until an accurate diagnosis is established. In cases of severe obstruction, it may be necessary to obtain delayed films at 24 to 48 hours. If an umbilical arterial line is present, part of the contrast material may be injected through this line and a film taken during injection to visualize the renal arteries. An inferior venacavogram may be obtained by injecting the contrast material into a dorsal vein of either foot, preferably the right. It may occasionally be necessary to perform an antegrade pyelogram to visualize the collecting system and show the site of the obstruction.

The excretory urogram evaluates renal function and determines precise anatomical detail of the kidney and collecting system. However, several other diagnostic procedures are available for pediatric patients with suspected renal abnormalities. These may be used in the appropriate clinical context. An excellent noninvasive method for evaluating renal function or the site of obstruction is a technetium renal scan. However, gray-scale ultrasonography is the easiest, most noninvasive and best screening procedure available today.

ULTRASONIC TECHNIQUE

Transverse and longitudinal scans of both kidneys are obtained with the patient in prone, supine and lateral decubitus positions using a 3.5- or 5.0-MHz transducer. Normally, the collecting system is seen as a somewhat linear band of dense echogenicity surrounded by the more homogeneous, less echogenic renal parenchyma with a sharp outer cortical margin. The corticomedullary function is often identified. With mild hydronephrosis, these dense, central echoes are separated by small ovoid or elongated lucencies. With more severe hydronephrosis, these sonolucencies become larger and may coalesce. In the most severe form, the major portion of the kidney is replaced by a sonolucent sac.

Ultrasonography is an excellent screening procedure in suspected cases of hydronephrosis as it only has a 2% false negative rate. However, there is a 26% false positive rate; therefore, any patient with an abnormality detected by ultrasound should have an excretory urogram.

CLASSIFICATION

Berdon et al. (1970) have categorized hydronephrosis into 4 grades based on the urographic appearance:

Grade I

The pelvicalyceal system initially appears lucent because it contains unopacified urine surrounded by a normal amount of functioning renal parenchyma (negative pyelogram). It then becomes progressively more dense as more contrast is excreted but remains less dense than the normal side because of the larger amount of unopacified urine. The contrast material eventually diffuses throughout the obstructed collecting system, identifying the point of obstruction.

Grade II

This shows a less than normal but adequate amount of functioning renal parenchyma during the nephrographic phase. However, the contrast material that is initially excreted into the collecting system lines the walls of the dilated calyces, producing a continuous, thin, dense, scalloped line, with the remainder of the calyces and pelvis appearing lucent (rim sign). Again, the collecting system proximal to the point of obstruction gradually becomes more opaque.

Grade III

A smaller amount of functioning renal parenchyma is present and develops a dense crescent as the result of concentration of the contrast material in dilated collecting ducts adjacent to the hydronephrotic calyces. This has been termed Dunbar's "crescent sign." Later there is gradual opacification of the hydronephrotic calyces and pelvis.

Grade IV

Only a thin rim of renal parenchyma surrounds the markedly enlarged nonopaque hydronephrotic calyces. This has been termed the shell "nephrogram" and is seen only during the nephrographic phase. Renal function is markedly impaired, to the point that there is no further visualization of the collecting system, although a small amount of contrast material is excreted.

In summary, this grading system is based on several factors: the amount of functioning renal parenchyma, the severity of the obstruction and the prognostic significance. The grading system represents a spectrum of hydronephrosis, with grade I having excellent surgical results and grade IV having very poor surgical results.

ACUTE OBSTRUCTION

Since acute ureteral obstruction is usually due to an impacted stone, and renal lithiasis is much less frequent in children than adults, it is uncommon in childhood. In 54% of the patients, no known cause is found. However, 30% of patients have associated renal anomalies, 10% have underlying metabolic disorders and in 6% the obstruction is a complication of a neurogenic bladder, prolonged recumbency or a foreign body. Other rare causes of renal stones in children include pyloric stenosis, burns, leukemia, heavy metal poisoning, vitamin D intoxication, sarcoidosis, hyperparathy-roidism, Cushing's syndrome, renal tubular acidosis and idiopathic hypercalcemia.

The urographic findings are similar to those seen in adults. Following contrast injection, there is a delayed and prolonged nephrogram with a temporary increase in density on the affected side. The kidney usually enlarges slightly. The pyelographic phase is delayed and the calyces become slightly blunted. The renal pelvis and ureter appear less radiopaque than on the normal side due to the admixture of contrast material and urine. Rarely, a striated appearance is seen in the renal pyramids due to contrast material in dilated tubules.

In addition to the sonographic abnormalities described previously, a dilated proximal ureter can usually be identified. If the obstruction is at the ureterovesical junction, scans of the pelvis may show the dilated distal ureter.

CHRONIC OBSTRUCTION

The urographic findings in chronic obstruction are similar to acute obstruction. However, because of the long-standing obstruction, there may be associated generalized parenchymal loss with an abnormal corticomedullary junction. If there is associated pyelonephritis (a common accompanying feature), focal and segmental parenchymal loss may be seen.

ETIOLOGY OF OBSTRUCTIVE UROPATHY

As previously mentioned, it is important to differentiate obstructive from nonobstructive causes of abnormal dilatation of the renal collecting system. Obstructive causes will be discussed according to their anatomical location; the nonobstructive causes will then be discussed.

CALYCEAL DILATATION

Abnormal calyceal dilatation can be seen in various conditions including hydrocalycosis, megacalycosis, back-pressure atrophy, renal vein thrombosis, papillary necrosis and reflux with infection.

Hydrocalycosis indicates calyceal dilatation secondary to infundibular obstruction. Both congenital and acquired abnormalities can cause this condition. Congenital lesions can be subdivided into intrinsic (stenosis) or extrinsic (compression by the renal artery anteriorly and vein posteriorly, Fraley's syndrome) abnormalities. Acquired lesions (such as tuberculosis, neoplasms and trauma) produce extrinsic infundibular obstruction.

Megacalycosis, on the other hand, is a congenital dilatation of the calyces without infundibular obstruction. In this condition, the kidney is usually enlarged and contains more than 20 calyces.

The other conditions mentioned above in the differential diagnosis are related in that they have a common denominator in their pathogenesis, i.e., impaired blood flow to the papillary portions of the kidney with resultant ischemia.

PELVIURETERIC JUNCTION OBSTRUCTION

Pelviureteric junction obstruction is the most common congenital obstruction of the urinary tract. Conditions necessary for development of the pelviureteric junction obstruction are a renal pelvis and an anatomical pelviureteric junction. Both of these are absent in the upper moiety of a duplex kidney so that, for practical purposes, if a pelviureteric junction obstruction occurs in a duplex kidney it will involve the lower-pole moiety. A few cases of "pelviureteric junction obstruction" involving the upper-pole moiety have been reported but are not anatomically explained. Pelviureteric junction obstruction of the lower-pole moiety may mimic Wilms' tumor in the early phase of an excretory urogram.

In infants under 1 year of age, pelviureteric junction obstruction is often bilateral, more frequent in males, and often associated with other significant anomalies of the urinary tract and other organs. These associations are usually not present in older infants and children.

The most common clinical presentation of pelviureteric junction obstruction is a palpable abdominal mass or abdominal enlargement. However, there may be diverse clinical manifestations of pelviureteric junction obstruction in children, particularly those simulating gastrointestinal disorders and intermittent obstruction with high urinary output. The diagnosis may be delayed in these patients for a significant period of time. An accurate and early diagnosis is obviously essential to prevent secondary effects on the kidney and can be made only if the child has a urographic examination while symptomatic.

The etiology of pelviureteric junction obstruction remains obscure. Multiple factors may play a role: a localized area of ischemia in utero, abnormal spatial orientation of the pelviureteric junction, infolding of the ureteral mucosa, a localized area of deficient neuromuscular innervation or aberrant vessels supplying the lower pole of the kidney.

The major differential diagnoses are ureteral polyps and major vesicoureteral reflux. Therefore, all patients suspected of having pelviureteric junction obstruction should have a voiding cystourethrogram to exclude vesicoureteral reflux. Excretory urography is then needed to evaluate function and demonstrate anatomical detail. The Lasix test may then be needed to ascertain whether obstruction is present. Pelviureteric junction obstruction needs surgical correction to prevent further renal damage.

MIDURETERAL OBSTRUCTION

Midureteral dilatation or obstruction may be categorized into congenital and acquired causes. Congenital causes include congenital ureteral stricture, which occurs in the lower lumbar region and in most cases is associated with a contralateral multicystic kidney; ureteral valves, which can occur anywhere but are usually located near the pelviureteric or ureterovesical junction (these valves are seen as a transverse filling defect in the ureter on the excretory urogram); and retrocaval ureter, which is a congenital anomaly in the development of the inferior vena cava. The right ureter abruptly deviates medially at the level of L3–4, causing partial obstruction and dilatation of the proximal part of the ureter. The distal part of the ureter courses inferiorly and overlies the right vertebral pedicles and is not abnormally dilated. Other uncommon causes include retroiliac ureter and obstruction due to persistence of the umbilical branch of the hypogastric artery.

Acquired causes include inflammatory lesions (such as tuberculosis, Crohn's disease or appendicitis), hydrometrocolpos, postoperative adhesions, and neoplasms (ovarian lesions, lymphoma and neuroblastoma).

There is, on occasion, a transient dilatation of the right ureter at the pelvic rim that occurs as a normal variation and should not be confused with a true obstruction.

Occasionally, abnormal peristalsis in a bifid ureter can also cause transient dilatation.

DISTAL URETERAL OBSTRUCTION (URETEROVESICAL JUNCTION OBSTRUCTION)

It is imperative to differentiate obstructive from nonobstructive causes (such as reflux) of ureteral dilatation, as mentioned previously. One must remember, however, that these 2 conditions may coexist, which necessitates careful fluoroscopic examination of the distal part of the ureter on voiding cystourethrography. Friedland (1978) divides the most important causes of distal ureteral obstruction into the following categories: I. congenital: (1) primary megaureter, (2) primary megaureter with coexisting reflux, (3) primary megaureter with coexisting bladder saccule, (4) simple ureterocele and (5) ectopic ureter and ectopic ureterocele; II. acquired: (1) following ureteral reimplantation, (2) following infection (tuberculosis, schistosomiasis), rare in children, and (3) stricture following passage of stones. The latter two are rare in children.

Primary megaureter, which is usually seen in male infants, commonly involves the left side and is bilateral in 20% of the patients. Genitourinary anomalies (such as agenesis of the kidney) and anomalies of other organ systems are commonly associated. Abnormal peristaltic activity of the distal ureter with associated fibrosis is the likely cause with the proximal dilated ureter either straight or tortuous. The condition may coexist with vesicoureteral reflux or bladder saccule without reflux.

A simple ureterocele (cystic dilatation of the intramural portion of the distal ureter) usually presents in an infant or young child as a unilateral flank mass. The diagnosis is established by excretory urography and cystography. A smoothly marginated filling defect is seen in the bladder with cystography. This defect then opacifies with excretory urography leaving a lucent "halo" around the dilated distal ureter representing ureteral and bladder mucosa (cobra-head sign). A ureterocele is often associated with ectopic insertion of a ureter (ectopic ureterocele). This often involves the ureter draining the upper-pole moiety of a duplex collecting system and is more common in females. About 50% of patients have a duplicated collecting system on the opposite side. In males, an ectopic ureterocele can occur without duplication and may be associated with a posterior urethral valve.

Since the ureter arises from the wolffian duct, which becomes the vas deferens in males (and Gartner's duct in females), the orifice of the ectopic ureter never inserts distal to the orifice of the vas deferens. Since this is proximal to the external sphincter, it is not associated with urinary incontinence in males. However, the ureter can insert anywhere along Gartner's duct. Therefore, this entity may be associated with urinary incontinence in females since the ureter can insert proximal or distal to the external sphincter. The main morphological types of ectopic ureteroceles are stenotic, sphincteric, cecoureterocele (analogous to cecum), blind and wide-mouth.

An excretory urogram and voiding cystourethrogram are the most important examinations to diagnose a duplex collecting system with or without an ectopic ureterocele. On excretory urography, the hydronephrotic upper pole will act as a mass displacing the lower-pole collecting system inferiorly and rotating its axis. This may simulate an adrenal mass. If an ectopic ureterocele is present, a filling defect is seen in the bladder that may obstruct the ureter draining the ipsilateral lower-pole or the contralateral ureter or both. Alternatively, the ipsilateral lower-pole ureter may be dilated secondary to vesicoureteral reflux rather than obstruction.

Ultrasonography is highly accurate in diagnosing this condition. Sonograms of the abdomen will demonstrate the hydronephrotic upper pole and possibly the dilated ureter. Scans of the pelvis with a distended bladder will demonstrate the ectopic ureterocele beneath the bladder mucosa. If the ureterocele is large, it may simulate a normal bladder. In this situation, another examination after voiding will ensure the correct diagnosis.

Bladder abnormalities may also cause distal ureteral obstruction, and include bladder neck obstruction secondary to fibromuscular hypertrophy (Marion's disease), an extremely rare condition found only in males; saccules and diverticula of the bladder, which can also cause reflux; duplication of the bladder; and trigonal cysts.

URETHRAL OBSTRUCTION IN MALES

A posterior urethral valve is the most common cause of severe urinary tract obstruction in male infants. Almost 75% are discovered during the first year of life; they may present in older children and rarely in adults. The initial symptoms vary considerably and are dependent on age. Infants usually are admitted with probable abdominal mass (abnormally distended bladder) and a poor voiding stream. If there is associated severe muscular hypertrophy of the bladder, the infant may void normally or even stronger than normal. These infants may also have a palpable flank mass (hydronephrosis), abdominal distention (urine ascites or intestinal ileus) or respiratory problems (urinothorax, renal failure or pneumothorax).

In children, the most common symptoms are suprapubic pain or dysuria, straining and hematuria.

The usual form of a posterior urethral valve consists of a mucosal flap originating from the verumontanum (previously called type I). Rarely is the valve a mucosal diaphragm with single or multiple openings (previously called type III). Type II used in the old classification probably does not exist.

The diagnosis is made with a voiding cystourethrogram, via either a suprapubic catheter or a feeding tube (no.5 or no.8 French) inserted through the ure-thra. The patient should be positioned in a steep oblique or lateral position and micturition should be recorded continuously on videotape. About 40% of patients will have associated vesicoureteral reflux that is usually due to a periureteral diverticulum. Fifteen percent of patients have an associated dysplastic kidney that almost always is associated with vesicoureteral reflux.

Other causes of posterior urethral obstruction include a müllerian duct cyst, postsurgical stenosis following repair of the rectourethral fistula, strictures following pelvic trauma or surgery, congenital urethral polyps and neoplasms such as rhabdomyosarcomas.

Anterior urethral obstruction in males is uncommon but may be secondary to strictures (congenital, inflammatory or traumatic), diverticula (congenital valve or posttraumatic) or urethral duplication.

URETHRAL OBSTRUCTION IN FEMALES

Urethral obstruction in females is rare but may be seen in cloacal or female intersex anomalies.

NONOBSTRUCTIVE CAUSES OF URINARY TRACT DILATATION

Urinary tract infection is the most common abnormality of the urinary tract in children. Following the 1st urinary tract infection, every infant and child should have an excretory urogram and voiding cystourethrogram. The patient's urine must be sterile for at least 2 weeks prior to the voiding cystourethrogram so that if vesicoureteral reflux is present, infected urine is not refluxed during the diagnostic study.

Urinary tract infections are usually caused by bacteria from fecal contamination of the perineum. Reflux, scarring, lithiasis or obstruction per se do not cause infection. However, when a bladder infection is present, major reflux (grades 2 and 3) may infect the kidneys.

The urographic manifestations of acute pyelonephritis are delayed function and renal enlargement on the involved side secondary to the inflammation and edema. Hydronephrosis may or may not be present. Striation of the renal pelvis and/or ureter secondary to the reflux of infected urine also may be seen. This is often optimally demonstrated on the early films of the excretory urogram.

The renal enlargement, edema and hydronephrosis may also be diagnosed by ultrasonography. This is especially useful in patients with a known sensitivity to urographic contrast agents. Comparison with the opposite kidney will show the disproportionate enlargement and relatively less echogenicity on the involved side. The collecting system dilatation is seen as previously described. A renal scan using ^{99M}Tc-glucoheptonate can then be used to evaluate and demonstrate the decreased renal function.

Chronic pyelonephritis will cause patchy calyceal clubbing and renal scarring, especially in the polar regions. The normal areas of the kidney may hypertrophy as pseudomass lesions to compensate for the focal loss of renal tissue. Eventually, the kidneys become abnormally small secondary to progressive parenchymal loss.

VESICOURETERAL REFLUX

Reflux without distal obstruction may cause urinary tract dilatation. This is graded as follows: grade 0, no reflux; grade 1, reflux into the ureter but not the renal pelvis; grade 2, reflux into the ureter and renal pelvis without any dilatation; grade 3, reflux into the ureter and renal pelvis with dilatation of both.

Not only is it important to grade the reflux, as outlined above, but the presence or absence of intrarenal reflux (pyelotubular backflow of the contrast material into the renal parenchyma) should be carefully evaluated.

Vesicoureteral reflux may be associated with focal renal scarring (chronic atrophic pyelonephritis), generalized scarring involving all the renal papillae (similar to that seen in prolonged obstruction), segmental renal hypoplasia and Ask-Upmark kidney. All of these changes may be grouped under the generic heading of reflux nephropathy.

The pathogenesis of reflux nephropathy is probably best explained on the basis of intrarenal reflux. When intrarenal reflux is associated with a high bladder voiding pressure, reflux nephropathy (focal fibrosis) will develop even with sterile urine. When intrarenal reflux is associated with infection it may result in a more severe degree of reflux nephropathy even when the bladder voiding pressure is low. However, intrarenal reflux with a low bladder voiding pressure and vesicoureteral reflux without intrarenal reflux are unlikely to produce any change of reflux nephropathy in the absence of infection.

NEUROGENIC BLADDER

Myelodysplasia is the most common cause of a neurogenic bladder in infants and children. Most of these patients have a mixed upper and lower motor neuron lesion. Since almost all of these patients have normal kidneys at birth, developing urinary tract dilatation is difficult to evaluate clinically; all patients with myelodysplasia should have an excretory urogram after the first week of life. (This allows the postnatal development of renal concentrating ability and the development of the dilatation.)

Another condition that may be overlooked clinically is partial sacral agenesis, especially if the lesion is a low one. Since innervation of the hips and legs is primarily lumbar and innervation of the bladder primarily sacral, one can have severe neurogenic bladder dysfunction with little or no musculoskeletal abnormality. Therefore, in patients who have an upper motor neuron lesion, an excretory urogram shows dilated ureters and some opaque urine in the posterior urethra because of bladder spasm. The voiding cystourethrogram shows a trabeculated bladder and spasm of the external sphincter causing relative obstruction and narrowing of the urethra as it courses through the urogenital diaphragm. If hydronephrosis develops, despite conservative management, insertion of an artificial sphincter or urinary diversion should be considered. Regular follow-up at periodic intervals is essential. Frequent ultrasonographic examination to detect urinary tract dilatation or obstruction and monitor bladder emptying may be interspersed with excretory urography to evaluate renal function.

FLOW UROPATHY

Patients with diabetes insipidus manifest this phenomenon. The dilatation of the urinary tract is secondary to 2 factors: (1) a high urinary flow rate and (2) bladder dilatation. The high urinary flow rate decreases ureteral peristalsis. The increased volume of urine delivered to the bladder results in its dilatation. The bladder dilatation may then cause ureterovesicle obstruction with subsequent urinary tract dilatation. Secondary changes in the kidneys (back-pressure atrophy) may be seen in severe cases.

GENERAL ABNORMALITIES OF THE URETERAL MUSCULATURE

Dilatation of the ureters or bladder may be due to an insufficient amount of muscle in the ureter or the muscle that is present may be structurally abnormal. It may be seen in patients with ectopic kidneys, but the most common condition demonstrating this abnormality is the prune-belly syndrome. Other synonyms for this syndrome are absent abdominal musculature syndrome, Eagle-Barrett syndrome or the triad syndrome.

Three main components are (1) abdominal muscular deficiency of varying degrees, (2) cryptorchidism and (3) nonobstructive dilatation of the bladder and ureters. The prune-belly syndrome can be divided into 3 groups. Patients in the 1st group have urethral obstruction (from a valve or atresia) associated with renal dysplasia. Pulmonary hypoplasia secondary to oligohydramnios leads to severe respiratory insufficiency. The infants are stillborn or die in the neonatal period.

Patients in the 2d group have severe neonatal and infantile urinary tract involvement. The lungs can sustain life as there is no oligohydramnios in utero. The kidneys, however, appear bizarre with lobulated contours, one smaller than the other, with random dilatation of asymmetrically arranged calyces emptying directly into the renal sinus. The renal pelvis appears normal but leads to a wandering ureter that varies in caliber from normal to far in excess of that seen with obstructive uropathies. The bladder is large with an unusual contour. Often there is a cystic urachal remnant, a wide bladder neck, elongation of the posterior urethra and vesicoureteral reflux.

Patients in the 3d group are less severely affected and present with cryptorchidism, a wrinkled abdominal wall and diastasis of the rectus musculature. The excretory urogram ranges from normal to the typical appearance described in group 2.

REFERENCES

Albertson, K. W., et al.: Valves of the ureters, Radiology 103:91, 1972.

Alton, D. J.: Urinary obstruction in the neonatal infant, Radiol. Clin. North Am. 14:343, 1975.

Alton, D. J.: Pelviureteric obstruction in childhood, Radiol. Clin. North Am. 15:61, 1977.

Barbaric, Z. L.: Pelvocalyceal wall opacification: A new radiological sign, Radiology 123:587, 1977.

Barratt, T. M., et al.: Obstructive uropathy in infants, Proc. R. Soc. Med. 63:42, 1970.

Beck, A. D.: The effect of intra-uterine urinary obstruction upon the development of the fetal kidney, J. Urol. 105:784, 1971.

Berdon, W. E., et al.: Hydronephrosis in infants and children: Value of high-dosage excretory urography in predicting renal salvageability, A.J.R. 109:380, 1970.

Berdon, W. E., et al.: The radiologic and pathologic spectrum of the prune-belly syndrome: The importance of urethral obstruction in prognosis, Radiol. Clin. North Am. 15:83, 1977.

Bigongiari, L. R., et al.: Visualization of the medullary rays on excretory urography in experimental ureteric obstruction, A.J.R. 129:89, 1977.

Cacciarelli, A. A., et al.: Gray-scale ultrasonic demonstration of nephrocalcinosis, Radiology 128:459, 1978.

Colodny, A. H.: Evaluation and management of infants and children with neurogenic bladders, Radiol. Clin. North Am. 15:71, 1977.

Cremin, B. J., et al.: Ectopic ureterocele in single non-duplicated collecting system: Diagnosis by radiography, Urology 5:154, 1975.

Crosse, J. E. W., et al.: Nonobstructive circumcaval (retrocaval) ureter: A report of 2 cases, Radiology 116:69, 1975.

Daeschner, C. W., et al.: Urinary tract calculi and nephrocalcinosis in infants and children, J. Pediatr. 57:721, 1960.

Davis, H.: Metabolic causes of renal stones in children, J.A.M.A. 171:2199, 1959.

Dunbar, J. S.: Excretory urography in the first year of life, Radiol. Clin. North Am. 10:367, 1972.

Edell, S., et al.: Ultrasonic evaluation of renal calculi, A.J.R. 130:261, 1978.

Ellenbogen, P. H., et al.: Sensitivity of gray-scale ultrasound in detecting urinary tract obstruction, A.J.R. 130:731, 1978.

Friedland, G. W.: Recurrent urinary tract infections in infants and children, Radiol. Clin. North Am. 15:19, 1977.

Friedland, G. W.: Hydronephrosis in infants and children: Part I. Curr. Probl. Diag. Radiol. 7:1, 1978.

Friedland, G. W.: Hydronephrosis in infants and children: Part II. Curr. Probl. Diag. Radiol. 7:1, 1978.

Friedland, G. W., et al.: Neonatal "urinothorax" associated with posterior urethral valves, Br. J. Radiol. 44:471, 1971.

Friedland, G. W., et al.: The elusive ectopic ureteroceles, A.J.R. 116:792, 1972.

Friedland, G. W., et al.: Ascites due to spontaneous rupture of the renal pelvis in an 11-month-old infant with ureteropelvic junction obstruction, Pediatr. Radiol. 2:263, 1974.

Griscom, N. T., et al.: Visualization of individual papillary ducts (ducts of Bellini) by excretory urography in childhood hydronephrosis, Radiology 106:385, 1973.

Harrison, R. B., et al.: Alkaline encrusting cystitis, A.J.R. 130:575, 1978.

Hedman, P. J. K., et al.: Measurement of vesicoureteral reflux with intravenous 99mTc-DTPA compared to radiographic cystography, Radiology 126:205, 1978.

Hodson, J., et al.: Reflux nephropathy, Kidney Int. 4 (suppl.): 550, 1975.

Johnston, J. H.: The neurogenic bladder in the newborn infant, Paraplegia 6:157, 1968.

Johnston, J. H., et al.: Megalourethra, J. Pediatr. Surg. 5:304, 1970.

Johnston, J. H., et al.: Intrarenal vascular obstruction of the superior infundibulum in children, J. Pediatr. Surg. 7:318, 1972.

Kay, C. J., et al.: Ultrasonic characteristics of chronic atrophic pyelonephritis, A.J.R. 132:47, 1979.

Kelalis, P. P., et al.: Ureteropelvic obstruction in children: Experiences with 109 cases, J. Urol. 106:418, 1971.

Kirchner, P. T., et al.: Patterns of excretion of radioactive chelates in obstructive uropathy, Radiology 114:655, 1975.

Koontz, W. W., et al.: Agenesis of the sacrum and the neurogenic bladder, J.A.M.A. 203:139, 1968.

Korobkin, M., et al.: Diminished radiopacity of contrast material: A urographic sign of ureteral calculus, A.J.R. 131:847, 1978.

Lebowitz, R. L., et al.: Neonatal hydronephrosis: 146 cases, Radiol. Clin. North Am. 15:49, 1977.

Lebowitz, R. L., et al.: Renal parenchymal infections in children, Radiol. Clin. North Am. 15:37, 1977.

Leonidas, J. C., et al.: Congenital urinary tract obstruction presenting with ascites at birth: Roentgenographic diagnosis, Radiology 96:111, 1970.

Mascatello, V. J., et al.: Ultrasonic evaluation of the obstructed duplex kidney, A.J.R. 129:113, 1977.

McLaughlin, A. P., et al.: The pathophysiology of primary megaloureter, J. Urol. 109:805, 1973.

Miyazaki, K.: Urological problems in children with spina bifida cystica and sacral defects, Paraplegia 10:37, 1972.

Nusbacher, N., et al.: Hydronephrosis of the lower pole of the duplex kidney: Another renal pseudotumor, A.J.R. 130:967, 1978.

Palubinskas, A. J.: Problem areas in uroradiology, Curr. Probl. Diag. Radiol. 6:1, 1976.

Pellman, C.: The neurogenic bladder in children with congenital malformations of the spine: A study of 61 patients, J. Urol. 93:472, 1965.

Pollack, H. M., et al.: Hernias of the ureter: An anatomic-roentgenographic study, Radiology 117:275, 1975.

Renert, W. A., et al.: Obstructive urologic malformations of the fetus and infant: Relation to neonatal pneumomediastinum and pneumothorax (air-block), Radiology 105:97, 1972.

Rusiewicz, E., et al.: The significance of isolated upper pole calyceal dilatation, J. Can. Assoc. Radiol. 19:179, 1968.

Siegel, M. J., et al.: Calyceal diverticula in children: Unusual features and complications, Radiology 131:79, 1979.

Sutton, T. J., et al.: Two unusual conditions simulating ectopic ureterocele, Radiology 117:381, 1975.

Weiss, R. M., et al.: Reflux and trapping, Radiology 118:129, 1976.

Whitaker, J., et al.: Urinary outflow resistance estimation in children: Theory, method, and results, Invest. Urol. 7:127, 1969.

Whitaker, R. H.: Investigating wide ureters with ureteral pressure flow studies, J. Urol. 116:81, 1976.

White, P., et al.: Exstrophy of the bladder, Radiol. Clin. North Am. 15:93, 1977.

Williams, D. I.: Hydrocalycosis: Report of 3 cases in children, Br. J. Urol. 40:541, 1968.

Williams, D. I.: *Urology in Childhood,* vol. 15 (suppl.), *Encyclopedia of Urology* (New York: Springer-Verlag New York, Inc., 1974).

Williams, G., et al.: Communicating cysts and diverticula of the renal pelvis, Br. J. Urol. 41:163, 1969.

Wilson, D. A., et al.: Ultrasound demonstration of diffuse cortical nephrocalcinosis in a case of primary hyperoxaluria, A.J.R. 132:659, 1979.

Wolf, E. L., et al.: Diagnosis of oligohydramnios-related pulmonary hypoplasia (Potter syndrome): Value of portable voiding cystourethrography in newborns with respiratory distress, Radiology 125:769, 1977.

Yoder, I. C., et al.: Radiology of colon loop diversion: Anatomical and urodynamic studies of the conduit and ureters in children and adults, Radiology 127:85, 1978.

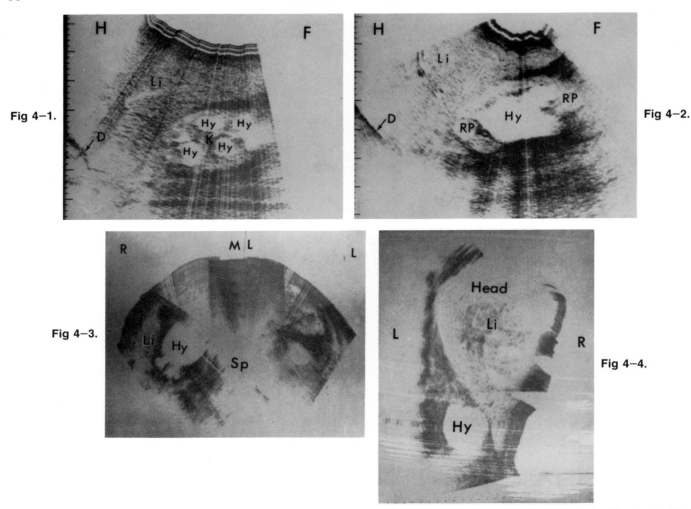

Figs 4–1 to 4–4.—Hydronephrosis: diagnosis and grad-ing. The major criterion for diagnosing hydronephrosis by ultrasonography is demonstration of fluid-containing areas within the renal sinus that conform anatomically to the renal collecting system. In standard longitudinal scans of kidney (Fig 4–1), individually dilated calyces can mimic normal re-nal pyramids if attention is not paid to through transmis-sion. However, if the specific gravity of the urine is high or if urinary sediment is present within the calyces, through transmission may not be significant. As a result, one must utilize multiple positions, particularly decubitus views, to demonstrate communication between peripheral dilated collecting system and central renal pelvis (Fig 4–2). This also aids in distinguishing variable degrees of hydrone-phrosis from various types of cystic disease.

Another important sonographic assessment is thickness of the remaining renal parenchyma. Although one cannot determine functional capacity of this tissue, the absence of any observable renal parenchyma (Figs 4–3 and 4–4) is highly suggestive of long-standing hydronephrosis and probable minimal renal function. H = head; F = feet; D = diaphragm; Li = liver; Hy = hydronephrosis; K = kidney; RP = renal parenchyma; ML = midline; Sp = spine; L = patient's left; R = patient's right.

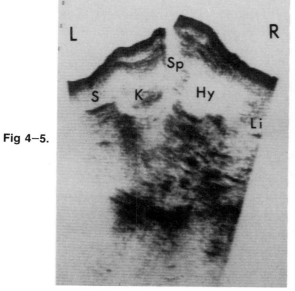

Fig 4–5.

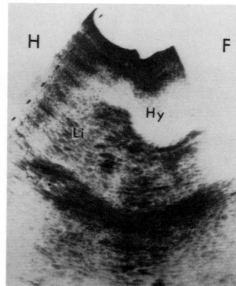

Fig 4–6.

Figs 4–5 and 4–6.—Hydronephrosis: diagnosis and grading. Another key feature of hydronephrosis on renal sonograms is the anteromedial bulging of fluid collection representing dilated renal pelvis (Figs 4–5 and 4–6). This is a fairly constant finding and is frequently best seen with ureteropelvic junction obstruction. When hydronephrosis is severe, it may be difficult to determine what portion of collecting system is dilated. L = left; R = right; H = head; F = feet; S = spleen; K = kidney; Sp = spine; Hy = hydronephrosis; Li = liver.

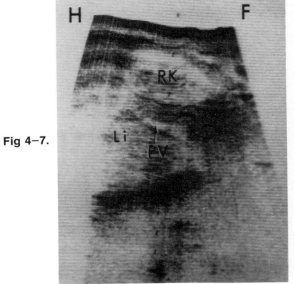

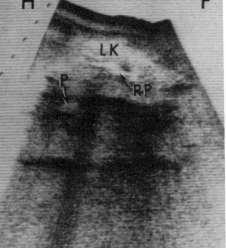

Fig 4–7.

Fig 4–8.

Figs 4–7 and 4–8.—Minimal hydronephrosis. It is often not possible to differentiate on ultrasonography the minimal fluid in a normal but slightly prominent renal pelvis from early or partial obstruction. Even though asymmetrical dilatation of a renal sinus may be more suggestive of mild hydronephrosis (Figs 4–7 and 4–8), it may occur normally. Consequently, when these minimal findings exist, and particularly if one cannot demonstrate dilatation of infundibula or calyces using multiple views, an excretory urogram is necessary to assess the functional state of the urinary tract. H = head; F = feet; RK = right kidney; LK = left kidney; Li = liver; PV = portal vein; P = pancreas; RP = renal pelvis.

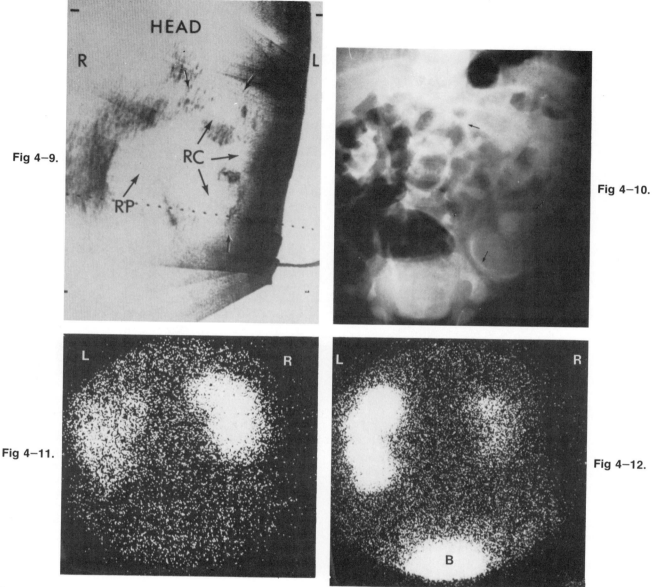

Fig 4–9.

Fig 4–10.

Fig 4–11.

Fig 4–12.

Figs 4–9 to 4–12.—Pelviureteric junction obstruction. Lateral decubitus scan (Fig 4–9) demonstrates marked hydronephrosis with pyelocaliectasis; small arrows point to remaining renal parenchyma. Excretory urography (Fig 4–10) shows normal functioning right kidney and enlargement of left kidney with grade 2 hydronephrosis *(arrows)*. A 20- to 30-second renal scintigram (Fig 4–11) shows de-creased function on left side. Later scan, taken at 18–20 minutes (Fig 4–12), shows marked hydronephrosis on left with no ureteral dilatation. This indicates obstruction at junction of ureter and pelvis. Notice normal washout of right kidney by 20 minutes. RP = renal pelvis; RC = renal calyces; B = bladder; R = patient's right; L = patient's left.

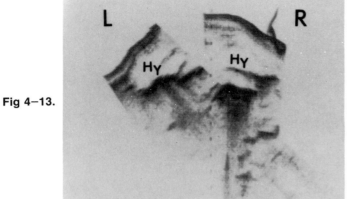

Fig 4–13.

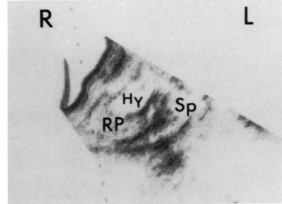

Fig 4–14.

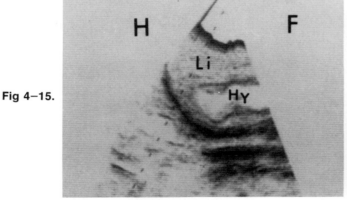

Fig 4–15.

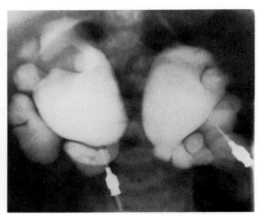

Fig 4–16.

Figs 4–13 to 4–16.—Bilateral pelviureteric junction obstruction. Multiple views of kidneys may be necessary to accurately diagnose hydronephrosis in any given patient. In transverse prone scan (Fig 4–13), abnormal fluid collection in both renal regions are evident; however, configuration is not necessarily typical of hydronephrosis. On transverse (Fig 4–14) and longitudinal (Fig 4–15) scans of right kidney, medial bulge secondary to hydronephrosis of renal pelvis as well as residual rind of renal parenchyma are optimally seen. Although bilateral nature of this process in this particular age group certainly favors hydronephrosis, these additional findings cinch the diagnosis. The site of obstruction was assessed using antegrade pyelography (Fig 4–16). This is a simple procedure and provides excellent anatomical detail. L = left; R = right; H = head; F = feet; Hy = hydronephrosis; Sp = spine; RP = renal parenchyma; Li = liver.

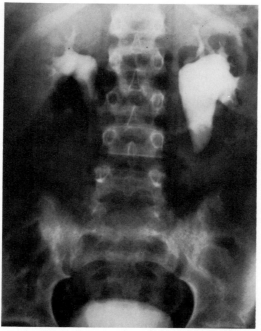

Fig 4–17.—Pelviureteric obstruction in duplex system. When pelviureteric obstruction is present in duplex collecting system, it characteristically involves lower-pole moiety; rarely, it may involve upper-pole moiety. Sonographically, dilatation of renal pelvis may obscure the fact that one is dealing with a duplex system. Also in the initial `phases of excretory urogram, this poorly functioning, dilated lower pelvis may simulate a Wilms' tumor.

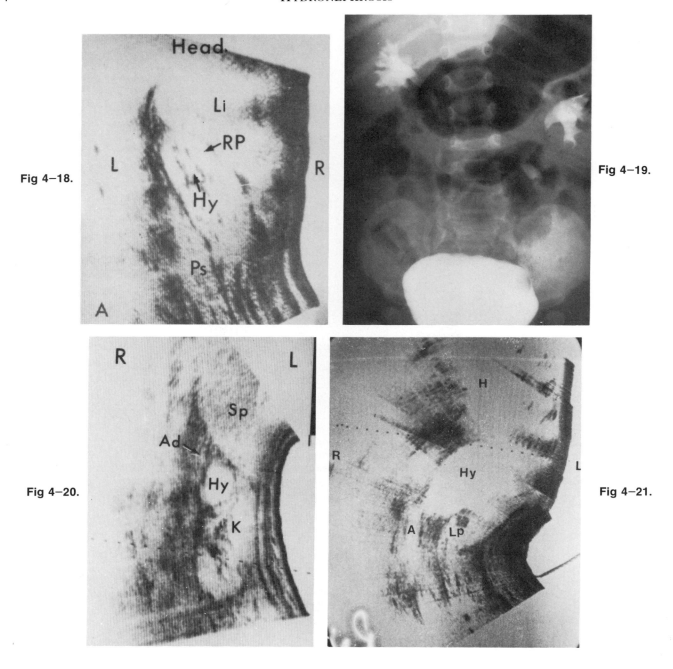

Fig 4–18.

Fig 4–19.

Fig 4–20.

Fig 4–21.

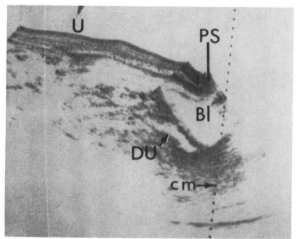

Fig 4–22.

Figs 4–18 to 4–22.—Hydronephrosis of duplicated collecting system. Hydronephrosis of duplicated collecting system usually affects upper-pole moiety (unlike pelviureteric obstruction, which involves lower-pole moiety) and is secondary to ectopic insertion of ureter with ureterocele. Such a complex of findings may lead to a variety of sonographic appearances, depending on amount of residual renal parenchyma and severity of obstruction. In some cases, there is only mild dilatation of collecting system in upper pole with normal renal axis and normal amount of renal parenchyma (Fig 4–18). In more severe cases, drooping-lily sign will be seen on excretory urography (Fig 4–19), and variable degrees of long-standing hydronephrosis of upper-pole moiety can be demonstrated on ultrasonograms (Figs 4–20 and 4–21). Usually straightening of renal axis or lateral deviation of upper pole will be demonstrated, and the more normal reniform nature of lower pole of the kidney can be appreciated. As in any case of suspected hydronephrosis, the pelvis should be examined for evidence of dilated ureter (Fig 4–22); occasionally a round, fluid-filled area within base of bladder indicating ectopic ureterocele can be demonstrated. H = head; L = left; R = right; Li = liver; RP = renal parenchyma; Hy = hydronephrosis; Ps = psoas muscle; U = umbilicus; PS = pubic symphysis; Bl = bladder; DU = dilated ureter; cm = centimeter marker; Sp = spleen; Ad = adrenal gland; K = kidney; A = aorta; Lp = lower pole of kidney.

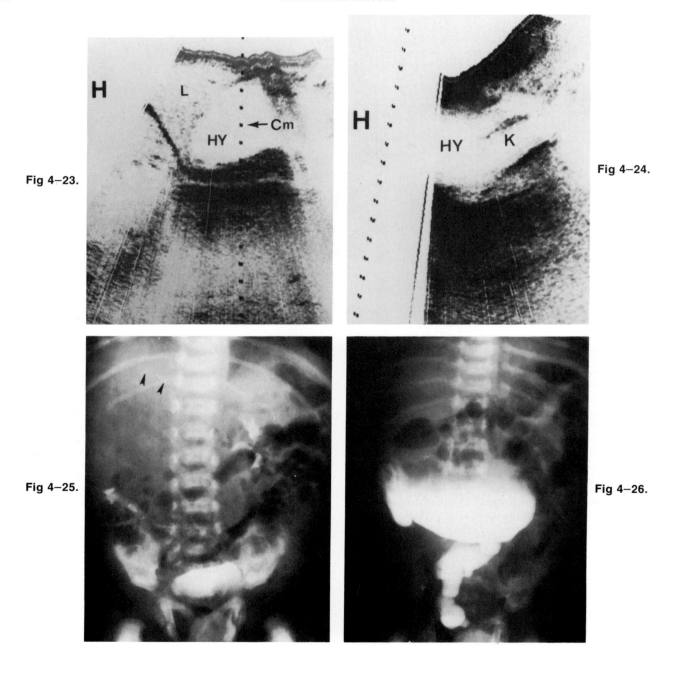

Fig 4–23.

Fig 4–24.

Fig 4–25.

Fig 4–26.

Figs 4–23 to 4–26. — Obstructed upper-pole collecting system. It is sometimes difficult to make an accurate diagnosis of obstructed duplex system on ultrasonography (Figs 4–23 and 4–24) since lower pole might be displaced over bony pelvis, which is difficult to scan. In this situation it may be necessary to scan the patient in prone position, with transducer angled to the side and caudad. Excretory urogram (Fig 4–25) demonstrates "shell nephrogram" of obstructed upper pole *(arrowheads)* and no further visualization, since remaining portion of right kidney and left kidney would excrete the contrast material. Because the ultrasonographic and urographic findings cannot totally exclude an adrenal cyst in this infant, direct puncture of the cystic structure (Fig 4–26) was done, which shows obstructed upper-pole system as a result of blind-end-type ureterocele. H = head; HY = hydronephrosis; K = kidney; L = liver; Cm = centimeter.

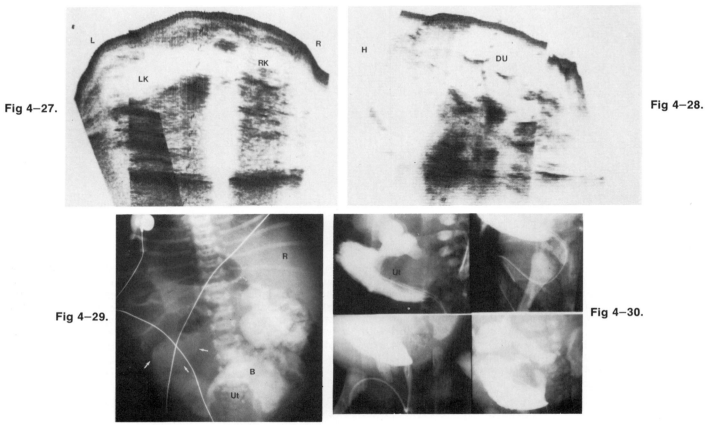

Fig 4–27.

Fig 4–28.

Fig 4–29.

Fig 4–30.

Figs 4–27 to 4–30. — Ureterocele. Transverse prone scan demonstrates bilateral hydronephrosis, which is more marked on left side (Fig 4–27). Longitudinal scan (Fig 4–28) demonstrates tortuous dilated ureter in lower abdomen. excretory urogram (Fig 4–29) in prone position shows marked hydronephrosis with minimal function on left side *(arrows)* and severe hydronephrosis on right side. Bladder is displaced, and there is large filling defect in bladder as result of ureterocele. Voiding cystourethrogram (Fig 4–30) demonstrates vesicoureteral reflux on right side and large filling defect in bladder as result of ureterocele. L = left; R = right; H = head; LK = left kidney; RK = right kidney; B = bladder; Ut = ureterocele; Du = dilated ureter.

Fig 4–31.

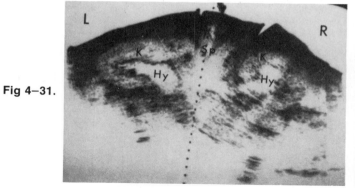

Fig 4–32.

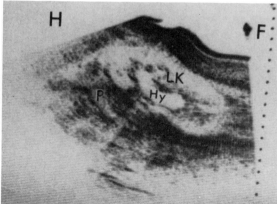

Fig 4–33.

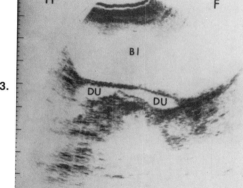

Figs 4–31 to 4–33.—Posterior urethral valve with mild hydronephrosis. Mild hydronephrosis can be distinguished from prominent renal pelvis by utilizing multiple scans to demonstrate not only fluid within renal pelvis but its communication with collecting system (Figs 4–31 and 4–32). Generally, prominent renal pelvis will not show calyceal dilatation.

Again, if hydronephrosis is present, the pelvis should be examined with full bladder (Fig 4–33). In patients with distal obstruction, dilated ureters may be demonstrated coursing through the pelvis, as in this case of bilateral hydronephrosis secondary to posterior urethral valve. L = left; R = right; H = head; F = feet; K = kidney; Sp = spine; Hy = hydronephrosis; LK = left kidney; P = pancreas; Bl = bladder; DU = dilated ureter.

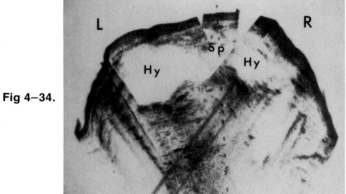

Fig 4—34.

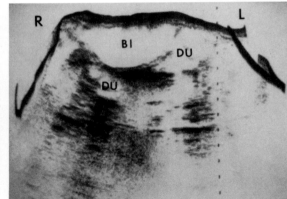

Fig 4—35.

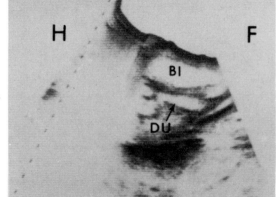

Fig 4—36.

Figs 4—34 to 4—36. — Bilateral hydronephrosis and posterior urethral valve. Degree of hydronephrosis in each kidney may be quite asymmetrical (Fig 4—34). Nevertheless, multiple scans will show typical sonographic configuration: medial bulging of dilated renal pelvis communicating with the ectatic infundibula and calyces. Scans of the pelvis with full bladder may demonstrate the dilated distal ureters (Fig 4—35). In addition, longitudinal scans frequently demonstrate a thickened bladder wall in cases of posterior urethral valve (Fig 4—36). L = left; R = right; Hy = hydronephrosis; Sp = spine; H = head; F = feet; Bl = bladder; DU = dilated ureter.

Fig 4–37.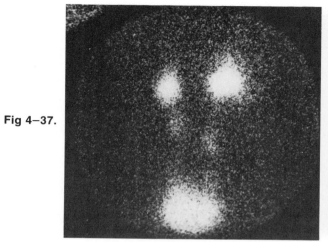

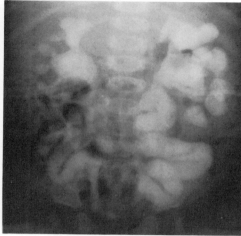 **Fig 4–38.**

Fig 4–39.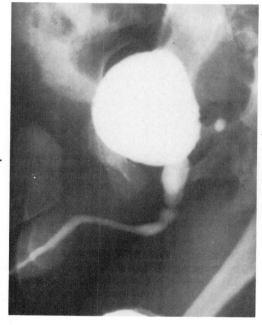

Figs 4–37 to 4–39.—Bilateral hydronephrosis. Renal scintiscan done in 18–20 minutes shows bilateral hydronephrosis and dilated ureters (Fig 4–37). This appearance might be seen as result of vesicoureteral reflux or in hydroureteronephrosis as a result of distal ureteral obstruction (Fig 4–38) and commonly is seen in posterior urethral valve such as in this patient (Fig 4–39).

Fig 4–40.

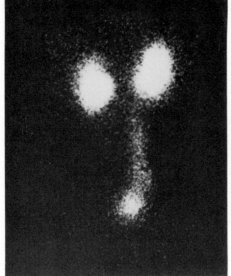

Fig 4–41.

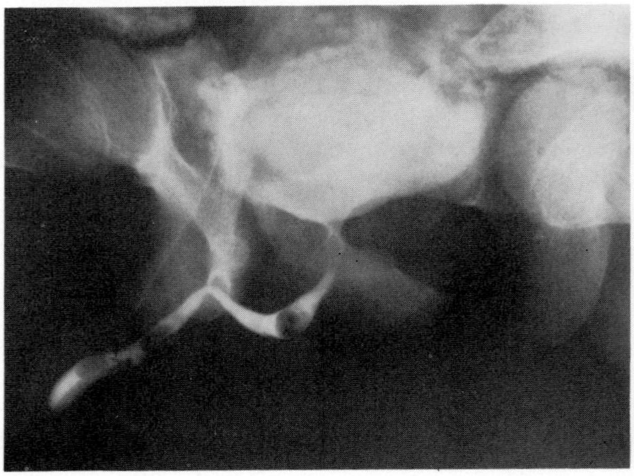

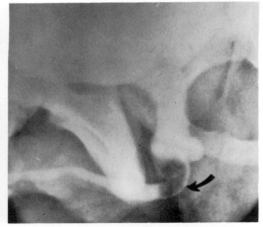

Fig 4–42.

Figs 4–40 to 4–42.—Vesicoureteral reflux. Scintiscan demonstrates bilateral hydroureteronephrosis (Fig 4–40). Again, differential diagnosis includes more common entities, such as posterior urethral valve or vesicoureteral re- flux; however, other rare causes should also be included, such as anterior urethral valve (Fig 4–41), especially if there is a markedly trabeculated bladder with no posterior ure- thral valve or urethral polyp (Fig 4–42, *arrow*).

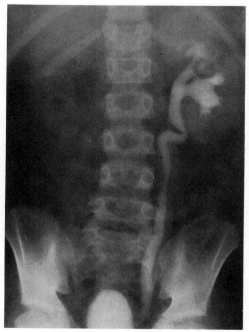

Fig 4–43.—Hydroureteronephrosis may be the result of infection. This is excretory urogram of patient with tuberculosis, with autonephrectomy on right side. There is evidence of left hydroureteronephrosis, irregularity of the ureter, small shrunken bladder, infundibular stenosis, cavitation and calyceal blunting. Sonographically, it may be difficult to differentiate obstructive from nonobstructive causes of hydronephrosis.

Fig 4—45.

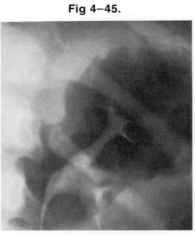

Fig 4—44.

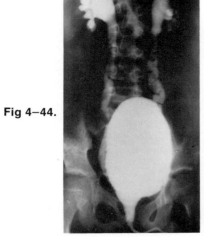

Fig 4—46.

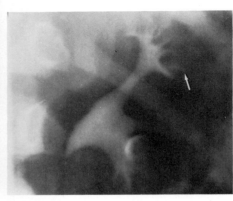

Figs 4—44 to 4—46.—Vesicoureteral reflux is another cause of hydroureteronephrosis that may be associated with posterior urethral valve (Fig 4–44). Commonly, however, vesicoureteral reflux is seen without evidence of ob- struction (Fig 4–45). In these patients it is extremely impor- tant to obtain a delayed film for evaluation of intrarenal reflux (Fig 4–46, *arrow*).

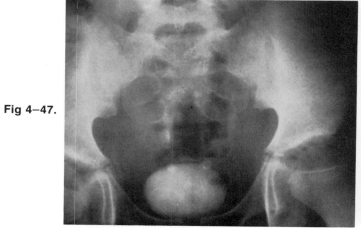

Fig 4–47.

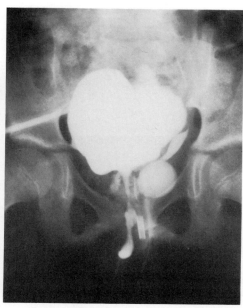

Fig 4–48.

Figs 4–47 and 4–48.—In children, urinary tract dilatation is rarely the result of urinary tract stones. Figure 4–47 shows nonobstructing large bladder stone. Dilatation of urinary tract may also be result of neurogenic bladder, which may be associated with reflux. In these patients, urinary continence may be achieved with an artificial sphincter (Fig 4–48).

Fig 4–49.

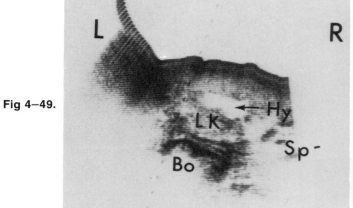

Fig 4–50.

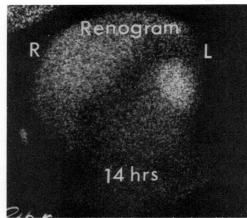

Fig 4–51.

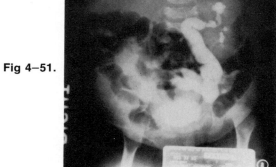

Figs 4–49 to 4–51.—Prune-belly syndrome. Transverse scan in prone position (Fig 4–49) shows mild hydronephrosis on left side. There was no visible right kidney. A renal scintigram of the same patient shows mild hydronephrosis of the left kidney at 14 hours with no function on right side (Fig 4–50). Excretory urogram (Fig 4–51) shows mild dilatation of calyces and random distribution of them on left side, with marked dilatation of ureter. L = left; R = right; LK = left kidney; Hy = hydronephrosis; Bo = bowel; Sp = spine.

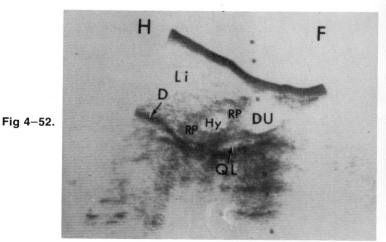

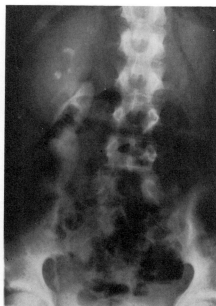

Fig 4–52.

Fig 4–53.

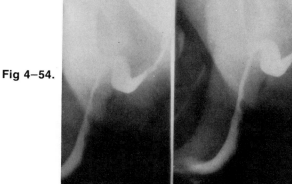

Fig 4–54.

Figs 4–52 to 4–54. — Prune-belly syndrome. Longitudinal scan on right side (Fig 4–52) demonstrates mild hydronephrosis and marked dilatation of ureter. This discrepancy in size between the ureter and pelvis is typical of the prunebelly syndrome. Excretory urogram of same patient (Fig 4–53) shows marked dilatation of the right ureter, with minimal dilatation of randomly distributed calyces. There is no evidence of functioning left kidney. Voiding cystourethrogram (Fig 4–54) demonstrates elongated urethra with areas of narrowing and dilatation. There is no evidence of posterior urethral valve. H = head; F = foot; D = diaphragm; Li = liver; RP = renal parenchyma; Hy = hydronephrosis; DU = dilated ureter; QL = quadratus lumborum muscle.

Fig 4–55.

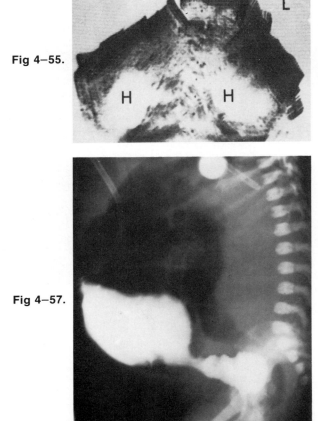

Fig 4–56.

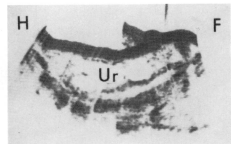

Fig 4–57.

Figs 4–55 to 4–57. — Prune-belly syndrome with posterior urethral valve. Prone scan in this newborn (Fig 4–55) demonstrates bilateral hydronephrosis. Longitudinal scan (Fig 4–56) demonstrates marked dilatation of ureter. Lateral view of voiding cystourethrogram (Fig 4–57) demonstrates posterior urethral valve. Note high location of bladder and patent urachus. This is the most severe form of the prune-belly syndrome. H = hydronephrosis (in Fig 4–55) and head (in Fig 4–56); L = left; F = foot; Ur = ureter.

5

Cystic Diseases of the Kidney

NUMEROUS CLASSIFICATIONS HAVE BEEN PROPOSED to define and encompass cystic diseases of the kidney. Two of these classifications are shown in Tables 5–1 and 5–2. Table 5–1 is a classification by Osathanondh and Potter (1964). The microdissection studies by the authors are the basis for this classification and provide valuable information about the pathogenesis of renal cystic diseases. Table 5–2 is a modified form of the classification described by Elkin et al. (1969) and will be used in this chapter. In this classification, well-accepted entities such as the dysplasias and polycystic diseases are grouped respectively. Those entities with an unknown or poorly understood pathogenesis are grouped according to their anatomical location, e.g., cortex or medulla. The remaining unusual intrarenal cystic lesions are grouped under a miscellaneous category, which includes renal cysts associated with in-flammatory, neoplastic and traumatic lesions of the kidneys.

Several diagnostic modalities are now available for evaluation of renal diseases. The specific technique of excretory urography in children is described in chapter 4. Ultrasonography has become a very useful screening modality for these diseases and is described in the figure legends. Computerized tomography, nuclear scintigraphy and angiography will be discussed in their appropriate contexts as they apply to specific diseases.

RENAL DYSPLASIA

The kidneys require a normal progression and branching of the ureteric bud and ampullae (the expanded forward portion of the dividing tubule) to prop-

TABLE 5-1.—OSATHANONDH AND POTTER CLASSIFICATION OF POLYCYSTIC KIDNEYS

TYPE	MECHANISM OF PRODUCTION	CLINICAL ENTITIES
1	Hyperplasia of interstitial portions of collecting ducts	Infantile polycystic kidneys
2	Inhibition of the activity of the ampullary portion of ureteric bud	Multicystic kidney Multilocular cyst Aplastic kidney
3	Scattered abnormalities of collecting ducts and nephrons	Adult-type polycystic kidneys Cyst in trisomy Cyst in tuberous sclerosis Medullary sponge kidney
4	Injury to the ampullary portion of ureteric bud from pressure due to distal urinary tract obstruction	Renal cysts in infants with posterior urethral valves or urethral atresia

Data from Osathanondh and Potter.

89

I. Renal dysplasia
   A. Multicystic kidney
   B. Multiple cysts associated with lower urinary tract
      obstruction
II. Polycystic disease
   A. Polycystic disease of the young
      1. Polycystic disease of the newborn
      2. Polycystic disease of childhood
   B. Adult-type polycystic disease
III. Cortical cysts
   A. Trisomy syndromes
   B. Tuberous sclerosis
   C. Simple cyst (solitary or multiple, unilateral or bilateral)
   D. Multilocular cyst
IV. Medullary cysts
   A. Medullary sponge kidney
   B. Medullary cystic disease (uremic)
   C. Medullary necrosis
   D. Pyelogenic cyst
V. Miscellaneous: Inflammatory, neoplastic, traumatic

°Modified from Elkin et al. (1969).

erly induce the metanephrogenic blastema to form nephrons. If this process is disturbed, maldevelopment will result. The following terms and definitions are offered to avoid confusion. *Plasia:* This originates from the Greek word *plassein,* meaning "to form." *Dysplasia:* This means abnormal formation. (Severe dysplasia is called *aplasia.*)

Multicystic Kidney

The basic defect in the pathogenesis of a multicystic kidney is abnormal development of the advancing ureteric bud. This causes abnormal induction of the nephrogenic tissue, with subsequent formation of primitive, dysplastic tissues. This maldevelopment occurs very early in embryonic life, resulting in atresia of the ureter, pelvis or both. There are 2 forms of multicystic kidney: pelviinfundibular atresia and hydronephrotic.

In the more common form, the atresia involves the pelviinfundibular region. As a result, the subsequent growth and branching of the ureteral bud is markedly altered. This severe renal disorganization is seen pathologically as "a cluster of grapes" with no resemblance to a normal kidney. Central cores of solid tissue

with recognizable dysplastic elements are surrounded by many cysts, ranging from a few millimeters to several centimeters in diameter. There is almost always an associated severe stenosis or atresia of the ureter. These cysts may or may not intercommunicate, depending on whether the proximal portion of the pelvis is present or obliterated.

In the hydronephrotic form of multicystic kidney, this atretic process involves only the ureter. The cysts in this form represent the dilated pelvicalyceal system, and they communicate via the dilated renal pelvis.

If one accepts the theory of an intrauterine obstruction as the major cause for development of a multicystic kidney, it is possible to explain focal and segmental forms of the disease: the focal form resulting in scattered areas of dysplasia secondary to collecting-duct obstruction; and the segmental form resulting in dysplasia of one moiety of a duplex collecting system.

Most multicystic kidneys manifest clinically as an abdominal mass in a healthy neonate, infant or child. In fact, a multicystic kidney is the most common cause of an abdominal mass in a neonate. Rarely, the mass is undetected until adult life and is discovered incidentally during a urological examination for an unrelated condition. In the adult, calcification may be seen in the walls of the cysts; this does not occur in children. No familial tendency has been described.

Up to one third of patients with a multicystic kidney have some form of obstructive uropathy involving the contralateral kidney. Therefore, it is essential to evaluate the entire urinary system with ultrasonography and excretory urography.

Ultrasonography usually demonstrates a large mass with multiple cystic areas of varying sizes separated by echogenic septae. There is no identifiable renal parenchyma or pelvicalyceal system, i.e., a well-defined ellipsoid and relatively sonolucent band of homogeneous echogenicity surrounding a linear, central, more echogenic band.

The flank mass may be identified on the scout film of the abdomen. During the total-body opacification phase of the excretory urogram, opacification of the cyst walls may be seen as a result of their vascular supply. Subsequently, during the early excretory phase, faint, thin, curvilinear densities (termed "calyceal crescents") appear as a result of stasis of the contrast material in compressed collecting tubules that lie adjacent to the cysts. On delayed films, irregular "puddled" opacification may be seen in the small or medium-sized cystic spaces, probably due to tubular reabsorption of water and therefore concentration of the contrast material. The renal artery is either very hypoplastic or absent. The bladder is normal.

Multiple Cysts Associated with Lower Urinary Tract Obstruction

In children with congenital urinary outlet obstruction, the kidneys usually have small cortical cysts as well as renal dysplasia. These renal cysts are probably the result of increased pressure on the ampullae during fetal development of the kidney. The most common cause in males is a posterior urethral valve. Other less common causes are an ectopic ureterocele or, rarely, urethral atresia. Patients present with advanced renal failure, bilateral flank masses (the hydronephrotic kidneys) and a lower abdominal mass (the dilated bladder).

Ultrasonography and excretory urography will demonstrate bilateral hydroureteronephrosis and a dilated, trabeculated bladder. The pelvicalyceal systems, although markedly dilated, are normally formed and communicate with the ureters.

The cause for the outlet obstruction is usually identified by a voiding cystourethrogram. With a posterior urethral valve, the prostatic urethra is markedly dilat-ed and the obstruction is at or just below the verumontanum. There is often associated vesicoureteral reflux. In a study done by Cussen (1971), all of the cystic kidneys demonstrated vesicoureteral reflux; however, reflux may be present without cystic changes in the ipsilateral kidney.

POLYCYSTIC DISEASE

Polycystic diseases of the kidney are divided into 2 major categories: polycystic disease in children and adult polycystic disease. It is generally accepted that these 2 forms are unrelated and represent distinct entities.

Polycystic Disease of the Young (Tubular Ectasia)

Polycystic disease of the young encompasses a spectrum of diseases that has at one end the newborn type and at the other end the childhood type (Table 5–3). It is best to consider polycystic disease of the young a two-organ disease, with the kidneys and liver involved in all patients. Multiple epithelial hepatic cysts, dilated bile ducts and periportal fibrosis are invariably present. There is an inverse relationship between the kidney and liver with respect to the degree of involvement with the polycystic disease, depending on the patient's age at the manifestation of the disease. In younger children, the kidneys are more severely involved; in older children the liver is more severely involved. Both types are genetically inherited as an autosomal recessive disease occurring in siblings. There is no crossover between the different

TABLE 5-3.—POLYCYSTIC DISEASE OF THE YOUNG

	CLINICAL PRESENTATION/ CAUSE OF DEATH	KIDNEY INVOLVEMENT (TUBULAR ECTASIA)	LIVER INVOLVEMENT (PERIPORTAL FIBROSIS)
Newborn type			
Group 1	Respiratory disease/ renal failure	++++	+
Group 2	Renal failure	+++	++
Childhood type			
Group 3	Related to liver involvement	++	+++
Group 4	Related to liver involvement	+	++++

types of polycystic disease of the young. Therefore, if the disease presents early in life (the newborn type) and the child dies at an early age, all affected children in that family do the same. If, in another family, the disease presents later in life (the childhood type), all affected children show this later onset of the disease and survive longer.

Pathologically, the kidneys are enlarged but maintain their reniform shape with a smooth cortical surface and normal fetal lobulation. There are numerous small cysts a few millimeters in diameter scattered throughout the kidney, giving it a spongy appearance. Gross inspection of the sectioned kidney shows dilated tubular channels oriented perpendicular to the cortical surface and extending to it. Most of the cysts represent dilated tubules (tubular ectasia), but some represent dilated nephrons. There is no dysplastic tissue present. There may also be cysts in other organs, such as the ovaries, pancreas and lungs. The bladder and ureter are normal.

It is theorized that initially the ureteric bud and metanephrogenic blastema develop normally and give rise to normal nephrons. But at some time during the last half of intrauterine life, the proximal collecting tubules develop large saccules and diverticula, and the more terminal tubules become enlarged, leading to Potter's term "tubular gigantism."

The clinical presentation and cause of death depend on the type of polycystic disease of the young. Early in life (newborn type), patients have a protuberant abdomen and bilateral abdominal masses. The infant has a "Potter facies." The most common cause of death in the first few days of life is respiratory failure secondary to pulmonary hypoplasia, congestive heart failure, pneumonia or pneumothorax. The lungs are hypoplastic as a result of the compressive mechanical pressure exerted on the lungs by the fetal abdominal contents and the uterus (associated maternal oligohydramnios). Following assisted ventilation, the alveoli can easily rupture, leading to pneumothorax.

In those patients with adequate pulmonary development who survive the first few days, progressive renal failure develops.

The childhood form of the disease presents somewhat later, at 4 or 5 years of age, with the major symptoms related to periportal fibrosis, i.e., gastrointestinal hemorrhage secondary to esophageal varices or jaundice secondary to severe liver disease. The cause of death is usually related to these complications.

Roentgenographic Findings

Roentgenograms of the abdomen show enlarged kidneys bilaterally. The kidney function depends on the degree of renal involvement by the polycystic disease. In the newborn type, there is very poor renal function and the collecting systems are usually not seen satisfactorily. The nephrographic phase is often prolonged, as long as a week, and shows a radiolucent mottled appearance, which is the result of numerous small cysts. The dilated tubules may be visualized, appearing as a "brush border" perpendicular to the surface of the kidney. The diagnosis is obvious in this form of polycystic disease of the young.

In the childhood type, there is better renal function. Medullary tubular ectasia leads to stasis of the excreted contrast material in the dilated ducts and gives a "brush border" appearance. The pelvicalyceal systems and ureters appear normal. The differentiation from the adult form of polycystic disease presenting in childhood may be difficult by excretory urography. However, the demonstration of periportal fibrosis by ultrasonography or liver biopsy favors the diagnosis of the childhood type of polycystic disease of the young.

Ultrasonographic Findings

The nephromegaly and multiple small uniform cysts, which give the kidney an increased echogenicity, are identified by gray-scale ultrasonography. The normal central echoes of the pelvicalyceal system are not seen. However, the most important aid provided by ultrasonography in this disease is the evaluation of the liver. The demonstration of liver cysts and/or periportal fibrosis assures the proper diagnosis. The liver cysts appear as simple cysts, but the periportal fibrosis imparts a highly echogenic character to the liver.

Polycystic Disease of the Adult

The adult form of polycystic disease is clearly a different entity than polycystic disease of the young. Adult polycystic disease is inherited as an autosomal dominant and is much more common than polycystic disease of the young.

In most patients, the disease is manifested in the 4th or 5th decade. Rarely, the adult form of polycystic disease, pathologically speaking, presents in childhood. There are 3 clinical presentations that may progress into one another: (1) an asymptomatic presentation with the diagnosis made only incidentally, (2) a symptomatic presentation with the patient having abdominal pain, hematuria and hypertension or (3) a uremic presentation, with progressive renal failure associated with proteinuria. Symptoms are related to the size of the cysts.

Pathologically, any portion of the nephron or collecting tubule may be enlarged and cystic, and, therefore, cysts are distributed throughout both the cortex and the medulla. The kidneys are bilaterally but often asymmetrically involved. In some instances, involvement of a kidney may be below the resolution of the diagnostic modality used, e.g., excretory urography, ultrasonography, computerized axial tomography or angiography.

The most frequent complications are infection and calculi (as much as 20%) secondary to urinary stasis within the ectatic collecting tubules. Other associated conditions may be present and include hepatic cysts, seen in up to one third of patients but without associated periportal fibrosis or portal hypertension; cysts in other organs, such as the pancreas, lung, spleen, ovaries, testes, thyroid and uterus; intracranial berry aneurysms, seen in 10–20% of patients; carcinoma of the kidney; and neurofibromatosis.

Roentgenographic Findings

Roentgenograms of the abdomen show bilateral renal enlargement. Occasionally, calculi, "milk of calcium" or, rarely, arcuate or amorphous calcification may be seen in the kidneys, liver or spleen. Excretory urography with nephrotomography usually demonstrates multiple lucent masses with distortion of the pelvicalyceal system. Retrograde pyelography shows distortion and displacement of the pelvicalyceal system by the large cysts. Angiography will show stretching of the intrarenal arteries and multiple large and small cysts in the cortex and medulla in the nephrographic phase. Visualization of these small cortical cysts, which give an inhomogeneous nephrographic appearance, in addition to the larger cysts, will differentiate this entity from multiple simple cysts, which show a homogeneous nephrogram with no evidence of multiple small cortical cysts. Lack of visualization of these small cysts does not exclude the diagnosis of adult polycystic disease. The demonstration of cysts in other organs, such as the liver, is strong evidence for the diagnosis of polycystic disease.

Ultrasonographic Findings

Ultrasonography will show, in addition to the nephromegaly, multiple discrete cysts, which are larger than the infantile type, distributed throughout the kidney. The normal central echogenic pelvicalyceal system is distorted by the adjacent cysts. Other organs that may also be involved, such as the liver, spleen, ovaries, uterus, pancreas and bladder, are easily surveyed.

CORTICAL CYSTS

Cystic lesions occurring primarily in the cortex are classified as follows: cysts associated with trisomy syndromes or tuberous sclerosis, simple cysts and multilocular cysts.

Cysts associated with the trisomy syndrome are very small cysts seen only histologically and have no clinical or roentgenographic importance.

Although renal masses in patients with tuberous sclerosis are usually hamartomas (angiomyolipomas), renal cysts do occur in this entity and may enlarge to the extent of markedly impairing renal function. Accurate diagnosis is usually accomplished following excretory urography, ultrasonography and angiography.

Simple (serous) renal cysts can be solitary or multiple and are very likely acquired lesions. Although simple cysts are primarily lesions of adults, they can occur in childhood and even in neonates. They contain serous fluid and do not (inherently) communicate with the collecting system, although they may rupture into it.

Excretory urography shows a round radiolucent mass usually bulging from a border of the kidney. Nephrotomography will demonstrate a thin rim surrounding the cyst, and the "beak sign," which is a result of compression of normal renal parenchyma by the slow-growing lesion. Ultrasonography will show a round sonolucency without internal echoes, a sharply defined, smooth border and an increased through transmission.

Since the possibility of a hypovascular cystic Wilms' tumor always exists and true simple cysts are rare in children, a cyst puncture under sonographic or fluoroscopic guidance is necessary for laboratory analysis of the fluid. At the same time, contrast material can be injected into the cyst and the entire wall carefully evaluated by multiple cross-table roentgenograms with the patient in prone, supine and both decubitus positions. Following these procedures, if there is still suspicion concerning the nature of the lesion, exploratory surgery is indicated to avoid misdiagnosing a cystic Wilms' tumor as a simple cyst.

Multilocular cysts are the least common of all congenital cystic lesions of the kidney. The etiology of the lesion is not known. This entity has been classified by some authors as a cystic hamartoma and by others as a benign multilocular cystic nephroma (benign form of Wilms' tumor). It usually is manifested in childhood as an asymptomatic abdominal mass discovered during a routine physical examination. It is a unilateral lesion involving only a portion of the kidney and sharply demarcated from the normal remaining renal parenchyma by a fibromuscular capsule. Pathologically, the lesion is composed of multiple loculi varying in size and separated from one another by septi composed of compact fibrous and smooth muscle tissue. There is no communication among the locules or with the renal pelvis.

The excretory urogram identifies the lesion as a sharply demarcated lucent area displacing the pelvicalyceal system. Angiographically, the lesion is relatively avascular, but vessels within the cyst may opacify, simulating a neoplasm.

MEDULLARY CYSTS

Cystic lesions occurring primarily in the medulla include medullary sponge kidney, medullary cystic disease, pyelogenic cysts and papillary necrosis (medullary type).

Medullary Sponge Kidney (Renal Tubular Ectasia)

Medullary sponge kidney is a developmental abnormality of the kidney limited to the medulla. The disease has no significant familial incidence and is usually discovered in the 3d or 4th decade of life because of the associated complication of infection, hematuria or calculus formation. There have been reports of association of medullary sponge kidney with hemihypertrophy, Ehlers-Danlos syndrome, congenital hypertrophic pyloric stenosis and Caroli's disease.

Pathologically, the collecting ducts in the renal pyramids are ectatic and associated with small cysts, 1–3 mm in diameter, that communicate with the collecting ducts and may be considered as "offshoots" or segmentally dilated portions of the ducts.

Roentgenographic Findings

Nephrocalcinosis (calcification in the renal pyramids) may be present on abdominal roentgenograms and is seen in up to 50% of patients with medullary sponge kidney. The excretory urogram shows typical streaks (and rounded collections) of opacified urine in the ectatic collecting ducts (and cysts) in the renal pyramids. These roentgenographic findings are present bilaterally in 60–80% of patients. In the remaining 20–40% of patients, the roentgenographic abnormalities are limited to 1 kidney or even to a single pyramid. However, the pathological changes are present throughout the kidneys bilaterally but are too small to be detected roentgenographically. The tubular ectasia may lead to overall enlargement of the pyramids, with a roentgenographic appearance of papillary hypertrophy manifested by splaying and elongation of the calyces. The kidneys are usually normal in size but may be slightly enlarged and, in the absence of complications, function normally. On the other hand, with loss of renal parenchyma due to infection or obstruction by renal calculi, the kidneys may be small and have decreased function.

It is often difficult on the excretory urogram to differentiate minimal tubular ectasia from the normal pyramidal blush seen with high-dose urography. In those instances in which discrete collections or streaks of contrast material even though few, can be demonstrated, the diagnosis of medullary sponge kidney is more likely since the normal pyramidal blush tends to be indistinct.

Although ultrasonography may show scattered areas of dense echogenicity representing the nephrocalcinosis, and possibly the small cysts, accurate diagnosis will be established by the excretory urogram.

Medullary Cystic Disease (Juvenile Nephronophthisis)

Medullary cystic disease of the kidney is probably a familial disease, although the mode of genetic transmission is not well defined. A higher incidence is seen in patients with blond or red hair. The disease usually presents in a teenager or young adult and is characterized by anemia, salt wasting, progressive azotemia and polyuria. The patients are invariably normotensive until the terminal stage of the disease, when hypertension may develop. Secondary hyperparathyroidism and renal osteodystrophy are relatively common complications.

Pathologically the kidneys are small, contain numerous cysts ranging in diameter from less than a millimeter to a few centimeters, and are located predominantly at the corticomedullary junction. Microscopically, there is interstitial fibrosis, periglomerular fibrosis and proximal tubular dilatation without calcific foci.

Medullary Necrosis

Renal papillary necrosis is the result of ischemia to portions of the pyramids from whatever cause. Conditions associated with papillary necrosis are diabetes mellitus, long-term phenacetin ingestion, shock, renal trauma, sickle cell anemia or trait, ureteral obstruction and pyelonephritis.

Papillary necrosis can be divided into three categories: (1) total papillary sloughing or "papillary necrosis," (2) partial papillary sloughing or "medullary necrosis" and (3) necrosis in situ. The medullary type of renal papillary necrosis enters into the differential diagnosis of renal cystic disease.

Pyelogenic Cysts (Calyceal Diverticulum)

A pyelogenic cyst is a small cavity in a renal column, frequently located medial to the corticomedullary junction. The cyst is connected to the adjacent calyx by an isthmus. The pathogenesis of this lesion is unknown; it may be congenital or acquired.

These cysts are usually asymptomatic; however, complications such as infection and calculus formation may occur. Of all the cystic lesions of the kidney, "milk of calcium" is found most commonly in a calyceal diverticulum. At excretory urography, the cyst opacifies after visualization of the pelvicalyceal system. The connecting isthmus may or may not be visualized.

REFERENCES

Ahmann, T. H., et al.: Transitional cell carcinoma in bilateral multiple renal cystic disease, J. Urol. 109:179, 1973.

Ahmed, S.: Simple renal cysts in childhood, Br. J. Urol. 44:71, 1972.

Arey, L.: *Developmental Anatomy* (7th ed.; Philadelphia: W. B. Saunders Co., 1965).

Ariyan, S., et al.: Ectopic multicystic kidney with hydronephrosis in a 7-year-old boy, J. Pediatr. Surg. 8:953, 1973.

Aterman, K., et al.: Solitary multilocular cyst of the kidney, J. Pediatr. Surg. 8:505, 1973.

Babka, J. C., et al.: Solitary intrarenal cyst causing hypertension, N. Engl. J. Med. 291:343, 1974.

Baldauf, M. C., et al.: Multilocular cyst of the kidney: Report of 3 cases with review of the literature, Am. J. Clin. Pathol. 65:93, 1976.

Barbaric, Z. L., et al.: Urinary tract obstruction in polycystic renal disease, Radiology 125:627, 1977.

Bearman, S. B., et al.: Multicystic kidney: A sonographic pattern, Radiology 118:685, 1976.

Becker, J. A., et al.: Simple cyst of the kidney, Semin. Roentgenol. 10:103, 1975.

Bernstein, J., et al.: Parenchymal Maldevelopment of the Kidney, in *Brennemann's Practice of Pediatrics*, vol. 3 (Hagerstown, Md.: Harper & Row Publishers, Inc., 1973).

Betkerur, U., et al.: Pleural effusion in Wilms' tumor, J. Pediatr. Surg. 12:523, 1977.

Blyth, H., et al.: Polycystic disease of kidneys and liver presenting in childhood, J. Med. Conct. 8:257, 1971.

Bosniak, M. A., et al.: Polycystic kidney disease, Semin. Roentgenol. 10:133, 1975.

Butler, M. R., et al.: Medullary sponge kidney: Review of the literature and presentation of 33 cases, Ir. Med. Assoc. J. 66:5, 1973.

Cole, A. T., et al.: Dual renal cell carcinomas in a unilateral polycystic kidney, J. Urol. 109:182, 1973.

Cooperman, L. R.: Delayed opacification in congenital multicystic dysplastic kidney, an important Roentgen sign, Radiology 121:703, 1976.

Cussen, L. J.: Cystic kidneys in children with congenital urethral obstruction, J. Urol. 106:939, 1971.

Devine, C. J., et al.: Calyceal diverticulum, J. Urol. 101:8, 1969.

DuMee, F. G. L.: Multilocular cysts of the kidney, Arch. Chir. Neerl. 25:293, 1973.

Eisenberg, R. L., et al.: Medullary sponge kidney associated with congenital hemihypertrophy (asymmetry): A case report and survey of the literature, A.J.R. 116:773, 1972.

Ekstrom, T., et al.: *Medullary Sponge Kidney: A Roentgenologic, Clinical, Histopathologic, and Biophysical Study* (Stockholm: Almquist and Wiksel, 1959).

Elkin, M.: Renal cystic disease: An overview, Semin. Roentgenol. 10:99, 1975.

Elkin, M., et al.: Cystic diseases of the kidney: Radiological and pathological considerations, Clin. Radiol. 20: 65, 1969.

Fanconi, V. G., et al.: Die familiare juvenile nephronophthise (die idiopathische parenchymatose schrumpfniere), Helv. Paediatr. Acta 6:1, 1951.

Felson, B., et al.: The hydronephrotic type of unilateral congenital multicystic disease of the kidney, Semin. Roentgenol. 10:113, 1975.

Firstater, M., et al.: Simple renal cyst in a newborn, Br. J. Urol. 45:366, 1973.

Flanagan, M. J., et al.: Congenital unilateral multicystic disease of the kidney, Arch. Surg. 96:983, 1968.

Friday, R. O., et al.: Multilocular renal cyst: Angiographic, ultrasonic and cyst puncture findings, Urology 3:354, 1974.

Friedenberg, R. M., et al.: Miscellaneous acquired cystic lesions of the kidney and retroperitoneum, Semin. Roentgenol. 10:155, 1975.

Garrett, R. A., et al.: Milk-of-calcium in caliceal diverticulum, J. Urol. 109:927, 1973.

Gellman, A. C., et al.: Carcinoma of kidney: Benign-appearing calcified cyst, Urology 2:556, 1973.

Gibson, A. A. M., et al.: Nephronophthisis: Report of 8 cases from Britain, Arch. Dis. Child. 47:84, 1972.

Giselson, N., et al.: Renal medullary cystic disease or familial juvenile nephronophthisis: A renal tubular disease, Am. J. Med. 48:174, 1970.

Gleason, D. C., et al.: Cystic disease of the kidneys in children, A.J.R. 100:135, 1967.

Granberg, P. O., et al.: Renal function studies in medullary sponge kidney, Scand. J. Urol. Nephrol. 5:177, 1971.

Green, W. M., et al.: A reappraisal of sonolucent renal masses, Radiology 121:163, 1976.

Greene, L. F., et al.: Multicystic dysplasia of the kidney with special reference to the contralateral kidney, J. Urol. 105: 482, 1971.

Griscom, N. T., et al.: Pelvoinfundibular atresia: The usual form of multicystic kidney: 44 unilateral and 2 bilateral cases, Semin. Roentgenol. 10:125, 1975.

Grossman, H., et al.: Roentgenographic classification of renal cystic disease, A.J.R. 104:319, 1968.

Gwinn, J. L., et al.: Cystic diseases of kidneys in infants and children, Radiol. Clin. North Am. 6:191, 1968.

Hare, W. S. C., et al.: The radiology of renal papillary necrosis as seen in analgesic nephropathy, Clin. Radiol. 25: 423, 1974.

Harp, G. E., et al.: Bleeding solitary renal cysts, Urology 3: 649, 1974.

Hayt, D. B., et al.: Direct magnification intravenous pyelography in the evaluation of medullary sponge kidney, A.J.R. 119:701, 1973.

Hoeffel, J. C., et al.: Classification of renal cysts in children, Aust. Radiol. J. 14:302, 1970.

Igawa, K., et al.: Unilateral medullary sponge kidney: Report of a case with some observations on urine osmotic pressure, J. Urol. 112:556, 1974.

Jackman, R. J., et al.: Benign hemorrhagic renal cyst: Nephrotomography, renal arteriography and cyst puncture, Radiology 110:7, 1974.

Johanson, K. E., et al.: Management of intrarenal peripelvic cysts, Urology 4:514, 1974.

Johnson, D. E., et al.: Multilocular renal cystic disease in children, J. Urol. 109:101, 1973.

Kearney, G. P., et al.: B-mode nephrosonography in renal masses: Its use and some limitations, Urology 6:125, 1975.

Kelsey, J. A., et al.: Gray-scale ultrasonography in the diagnosis of polycystic kidney disease, Radiology 122:791, 1977.

Kendall, A. R., et al.: Congenital cystic disease of the kidney: Classification of manifestations, Urology 4:635, 1974.

Kerr, D. N. S., et al.: A lesion resembling medullary sponge kidney in patients with congenital hepatic fibrosis, Clin. Radiol. 13:85, 1962.

Koehler, P. R., et al.: Ultrasonic "B" scanning in the diagnosis of complications in renal transplant patients, Radiology 119:661, 1976.

Kutcher, R., et al.: Calcification in polycystic disease, Radiology 122:77, 1977.

Kyaw, M. M.: Roentgenologic triad of congenital multicystic kidney, A.J.R. 119:710, 1973.

Kyaw, M. M.: The radiological diagnosis of congenital multicystic kidney: "Radiological triad," Clin. Radiol. 25:45, 1974.

Kyaw, M. M., et al.: Value of aortography in the diagnosis of congenital multicystic kidney, J. Can. Assoc. Radiol. 25: 105, 1974.

Lalli, A. F., et al.: Urographic analysis of the development of polycystic kidney disease, A.J.R. 119:705, 1973.

Lang, E. K.: Roentgenologic assessment of medullary cysts, Semin. Roentgenol. 10:145, 1975.

Leopold, G. R., et al.: Renal ultrasonography: An updated approach to the diagnosis of renal cyst, Radiology 109:671, 1973.

Lieberman, E., et al.: Infantile polycystic disease of the kidneys and liver: Clinical, pathological and radiological correlation and comparison with congenital hepatic fibrosis, Medicine 50:277, 1971.

Lister, J., et al.: Pelvicalyceal cysts in children, J. Pediatr. Surg. 8:901, 1973.

McCroy, W.: Developmental Nephrology, in Commonwealth Fund Book (Cambridge, Mass: Harvard University Press, 1972).

McLaughlin, A. P., et al.: Spontaneous rupture of renal cysts into the pyelocaliceal system, J. Urol. 113:2, 1975.

Mena, E., et al.: Angiographic findings in renal medullary cystic disease, Radiology 110:277, 1974.

Meyers, M. A.: Uriniferous perirenal pseudocyst: New observations, Radiology 117:539, 1975.

Moore, K. L.: Developing Human Clinically Oriented Embryology (Philadelphia: W. B. Saunders Co., 1977).

Neustein, D. H., et al.: Müllerian duct cyst: With report of a case, Br. J. Urol. 40:72, 1968.

Newman, L., et al.: Unilateral total renal dysplasia in children, A.J.R. 116:778, 1972.

Nordlander, S., et al.: Differential diagnosis of space-occupying lesions in the kidneys with the scintillation camera, Acta Radiol. Diagn. 15:630, 1974.

Osathanondh, V., et al.: Pathogenesis of polycystic kidneys, Arch. Pathol. 77:466, 1964.

Palubinskas, A. J.: Renal pyramidal structure opacification in excretory urography and its relation to medullary sponge kidney, Radiology 81:963, 1963.

Pathak, I. G., et al.: Multicystic and cystic dysplastic kidneys, Br. J. Urol. 36:318, 1964.

Patten, B.: Human Embryology (3d ed.; New York: McGraw-Hill Book Co., 1968).

Pickens, R. L.: Early diagnosis of polycystic kidney disease, Urology 2:188, 1973.

Pollack, H. M., et al.: A systematized approach to the differential diagnosis of renal masses, Radiology 113: 653, 1974.

Potter, E. L.: Facial characteristics of infants with bilateral renal agenesis, Am. J. Obstet. Gynecol. 51:885, 1946.

Powell, T., et al.: Multilocular cysts of the kidney, Br. J. Urol. 23:142, 1951.

Raskin, M. M., et al.: Percutaneous management of renal cysts: Results of a 4-year study, Radiology 115:551, 1975.

Rayfield, E. J., et al.: Red and blonde hair in renal medullary cystic disease, Arch. Intern. Med. 130:72, 1972.

Reilly, B. J., et al.: Renal tubular ectasia in cystic disease of kidneys and liver, A.J.R. 84:546, 1960.

Risdon, R. A.: Renal dysplasia, J. Clin. Pathol. 24:57, 1971.

Roberts, P. F.: Medical memoranda: Bilateral renal carcinoma associated with polycystic kidneys, Br. Med. J. 3: 273, 1973.

Rockson, S. G., et al.: Solitary renal cyst with segmental ischemia and hypertension, J. Urol. 112:550, 1974.

Rosenfield, A. T., et al.: Gray-scale ultrasonography in medullary cystic disease of the kidney and congenital hepatic fibrosis with tubular ectasia: New observations, A.J.R. 129:297, 1977.

Rouiller, C.: *The Kidney: Morphology, Biochemistry, Physiology* (New York: Academic Press, 1969).

Rudhe, U., et al.: Congenital urethral diverticulae, Acta Radiol. 13:289, 1970.

Salvatierra, O., et al.: Polycystic renal disease treated by renal transplantation, Surg. Gynecol. Obstet. 137:431, 1973.

Scholtmeijer, R. J., et al.: Unilateral multicystic kidney and contralateral hydronephrosis in the newborn, Br. J. Urol. 47:176, 1975.

Smith, C. H., et al.: Congenital medullary cysts of the kidneys with severe refractory anemia, Am. J. Dis. Child. 69: 369, 1945.

Smith, D. W., et al.: A syndrome of multiple developmental defects including polycystic kidneys and intrahepatic biliary dysgenesis in 2 siblings, J. Pediatr. 67:617, 1965.

Spence, H. M., et al.: What is sponge kidney disease and where does it fit in the spectrum of cystic disorders? J. Urol. 107:176, 1972.

Spicer, R. D., et al.: Renal medullary cystic disease, Br. Med. J. 1:824, 1969.

Sprayregen, S., et al.: Medullary sponge kidney and congenital total hemihypertrophy, N. Y. State J. Med. 73:2768, 1973.

Steel, J. F., et al.: Spontaneous remission of peripelvic renal cysts, J. Urol. 114:10, 1975.

Stella, F. J., et al.: Medullary sponge kidney associated with parathyroid adenoma: A report of 2 cases, Nephron 10: 332, 1973.

Strass, M., et al.: *Diseases of the Kidney* (2d ed.; Boston: Little, Brown & Co., 1971).

Strauss, M. D., et al.: Medullary cystic disease and familial juvenile nephronophthisis: Clinical and pathological identity, N. Engl. J. Med. 277:863, 1967.

Stuppler, S. A., et al.: Medullary sponge kidney: Review of the literature and presentation of 4 cases, W. Va. Med. J. 69:167, 1973.

Swenson, R. S., et al.: Cystic disease of the renal medulla in the elderly, J.A.M.A. 288:1401, 1974.

Tegtmeyer, C. J., et al.: Angiographic diagnosis of renal tumors associated with polycystic disease, Radiology 126: 105, 1978.

Thaler, M. M., et al.: Congenital fibrosis and polycystic disease of liver and kidneys, Am. J. Dis. Child. 126:374, 1973.

Thornbury, J. R., et al.: Use of excretory urogram information in the solution of the renal cyst/tumor/cortical nodule problem, Radiology 118:575, 1976.

Towbin, R., et al.: Multilocular cystic dysplasia of half of a horseshoe kidney, J. Pediatr. Surg. 9:421, 1974.

Uson, A. C., et al.: Multilocular cysts of kidney with intrapelvic herniation of a "daughter" cyst: Report of 4 cases, J. Urol. 89:341, 1963.

Varma, K. R., et al.: Papillary carcinoma in wall of simple renal cyst, Urology 3:762, 1974.

Vuthibhagdee, A., et al.: Infantile polycystic disease of the kidney, Am. J. Dis. Child. 125:167, 1973.

Wallack, H. I., et al.: Polycystic kidneys: Indications for surgical intervention, Urology 3:552, 1974.

Woesner, M. E., et al.: Contralateral displacement of the kidney by solitary renal cyst, A.J.R. 116:766, 1972.

Wright, F. W., et al.: Polycystic kidneys, renal hamartomas: Their variants and complications, Clin. Radiol. 25:27, 1974.

Wright, F. W., et al.: The radiological diagnosis of "avascular" renal tumours, Br. J. Urol. 47:253, 1975.

Young, L. W., et al.: Delayed excretory urographic opacification: A puddling effect, in multicystic renal dysplasia, Ann. Radiol. 17:391, 1974.

Leading articles: Renal cysts and red hair, Br. Med. J. 1:631, 1973.

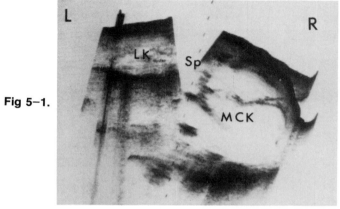 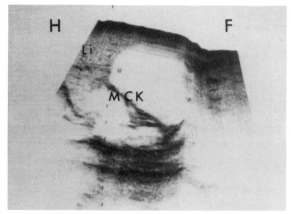

Fig 5–1.   **Fig 5–2.**

Figs 5–1 and 5–2. — Multicystic kidney disease. A multicystic kidney is one of the more common diseases affecting neonates and infants. The sonographic pattern ranges from a complex, mixed cystic and solid, mass to a more simple cystic mass. Involvement is usually unilateral, and the characteristic appearance of hydronephrosis previously described is not seen (Figs 5–1 and 5–2); the cystic mass does not necessarily bulge medially, and the normal rind of renal parenchyma cannot be demonstrated. H = head; F = feet; L = left; R = right; Li = liver; MCK = multicystic kidney; Lk = left kidney; Sp = spine.

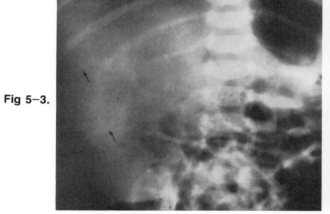

Fig 5–3.   **Fig 5–4.**

Figs 5–3 and 5–4. — Multicystic kidney disease. Excretory urogram (Fig 5–3) shows large mass on right side. Some contrast outlines septations of this multicystic kidney *(arrows).* Contrast injection of the surgically resected kidney (Fig 5–4) shows the cystic lobulation and demonstrates that there is no connection between these cysts and renal pelvis (pelviinfundibular atresia). Multicystic kidney may be large, as in this patient, or may appear as smaller mass.

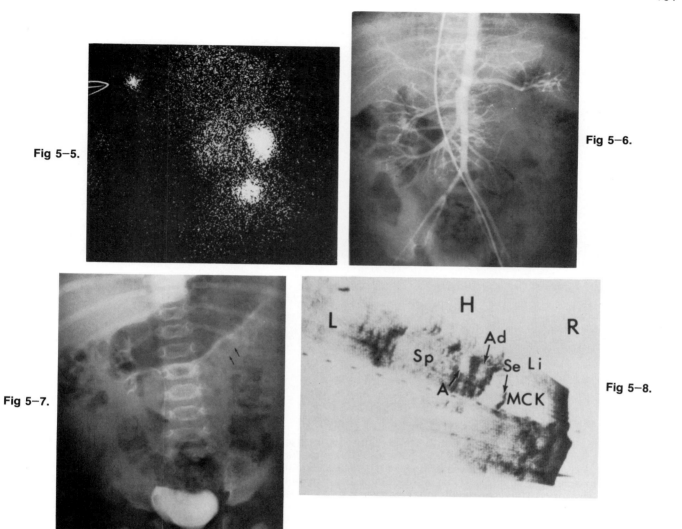

Fig 5–5.

Fig 5–6.

Fig 5–7.

Fig 5–8.

Figs 5–5 to 5–8.—Multicystic kidney disease on left side. Renal scintiscan (Fig 5–5) shows normally functioning right kidney and no evidence of function on left side. Delayed scans also failed to demonstrate any function on left side. Following contrast injection (Fig 5–6) there is visualization of aorta and normal right renal artery, with no evidence of left renal artery. A 12-minute excretory urogram (Fig 5–7) shows normally functioning right kidney and no function of left kidney. Arrows point to visualization of septum following injection of contrast material. The coronal sonogram also clearly demonstrates the multicystic kidney on left (Fig 5–8). L = left; R = right; H = head; Sp = spleen; A = aorta; Ad = adrenal gland; Li = liver; MCK = multicystic kidney disease; Se = septum.

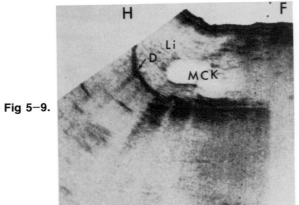

Fig 5–9.

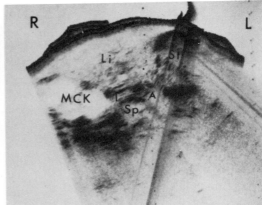

Fig 5–10.

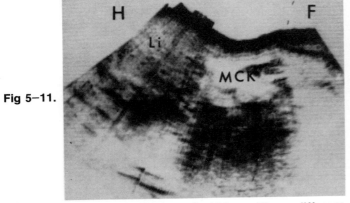

Fig 5–11.

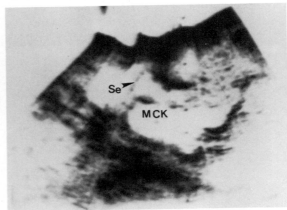

Fig 5–12.

Figs 5–9 to 5–12.—Multicystic kidney. Three different cases demonstrate the various sonographic features of this entity (case 1, Figs 5–9 and 5–10; case 2, Fig 5–11; case 3, Fig 5–12). In each case, multiple scans were obtained to demonstrate any form of normal renal parenchyma and to assess dilatation of renal pelvis and calyces. In no case could renal parenchyma be demonstrated. The cystic masses projected laterally and posteriorly rather than medially, as seen in hydronephrosis. These three cases demonstrate the variability of size, lobulation and septation in multicystic kidney disease. H = head; F = feet; R = right; L = left; Li = liver; D = diaphragm; MCK = multicystic kidney; I = inferior vena cava; A = aorta; Sp = spine; St = stomach; Se = septum.

Fig 5–13.

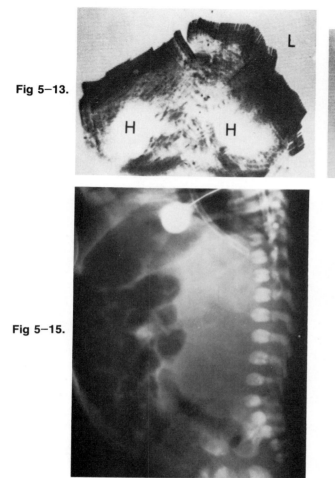

Fig 5–14.

Fig 5–15.

Figs 5–13 to 5–15.—Renal cystic dysplasia associated with lower urinary tract obstruction. Ultrasound with patient in supine (Fig 5–13) and longitudinal (Fig 5–14) positions shows marked dilatation and hydronephrotic appearance of both kidneys; however, there is no evidence of demonstrable renal parenchyma. Lateral film, following injection of contrast material (Fig 5–15), shows bilateral renal enlargement but no functioning renal tissue. This patient had posterior urethral valve (as well as prune-belly syndrome). This type of dysplasia has been classified by Potter as type 4 renal dysplasia. In this patient, the associated small cortical cysts are not visible ultrasonographically. L = left; F = feet; Li = liver; H = head (Fig 5–14) or dysplastic kidney (Figs 5–13 and 5–14).

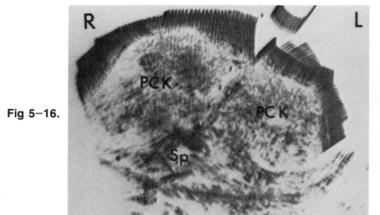

Fig 5–16.

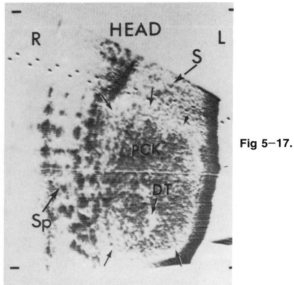

Fig 5–17.

Figs 5–16 and 5–17.—Infantile polycystic kidney disease. Infantile polycystic kidney disease represents a spectrum of associated abnormalities affecting the kidneys and liver. Kidneys are severely involved and bilateral renal enlargement is evident on ultrasonography (Figs 5–16 and 5–17). Since the cysts are anatomically located in the medullary portion of the kidney, a normal rind of cortical parenchyma is evident *(arrows)*. However, since cystic changes are below resolution of sound beam, they appear as echogenic expansion of the renal sinus and medulla. If significant tubular ectasia is present, dilated tubules (Fig 5–17) may be individually imaged. R = right; L = left; PCK = polycystic kidney; Sp = spine; S = spleen; DT = dilated tubules.

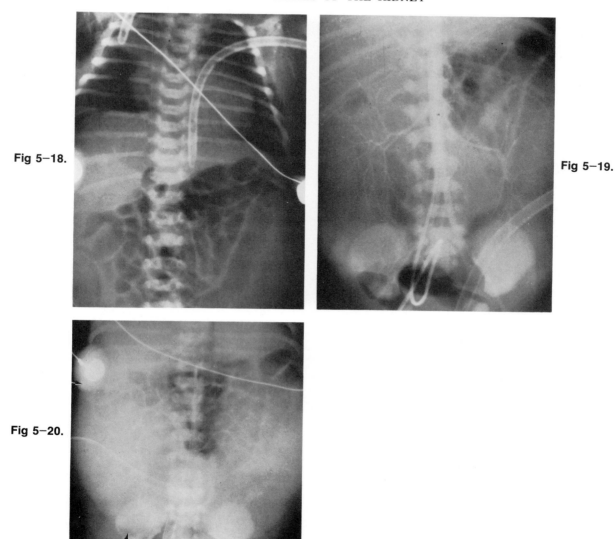

Fig 5–18.

Fig 5–19.

Fig 5–20.

Figs 5–18 to 5–20.—Infantile polycystic kidney disease. Chest and abdomen film of a newborn demonstrates bilateral pneumothoraces and displacement of bowel loops medially by bilateral renal masses (Fig 5–18). Presence of bilateral pneumothoraces with no detectable pulmonary disease should suggest severe renal disease. Injection of contrast material through umbilical arterial catheter (Fig 5–19) demonstrates both renal arteries and enlargement of both kidneys with splaying of the intrarenal arteries by numerous cysts. The 24-hour film (Fig 5–20) again demonstrates the enlarged kidneys and the typical "brush-border" appearance of contrast material in the dilated tubules characteristic of polycystic disease of the newborn.

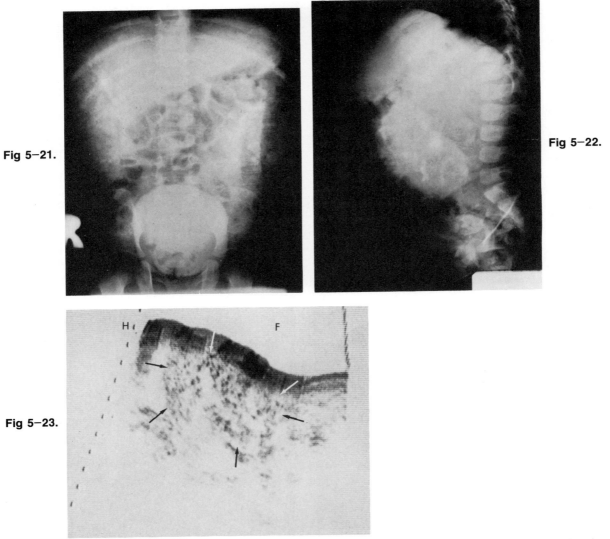

Fig 5–21.

Fig 5–22.

Fig 5–23.

Figs 5–21 to 5–23.—Polycystic disease of childhood. Frontal (Fig 5–21) and lateral (Fig 5–22) views of excretory urogram demonstrate enlarged kidneys. Visualized portions of calyces appear normal. The "brush-border" appearance is secondary to contrast in dilated tubules. This is a mild form compared to newborn type of polycystic disease. On ultrasonogram (Fig 5–23), kidney is enlarged *(arrows)* and acoustic texture pattern is totally distorted, with multiple tubular fluid areas located centrally. H = head; F = feet.

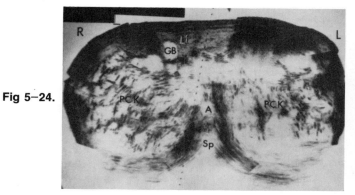

Fig 5–24.

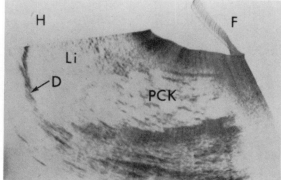

Fig 5–25.

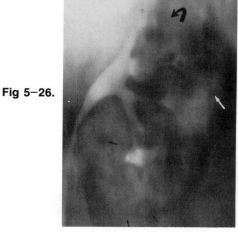

Fig 5–26.

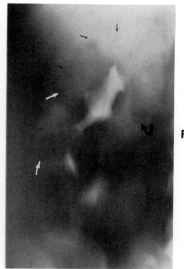

Fig 5–27.

Figs 5–24 to 5–27.—Adult polycystic kidney disease. In adult form of polycystic kidney disease, the cysts are seen in both cortical and medullary portions of kidney. On ultrasonography multiple cysts of varying size are present throughout the kidney (Figs 5–24 and 5–25). Nevertheless, kidney tends to maintain its reniform shape. Longitudinal and decubitus scans are particularly helpful in assessing the extent of cystic involvement of kidneys and liver. However, even with these views it may be difficult to ascertain if a cyst arises from liver or upper pole of kidney. With this form of polycystic disease, pancreas should also be examined since it too has significant but smaller incidence of cystic involvement. Figures 5–26 and 5–27 are tomograms of both kidneys during excretory urography which demonstrate numerous cysts of varying sizes *(arrows)* and small cortical cysts that differentiate polycystic kidney from multiple simple cysts. In any child with a urographic appearance similar to those of adult polycystic kidney disease, diagnosis of tuberous sclerosis should be considered; further studies are necessary to make correct diagnosis. R = right; L = left; PCK = polycystic kidney; Sp = spine; GB = gallbladder; A = aorta; H = head; F = foot; Li = liver; D = diaphragm.

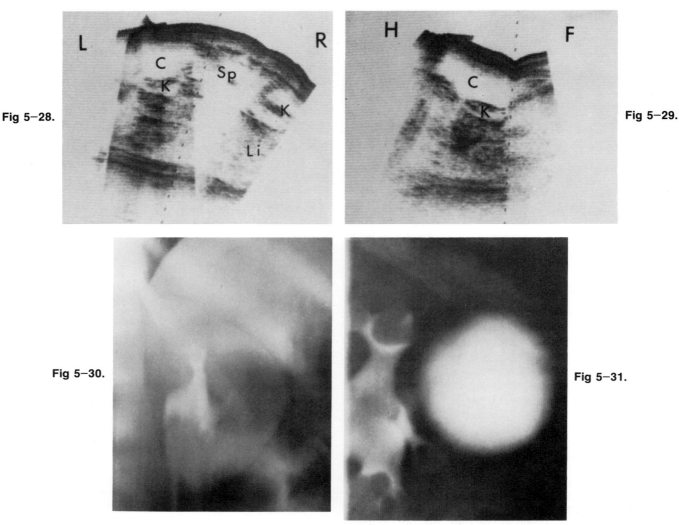

Fig 5–28.

Fig 5–29.

Fig 5–30.

Fig 5–31.

Figs 5–28 to 5–31.—Simple renal cyst. Simple renal cysts are uncommon in childhood. Since both Wilms' tumors and neuroblastoma may undergo significant cystic change, a confident diagnosis of a simple cyst of the kidney can be difficult. Rigid criteria must be applied: no internal echoes, increased through transmission and a sharp, well-defined posterior wall (Figs 5–28 and 5–29). In addition, adjacent renal parenchyma and renal sinus should be normal. However, in this age group, even with these findings, cyst aspiration is probably warranted.

A tomogram following intravenous injection of contrast material (Fig 5–30) demonstrates the renal cyst, which is relatively lucent compared to remaining renal parenchyma, in midportion of left kidney. Since a simple renal cyst is uncommon in this age group, cyst was punctured and contrast injected (Fig 5–31). The aspirated fluid was sent for laboratory analysis, which confirmed the diagnosis of simple cyst. L = left; R = right; H = head; F = feet; C = cyst; K = kidney; Sp = spine; Li = liver.

Fig 5–32.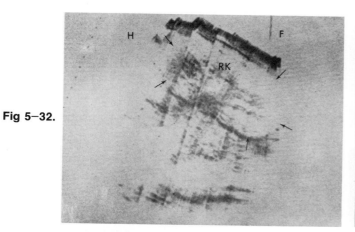

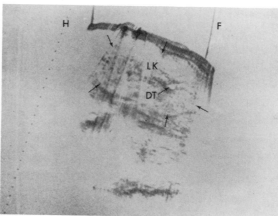 **Fig 5–33.**

Fig 5–34.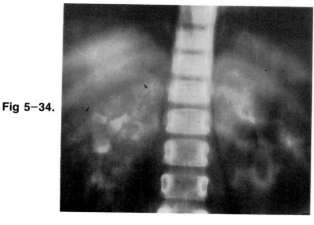

Figs 5–32 to 5–34.—Tubular ectasia (medullary sponge kidney). In tubular ectasia, renal acoustic texture is more normal than in other cystic diseases of the kidney. Kidneys may be somewhat enlarged (Figs 5–32 and 5–33, *arrows*); however, renal sinus-renal parenchyma ratio is close to normal. Fluid areas representing dilated tubules may be seen in renal sinus region.

Figure 5–34 is a tomogram following intravenous injection of contrast material that demonstrates enlarged kidneys and renal tubular ectasia *(arrows)*. H = head; F = feet; RK = right kidney; LK = left kidney; DT = dilated tubule.

Fig 5–35.

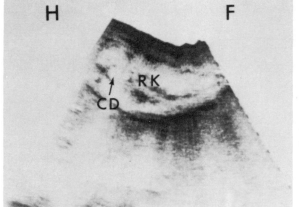

Fig 5–36.

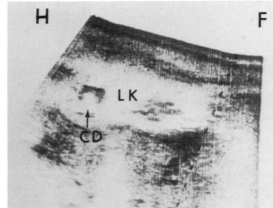

Fig 5–37.

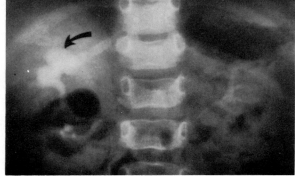

Figs 5–35 to 5–37.—Calyceal diverticulum. On ultrasonography, a calyceal diverticulum is a cystic area positioned within and separating a portion of dense echoes of the renal sinus (Figs 5–35 and 5–36). If large, it may be difficult to differentiate from minimally dilated upper-pole collecting system of duplicated kidney. Final diagnosis is usually made on excretory urography. Figure 5–37 is cone-down film of excretory urogram, with arrow pointing to calyceal diverticulum. H = head; F = feet; RK = right kidney; LK = left kidney; CD = calyceal diverticulum.

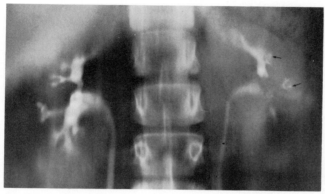

Fig 5–38.—Papillary necrosis. Papillary necrosis (medullary type) must be differentiated from other cystic diseases. The urographic appearance is usually characteristic, with a ring of contrast *(arrows)* surrounding the "cystic" lucency (papilla).

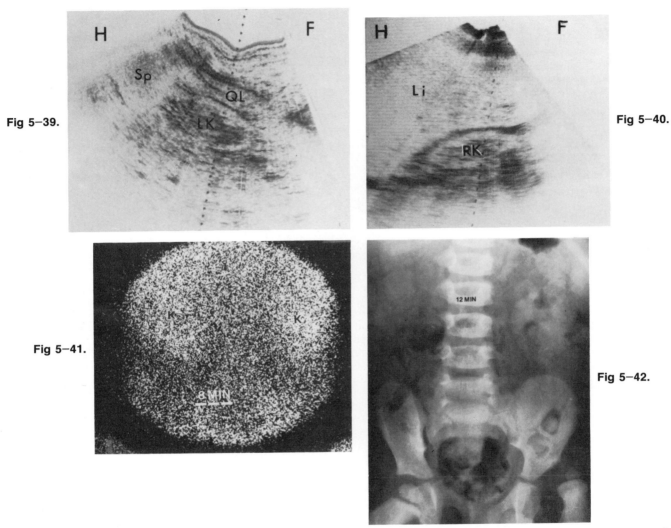

Fig 5–39.

Fig 5–40.

Fig 5–41.

Fig 5–42.

Figs 5–39 to 5–42.—Chronic renal disease secondary to medullary cystic disease of kidney. One form of chronic renal disease is secondary to medullary cystic disease. The sonographic abnormalities are a decrease in renal size with increased echogenicity of renal parenchyma secondary to fibrosis (Figs 5–39 and 5–40). Because kidney may have lobulated contour, margins may be difficult to delineate on ultrasonograms. In medullary cystic disease, although kidney is small renal sinus and medulla represent the major portion of kidney.

Figure 5–41 is renal scintiscan that shows very faint function of both kidneys. A 12-minute film from the excretory urogram (Fig 5–42) also demonstrates markedly decreased function of both kidneys. Bones are osteopenic. Findings on excretory urogram, renal scintiscan or sonogram are not diagnostic of medullary cystic disease and may be seen in any form of chronic renal disease such as chronic glomerulonephritis or Alport's syndrome. H = head; F = feet; Sp = spleen; Li = liver; QL = quadratus lumborum muscle; LK = left kidney; RK = right kidney; K = kidney.

6

Urinary Tract Neoplasms

IN CHILDREN, RENAL TUMORS are much more common than lower urinary tract neoplasms. The clinical presentation of renal masses includes a palpable abdominal mass (the majority of the patients), hypertension (particularly in Wilms' tumor), anemia and symptoms secondary to metastases.

WILMS' TUMOR (CONGENITAL NEPHROBLASTOMA)

Wilms' tumor is the most common intra-abdominal malignant tumor in childhood. This tumor originates from the metanephrogenic blastema. It may present at any age, but the peak incidence is 3–4 years, with equal sex predilection. The incidence of bilateral tumors ranges from 3 to 11%. A familial incidence has been reported, but it is uncommon (less than 1%). A higher incidence of bilateral Wilms' tumor is seen in these familial cases.

Tumors presenting in the neonatal period are more likely to be hamartomatous (congenital mesoblastic nephroma); these lesions are considered to be benign neoplasms. Although there is clear histopathological differentiation between fetal renal hamartoma and Wilms' tumor, it may be difficult to differentiate them roentgenographically. This differentiation is necessary because the vast majority of patients with fetal renal hamartomas are cured by nephrectomy alone, without need for radiation therapy or chemotherapy.

The Relationship of Wilms' Tumor to Nodular Nephroblastomatosis

The term "nodular nephroblastomatosis" refers to small nodules of primitive renal blastema (hamartomas) scattered diffusely or multifocally throughout the renal cortex. Renal tissue containing the multifocal form of nodular nephroblastomatosis is at high risk to dévelop Wilms' tumor(s). Stated differently, at least one third of patients with Wilms' tumor have associated nodular nephroblastomas in the renal cortex; this association is present in all patients with bilateral Wilms' tumors. These foci of primitive renal tissue may progressively enlarge (Wilms' tumorlet) and subsequently become a Wilms' tumor.

Associated Anomalies

Children with Wilms' tumors have an increased incidence of congenital anomalies. Associated anomalies that have been described include chromosomal abnormalities (trisomy 8 and trisomy 18), genitourinary tract anomalies (cryptorchidism, hypospadias, duplication of the urinary tract and horseshoe kidney), sporadic aniridia, the Beckwith-Wiedemann syndrome (organomegaly involving the kidney, adrenal cortex and liver) and congenital hemihypertrophy. This musculoskeletal hypertrophy may involve a segment or an entire side of the body. Hemihypertrophy has been also reported in association with adrenal cortical and hepatic tumors.

Prognosis

Several key factors play a role in the prognosis of patients with Wilms' tumor: (1) The histological pattern of the neoplasm. A histological classification, i.e., favorable vs. unfavorable, is determined by careful examination of multiple sections of the primary tumor (the absence of sarcomatous elements and the presence of some tissue differentiation yields a better prognosis). (2) The patient's age. The younger the patient at the time of diagnosis, the better the prognosis. (3) The extent of the disease. This is the most significant factor, as patients with more extensive spread of the disease have a poorer prognosis. Because of this, a staging classification is used as follows:

Stage I: The tumor is encapsulated and removed entirely.

Stage II: The tumor extends beyond the kidney but is completely resected.

Stage III: The tumor extends beyond the kidney but is incompletely resected.

Stage IV: There are metastases to the lungs, liver, brain or bones.

Stage V: There is bilateral renal involvement with the tumor.

It should be noted, however, that in a number of reports there has been a better long-term survival rate in patients with stages IV or V disease compared to stage III disease. It might be of value to stage each kidney separately if both are involved.

Wilms' tumors most often metastasize hematogeneously, with the lungs being the commonest site. Therefore, a chest x-ray is necessary in the initial evaluation of the patient and follow-up chest films should be obtained routinely every 1–2 months during the 1st year of therapy. Metastases to the liver (the 2d most common organ), brain, bone and other organs can be seen.

Treatment of Wilms' tumor includes surgical removal, radiation therapy (particularly in patients with stage II disease and higher) to the renal fossa and metastatic sites, and chemotherapy.

RENAL CELL CARCINOMA (HYPERNEPHROMA)

Renal cell carcinoma rarely occurs in children, with most reported patients being more than 5 years of age. Roentgenographically, these carcinomas have an appearance similar to Wilms' tumor but calcification is more frequent.

ANGIOMYOLIPOMA

Angiomyolipoma is a hamartoma containing vascular, fatty and muscular tissue. It occurs at all ages, particularly in patients with tuberous sclerosis (50% of renal lesions are in patients with tuberous sclerosis). As many as 80% of patients with tuberous sclerosis have renal involvement with hamartomas. It is a familial disorder, with hamartomatous lesions involving multiple organ systems including the kidneys, lungs, eyes, skeletal system, heart, brain and skin. The renal lesions are multiple and bilateral. They seldom cause symptoms until late childhood or adult life. Unilateral angiomyolipomas may occur without associated tuberous sclerosis but are usually seen in adults.

Other rare renal tumors that may be seen in childhood include rhabdomyosarcomas, leiomyosarcomas, hemangiomas, hemangiopericytomas, cystadenomas (also called multilocular cysts or lymphangiomas) and mucosal epithelial tumors.

Retroperitoneal mesenchymal tumors, such as teratomas and sarcomas, may be roentgenographically similar to Wilms' tumor (or neuroblastomas).

RENAL INVOLVEMENT SECONDARY TO OTHER NEOPLASMS

Of all neoplasms that secondarily involve the kidneys, leukemia and lymphoma are the most frequent. These usually cause nephromegaly but must be differentiated from other causes, such as renal vein thrombosis or glycogen storage disease.

Renal infiltration occurs in more than 30% of patients with malignant lymphoma. Nodular involvement is seen in approximately 60%. In 25% only one kidney is involved.

Renal enlargement due to leukemic infiltration occurs in 30–50% of patients with acute or chronic leukemia. The nephromegaly is usually diffuse and bilateral. Renal enlargement may also occur in the absence of significant infiltration for an unknown reason. Severe leukemic involvement of the kidneys may cause acute renal failure.

Of various types of leukemia and lymphoma that occur in childhood or adult life, 2 conditions stand out primarily as childhood diseases: lymphocytic leukemia and Burkitt's lymphoma.

NEOPLASTIC DISEASES INVOLVING THE LOWER URINARY TRACT IN CHILDREN

Rhabdomyosarcoma is the most common tumor involving the lower urinary tract in children. This is an embryonic sarcoma that may be found in the orbit, lungs and biliary tract in addition to the lower urinary tract. The tumor characteristically presents during the first 4 years of life, with a male predominance. The tumor occurs in 2 forms: polypoid (sarcoma botryoides) and solid. Sarcoma botryoides is a polypoid rhabdomyosarcoma with coarse lobulation, giving it a "grape-like" appearance, arising in the bladder or vagina. It is distinct from the solid form, which is more commonly seen arising in the bladder base, prostate, broad ligament or paratesticular tissues.

Other uncommon or rare tumors involving the lower urinary tract include transitional cell carcinoma, leukemic infiltration of the bladder, neurofibroma, myoma, simple fibromatous polyps, hemangioma and pheochromocytoma. Transitional cell carcinomas are exceptionally rare in childhood. Leukemic infiltration of the bladder, which is seen in advanced cases following prolonged chemotherapy, must be differentiated from cyclophosphamide-induced cystitis, which is more common.

Neurofibromatosis may affect the pelvic nerves, producing a mass, or involve the submucosal layer of the bladder. Myomas produce a solid polypoid filling defect within the bladder. Simple fibromatous polyps arise on a stalk in the region of the verumontanum and may cause urine retention. Occasionally they may prolapse into the urethra. Hemangiomas rarely involve the bladder and are associated with hemangiomas elsewhere in the body in about one third of the patients. Pheochromocytomas have been reported in the bladder but are extremely rare.

REFERENCES

Alford, B. A., et al.: Roentgenographic features of American Burkitt's lymphoma, Radiology 124:763, 1977.

Appleyard, W. J.: Hyperuricaemia and renal failure preceding the onset of acute lymphoblastic leukaemia, Proc. R. Soc. Med. 64:40, 1971.

Arey, J. B.: Tumors of the Kidney, in Vaughan, V. C., and McKay, R. J. (eds.): Nelson Textbook of Pediatrics (10th ed.; Philadelphia: W. B. Saunders Co., 1975).

Barakat, A. Y., et al.: Acute lymphoblastic leukemia diagnosed by renal biopsy, J. Urol. 118:103, 1977.

Beckwith, J. B., et al.: Histopathology and prognosis of Wilms' tumor, Cancer 41:1937, 1978.

Bekerman, C., et al.: Scintigraphic evaluation of lymphoma: A comparative study of ^{67}Ga-citrate and ^{111}In-bleomycin, Radiology 123:687, 1977.

Berry, C. L., et al.: Coincidence of congenital malformation and embryonic tumours of childhood, Arch. Dis. Child. 45:229, 1970.

Bishop, H. C., et al.: Survival in bilateral Wilms' tumor: Review of 30 national Wilms' tumor study cases, J. Pediatr. Surg. 12:631, 1977.

Bolande, R. P., et al.: Congenital mesoblastic nephroma of infancy: A report of 8 cases and the relationship to Wilms' tumor, Pediatrics 40:272, 1967.

Boldt, D. W., et al.: Computed tomography of abdominal mass lesions in children: Initial experience, Radiology 124:371, 1977.

Bond, J. V.: Wilms's tumour, hypospadias, and cryptorchidism in twins, Arch. Dis. Child. 52:243, 1977.

Bond, J. V., et al.: Pulmonary metastases in Wilms' tumour, Clin. Radiol. 27:191, 1976.

Bove, K. E., et al.: The Nephroblastomatosis Complex

and Its Relationship to Wilms' Tumor: A Clinicopathologic Treatise, in Rosenberg, H. S., and Bolande, R. P. (eds.): *Perspectives in Pediatric Pathology*, vol. 3 (Chicago: Year Book Medical Publishers, Inc., 1976).

Brantley, R. E., et al.: Angiography and histopathology of nephroblastomatosis, Radiology 120:151, 1976.

Braunstein, P., et al.: Scintiscan evaluation of prominent renal columns, Radiology 104:103, 1972.

Burke, J. F., et al.: Malignant lymphoma with "myeloma kidney" acute renal failure, Am. J. Med. 60:1055, 1976.

Cadman, E. C., et al.: Systemic methotrexate toxicity: A pharmacological study of its occurrence after intrathecal administration in a patient with renal failure, Arch. Intern. Med. 136:1321, 1976.

Cameron, K. M.: Neurofibromatosis of the bladder, Br. J. Urol. 36:77, 1964.

Carlson, D. H., et al.: Benign multilocal cystic nephroma, A.J.R. 131:621, 1978.

Cook, J. H., et al.: Ultrasonic demonstration of intrarenal anatomy, A.J.R. 129:831, 1977.

Cremin, B. J., et al.: Arteriography in Wilms' tumour: The results of 13 cases and comparison to renal dysplasia, Br. J. Radiol. 45:415, 1972.

Datnow, B., et al.: Polycystic nephroblastoma, J.A.M.A. 236:2528, 1976.

Dehner, L. P., et al.: Renal cell carcinoma in children: A clinicopathologic study of 15 cases and review of the literature, J. Pediatr. 76:358, 1970.

Duffy, P., et al.: Ultrasound demonstration of a 1.5 cm intrarenal angiomyolipoma, J. Clin. Ultrasound 5:111, 1977.

Engel, R. M. E.: Unusual presentation of Wilms' tumor, Urology 8:288, 1976.

Farah, J., et al.: Angiography of Wilms's tumor, Radiology 90:775, 1968.

Favara, B. E., et al.: Renal tumors in the neonatal period, Cancer 22:845, 1968.

Filly, R. A., et al.: The ultrasonographic spectrum of abdominal and pelvic Hodgkin's disease and non-Hodgkin's lymphoma, Cancer 38:2143, 1976.

Frei, E., et al.: Renal complications of neoplastic disease, J. Chronic Dis. 16:757, 1963.

Freimanis, A. K.: Ultrasonic imaging of neoplasms, Cancer 37:496, 1976.

Ganem, E. J., et al.: Benign neoplasms of the urinary bladder in children: Review of the literature and report of a case, J. Urol. 73:1032, 1955.

Garcia, M., et al.: Classification and prognosis in Wilms's tumor, Radiology 80:574, 1963.

Ghazali, S.: Embryonic rhabdomyosarcoma of the urogenital tract, Br. J. Surg. 60:124, 1973.

Goldstein, C., et al.: Multiple ossified metastases to the kidney from osteogenic sarcoma, A.J.R. 128:148, 1977.

Goldstein, H. M., et al.: Ultrasonic detection of renal tumor extension into the inferior vena cava, A.J.R. 130:1083, 1978.

Goswami, A. P.: Metastatic cancer to the ureter and kidney from malignant lymphoma: A review of the literature, J. Urol. 117:381, 1977.

Granmayeh, M., et al.: Sarcoma of the kidney: Angiographic features, A.J.R. 129:107, 1977.

Grosfeld, J. L., et al.: Pelvic rhabdomyosarcoma in infants and children, J. Urol. 107:673, 1972.

Grossman, H.: Observing the growth of Wilms' tumor, Radiology 121:697, 1976.

Hahn, F. J. Y., et al.: Renal lymphoma simulating adult polycystic disease, Radiology 122:655, 1977.

Hamanaka, Y., et al.: Fibroma of the kidney in the newborn, J. Pediatr. Surg. 4:250, 1969.

Hansen, G. C., et al.: Computed tomography diagnosis of renal angiomyolipoma, Radiology 128:789, 1978.

Hattery, R. R., et al.: Computed tomography of renal abnormalities, Radiol. Clin. North Am. 15:401, 1977.

Hendry, W. F., et al.: Haemangioma of bladder in children and young adults, Br. J. Urol. 43:309, 1971.

Hope, J. W., et al.: Abdominal tumors in infants and children, Med. Radiogr. Photogr. 38:1, 1962.

Jarman. W. D., et al.: Polypoid rhabdomyosarcoma of the bladder in children, J. Urol. 103:227, 1970.

Kalousek, D. K., et al.: Metastatic infantile Wilms' tumor and hydrocephalus: A case report with review of the literature, Cancer 39:1312, 1977.

Kasper, T. E., et al.: Urologic abdominal masses in infants and children, J. Urol. 116:629, 1976.

Kaufman, R. A., et al.: Calcification in primary and metastatic Wilms' tumor, A.J.R. 130:783, 1978.

King, D. L.: Renal ultrasonography, Radiology 105:633, 1972.

Knudson, A. G.: Genetics and the etiology of childhood cancer, Pediatr. Res. 10:513, 1976.

Kropp, K. A., et al.: Morbidity and mortality of renal exploration for cysts, Surg. Gynecol. Obstet. 125:803, 1967.

Lang, E. K.: Asymptomatic space-occupying lesions of the

kidney: A programmed sequential approach and its impact on quality and cost of health care, South. Med. J. 70:277, 1977.

Lee, K. R., et al.: Some important radiological aspects of the kidney in Hippel-Lindau syndrome: The value of prospective study in an affected family, Radiology 122: 649, 1977.

Leopold, G. R., et al.: Renal ultrasonography: An updated approach to the diagnosis of renal cyst, Radiology 109:671, 1973.

Levin, D. C., et al.: Reticular neovascularity in malignant and inflammatory renal masses, Radiology 120:61, 1976.

Loomis, R. C.: Primary leiomyosarcoma of the kidney: Report of a case and review of the literature, J. Urol. 107:557, 1972.

Lungberg, W. B., et al.: Renal failure secondary to leukemic infiltration of the kidneys, Am. J. Med. 62:636, 1977.

Lutz, H., et al.: Possibilities and limitations of ultrasonic diagnosis of space-occupying lesions in internal medicine, Ultrasonics 14:156, 1976.

McCullough, D. L., et al.: Renal angiomyolipoma (hamartoma): Review of the literature and report of 7 cases, J. Urol. 105:32, 1971.

Magilner, A. D., et al.: Computed tomography in the diagnosis of renal masses, Radiology 126:715, 1978.

Maklad, N. F., et al.: Ultrasonic characterization of solid renal lesions: Echographic, angiographic and pathologic correlation, Radiology 123:733, 1977.

Marks, W. M., et al.: CT diagnosis of tumor thrombosis of the renal vein and inferior vena cava, A.J.R. 131:843, 1978.

Merten, D. F., et al.: Wilms' tumor in adolescence, Cancer 37:1532, 1976.

Parker, J. A., et al.: Magnification renal scintigraphy in the differential diagnosis of septa of Bertin, Pediatr. Radiol. 4: 157, 1976.

Pendergrass, T. W.: Congenital anomalies in children with Wilms' tumor: A new survey, Cancer 37:403, 1976.

Peterson, N. E., et al.: Renal hemangioma, J. Urol. 105:27, 1971.

Pfister, R. C., et al.: Congenital asymmetry (hemihypertrophy) and abdominal disease: Radiological features in 9 cases, Radiology 116:685, 1975.

Pollack, H. M., et al.: A systematized approach to the differential diagnosis of renal masses, Radiology 113:653, 1974.

Pollack, H. M., et al.: Changing concepts in the diagnosis and management of renal cysts, J. Urol. 111:326, 1974.

Prevot, J., et al.: A case of EMG (exomphalos, macroglossia and gigantism) syndrome with associated renal tumor, J. Pediatr. Surg. 12:583, 1977.

Randall, R. E., et al.: Manifestations of systemic light chain deposition, Am. J. Med. 60:293, 1976.

Richards, M. J. S., et al.: Radical partial renal irradiation: An alternative to partial nephrectomy in bilateral Wilms' tumor, Cancer 38:2093, 1976.

Richmond, H., et al.: Neonatal renal tumors, J. Pediatr. Surg. 5:413, 1970.

Rosenfield, A. T., et al.: Gray-scale nephrosonography: Current status, J. Urol. 117:2, 1977.

Sagel, S. S., et al.: Computed tomography of the kidney, in Hodson, J. R., et al. (eds.): Renal Imaging (New York: Appleton-Century-Crofts, 1978).

Sagel, S. S., et al.: Computed Tomography of the Kidney, Radiology 124:359, 1977.

Sample, W. F., et al.: Gray-scale ultrasound in pediatric urology, J. Urol. 117:518, 1977.

Sanders, R. C.: Renal ultrasound, Radiol. Clin. North Am. 13:417, 1975.

Sanders, R. C., et al.: The ultrasonic characteristics of the renal pelvicalyceal echo complex, J. Clin. Ultrasound 5: 372, 1977.

Scheible, W., et al.: Lipomatous tumors of the kidney and adrenal: Apparent echographic specificity, Radiology 129: 153, 1978.

Seidelmann, F. E., et al.: Accuracy of CT staging of bladder neoplasms using the gas-filled method: Report of 21 patients with surgical confirmation, A.J.R. 130:735, 1978.

Shearn, M. A.: Sjogren's syndrome, Med. Clin. North Am. 61:271, 1977.

Shen, S. C., et al.: Leiomyosarcoma developing in a child during remission of leukemia, J. Pediatr. 89:780, 1976.

Siegel, M. B., et al.: Renal failure in Burkitt's lymphoma, Clin. Nephrol. 7:279, 1977.

Slovis, T. L., et al.: Wilms' tumor to the heart: Clinical and radiographic evaluation, A.J.R. 131:263, 1978.

Stanley, K. E.: Hemangioma-lymphangioma of the bladder in a child: Report of a case with associated hemangiomas of the external genitalia, J. Urol. 96:51, 1966.

Suki, W. N., et al.: The Kidney in Systemic Disease (New York: John Wiley & Sons, Inc., 1976).

Troup, C. W., et al.: Infiltrative lesion of the bladder presenting as gross hematuria in child with leukemia: Case report, J. Urol. 107:314, 1972.

Vallance, R., et al.: Grey-scale ultrasonic imaging of the kidney, Br. J. Radiol. 49:635, 1976.

Weiner, S. N., et al.: Renal oncocytoma: Angiographic features of 2 cases, Radiology 125:633, 1977.

Williams, D. I., et al.: Lower urinary tract tumours in children, Br. J. Urol. 36:51, 1964.

Williams, D. I.: Neoplastic Disease, the Kidney, in *Urology in Childhood*, vol. 15 (Suppl.), *Encyclopedia of Urology* (New York: Springer-Verlag New York Inc., 1974).

Williams. D. I.: Neoplastic Disease, the Lower Urinary Tract, in *Urology in Childhood* (New York: Springer-Verlag New York Inc., 1974).

Yeh, H. C., et al.: Ultrasonography of renal sinus lipomatosis, Radiology 124:799, 1977.

Leading articles: Wilms's tumor, Br. Med. J. 1:1166, 1976.

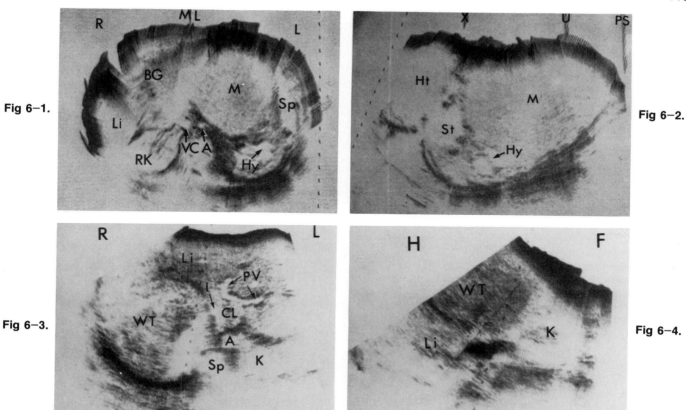

Fig 6–1.

Fig 6–2.

Fig 6–3.

Fig 6–4.

Figs 6–1 to 6–4.—Wilms' tumor. On ultrasonograms, Wilms' tumor of the kidney may have a variety of acoustical patterns. Acoustical textures may be related in part to the type of instrumentation used as well as the form of gray-scale assignment. Nevertheless, the more common pattern represents fairly homogeneous solid mass of variable echogenicity (Figs 6–1–6–4). Because these tumors may become quite bulky on any single cut, the mass may appear separate from kidney and other organs (Fig 6–1). However, multiple scans will usually demonstrate renal origin of the mass as well as any associated hydronephrosis in remaining normal portion of kidney (Figs 6–1 and 6–2). Some tumors may be relatively more echogenic than normal renal parenchyma and therefore similar to neuroblastomas (Figs 6–3 and 6–4). R = right; L = left; ML = midline; BG = bowel gas; M = mass; Sp = spleen (Fig 6–1) or spine (Fig 6–3); Li = liver; RK = right kidney; IVC or I = inferior vena cava; A = aorta; Hy = hydronephrosis; Ht = heart; St = stomach; WT = Wilms' tumor; PV = portal vein; K = kidney; PS = pubic symphisis; X = xyphoid; U = umbilicus; CL = caudad lobe of liver; H = head; F = foot.

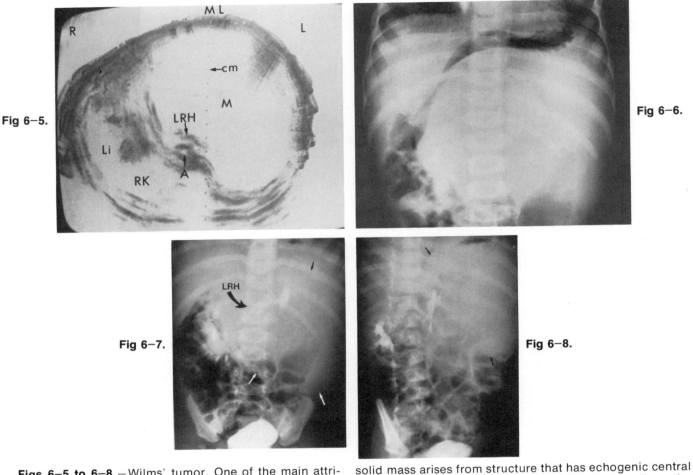

Fig 6–5.

Fig 6–6.

Fig 6–7.

Fig 6–8.

Figs 6–5 to 6–8. — Wilms' tumor. One of the main attributes of ultrasound in examination of palpable abdominal masses is assessment of organ of origin. Since it may not always be clear from physical findings what the origin is, a diagnostic modality that can image multiple abdominal organs is preferable as screening procedure.

Furthermore, even when other imaging modalities are utilized, it may be unclear from impressions or deviations of the organ whether it is truly the origin of the mass. In this case of Wilms' tumor (Fig 6–5), large homogeneous solid mass arises from structure that has echogenic central region. This is typical of the renal hilus and confirms the renal origin of the mass.

Excretory urography demonstrates large mass (Figs 6–6 to 6–8, *small arrows*) with distortion of renal collecting system and displacement of the left renal hilum medially *(curved arrow)*. The affected kidney commonly functions well. R = right; L = left; ML = midline; cm = centimeter marker; M = mass; LRH = left renal hilus; A = aorta; RK = right kidney; Li = liver.

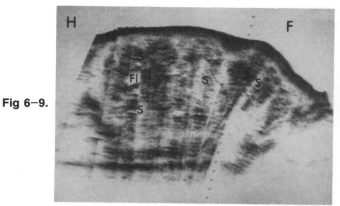

Fig 6–9.

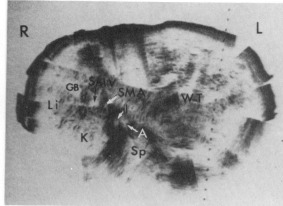

Fig 6–10.

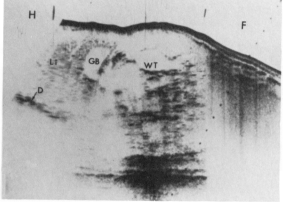

Fig 6–11.

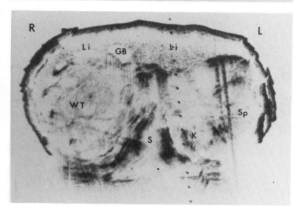

Fig 6–12.

Figs 6–9 to 6–12.—Wilms' tumor. Wilms' tumor may undergo variable cystic degeneration (Figs 6–9 to 6–12). Corresponding acoustical patterns will be demonstrated with ultrasonography, ranging from small fluid areas within predominantly solid echogenic masses to large, sometimes septated, fluid areas intermingled with solid components. Transverse and longitudinal scans in these two cases demonstrate the ability of ultrasound to demonstrate the re- lationship of frequently large masses to the prevertebral vessels as well as other nearby abdominal organs. H = head; F = feet; S = solid components (Fig 6–9) or spine (Fig 6–12); Fl = fluid components; Li = liver; GB = gall- bladder; SMV = superior mesenteric vein; SMA = superior mesenteric artery; I = inferior vena cava; A = aorta; WT = Wilms' tumor; K = kidney; Sp = spine (Fig 6–10) or spleen (Fig 6–12); D = diaphragm; R = right; L = left.

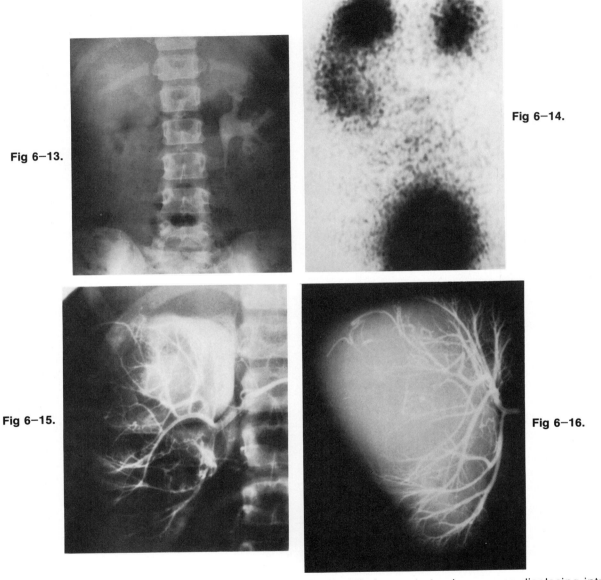

Figs 6–13.

Fig 6–14.

Fig 6–15.

Fig 6–16.

Figs 6–13 to 6–16.—Wilms' tumor. Excretory urogram (Fig 6–13) demonstrates faint visualization of right upper pole. Left kidney appears normal. A renal scintiscan (Fig 6–14) with patient in prone position demonstrates normal left kidney. Lower portion of right kidney is not visible, while the upper portion functions well. Late arterial phase (Fig 6–15) demonstrates large mass displacing intrarenal branches and neovascularity. Notice dense nephrogram seen in right upper pole, which is uninvolved portion of the kidney. Injection of the surgical specimen (Fig 6–16) demonstrates the extent of tumor involvement.

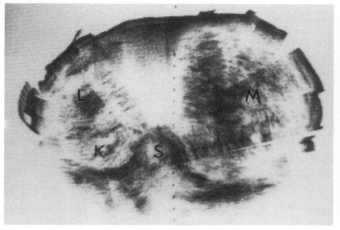

Fig 6–17.

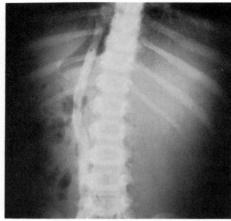

Fig 6–18.

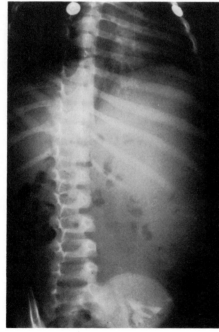

Fig 6–19.

Figs 6–17 to 6–19. — Wilms' tumor. Supine transverse scan demonstrates highly echogenic mass on left side (Fig 6–17). Since renal collecting system is displaced inferiorly overlying the bony pelvis, it cannot be seen sonographically. Injection of contrast material through dorsal vein of foot (Fig 6–18) demonstrates good visualization of inferior vena cava, which is displaced to right. A 24-hour film (Fig 6–19) demonstrates large mass, distorting left kidney with displacement of collecting system over bony pelvis. L = liver; K = kidney; S = spine; M = mass.

Fig 6—21.

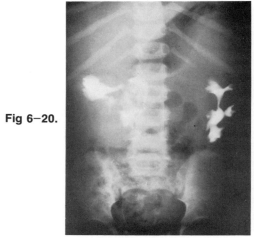

Fig 6—20.

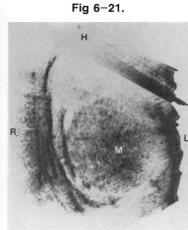

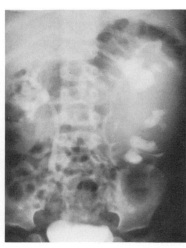

Fig 6—22.

Figs 6—20 to 6—22. — Grading of Wilms' tumor. Bilateral Wilms' tumor (Fig 6–20) has a bad prognosis and indicates grade 5. In contrast, tumors occurring in patients younger than 1 year of age are usually well encapsulated and have a good prognosis (Figs 6–21 and 6–22). Most lesions in this age group are considered benign fetal renal hamartomas. H = head; R = right; L = left; M = mass.

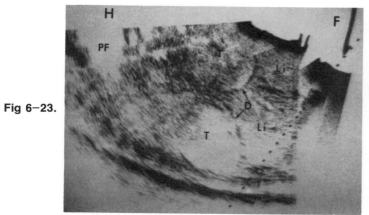

Fig 6–23.

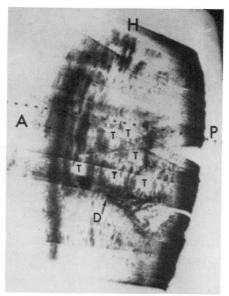

Fig 6–24.

Fig 6–23 and 6–24.—Wilms' tumor with metastases. Longitudinal scan in patient with Wilms' tumor (Fig 6–23) demonstrates intrathoracic metastases. Major portion of tumor appears solid. Scanning over thorax (Fig 6–24) clearly demonstrates that metastases to chest are solid. T = tumor; D = diaphragm; Li = liver; PF = pleural effusion; F = foot; A = anterior; P = posterior; H = head.

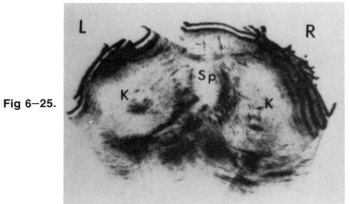

Fig 6–25.

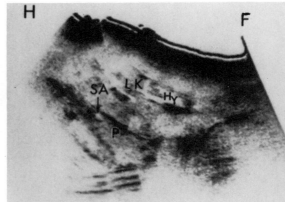

Fig 6–26.

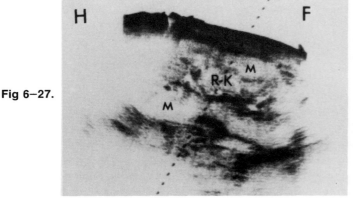

Fig 6–27.

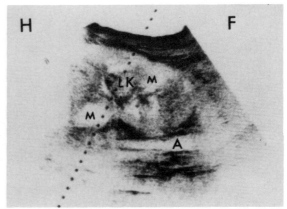

Fig 6–28.

Figs 6–25 to 6–28.—Renal lymphoma. Lymphomatous involvement of kidneys may be focal nodular in nature or diffuse. In these two cases, generalized (Figs 6–25 and 6–26) and focal nodular involvement (Figs 6–27 and 6–28) of kidneys is evident. However, texture patterns throughout renal parenchyma are inhomogeneous but clearly solid in nature. Variable degrees of regional hydronephrosis may be evident. Although this pattern may not be clearly differentiated from other benign infiltrative diseases of kidney, usually clinical correlation will help to suggest the diagnosis. L = left; R = right; K = kidney; Sp = spine; SA = splenic artery; P = pancreas; LK = left kidney; Hy = hydronephrosis; M = mass; RK = right kidney; A = aorta; H = head; F = feet.

Fig 6—29.

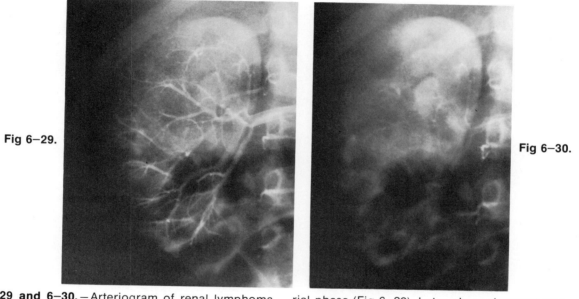

Fig 6—30.

Figs 6—29 and 6—30.—Arteriogram of renal lymphoma. Displacement of renal arterial branches is seen in late arterial phase (Fig 6—29). Later phase demonstrates numerous nodular masses in the kidney (Fig 6—30).

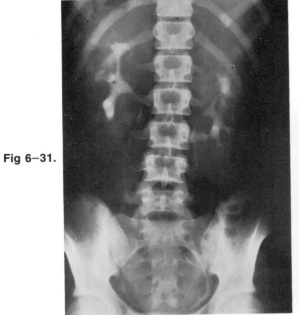

Fig 6–31.

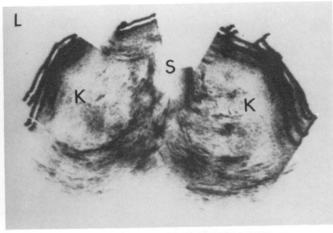

Fig 6–32.

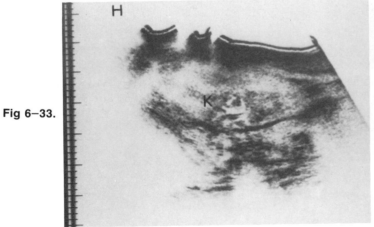

Fig 6–33.

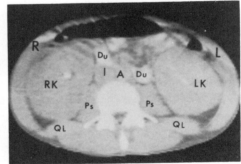

Fig 6–34.

Figs 6–31 to 6–34.—Renal lymphoma. In older children and adults, it may be difficult to differentiate between renal lymphoma (Fig 6–31) and adult polycystic disease on excretory urogram. However, in this patient no cysts can be identified and, as a result, solid renal process should be suspected. However, any time confusion arises, either ultrasonography or computerized tomography (Figs 6–32 to 6–34) can be utilized to demonstrate solid nature of the process. On ultrasonogram, inhomogeneous acoustical texture of renal parenchyma is evident. On computed tomography, at wide window setting, solid nature of the process is evident. L = left; H = head; K = kidney; S = spine; R = right; Du = duodenum; I = inferior vena cava; A = aorta; RK = right kidney; LK = left kidney; Ps = psoas muscle; QL = quadratus lumborum muscle.

128

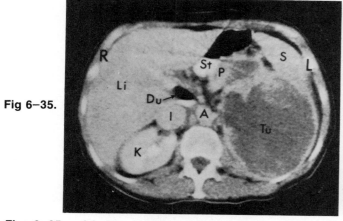

Fig 6–35.

Fig 6–36.

Figs 6–35 and 6–36.—Undifferentiated necrotic sarcoma of kidney. Undifferentiated large necrotic sarcoma of kidney, which displaces the ureter anteriorly and laterally, is clearly demonstrated on computerized tomography. R = right; L = left; Li = liver; Du = duodenum; St = stomach; P = pancreas; A = aorta; I = inferior vena cava; K = kidney; Tu = tumor; Ur = ureter; LN = lymph nodes; Ps = psoas muscle; S = spleen.

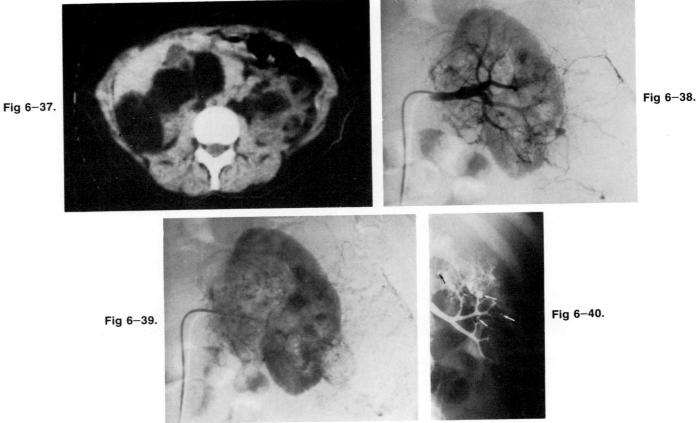

Fig 6–37.

Fig 6–38.

Fig 6–39.

Fig 6–40.

Figs 6–37 to 6–40. — Bilateral angiomyolipomas in patient with tuberous sclerosis. Computerized tomography demonstrates multiple renal masses bilaterally in older patient (Fig 6–37). Arteriographically (Figs 6–38 and 6–39), it is sometimes difficult to differentiate these tumors from other neoplastic processes. Visualization of small aneurysms are suggestive of the diagnosis. Figure 6–40 shows another patient with angiomyolipoma and visualization of aneurysms (arrows).

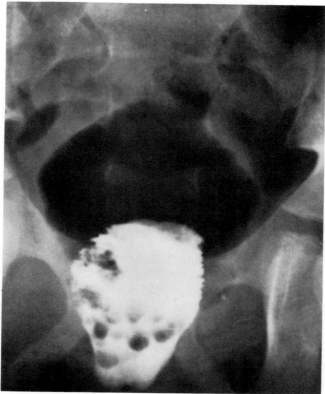

Fig 6–41.—Rhabdomyosarcoma of bladder in child. The bladder is small, with an irregular marginal contour and multiple polypoid filling defects characteristic of sarcoma botryoides. Notice that tumor has similar appearance to "bunch of grapes."

7

Adrenal Gland

EACH ADRENAL GLAND is situated anterior, medial and superior to the kidney. They are basically triangular in shape anatomically. However, sonographically they may appear crescentic or linear, depending on the imaging plane. The right adrenal gland is bordered medially by the right crus of the diaphragm, anteriorly by the inferior vena cava and laterally by the right lobe of the liver. The left adrenal gland is bordered medially by the left crus of the diaphragm, anteriorly by the tail of the pancreas and laterally by the spleen. The adrenal gland is grossly divided into 2 main anatomical regions, the cortex and medulla, that function in 2 different endocrine systems. Sympathetic neural elements invade the primordium of the adrenal cortex (mesoderm) to form the medulla. The medulla is derived from neuroectodermal tissue that resides within the base of the gland. Later these cells differentiate into chromaffin cells capable of synthesizing and storing catecholamines. Tumors arising from the medulla include neuroblastomas, ganglioneuromas and pheochromocytomas. The adrenal cortex is derived from the mesoderm, the major portion of which lies in the apex of the gland. The adrenal cortex secretes corticosteroids, including glucocorticoids (hydrocortisone), mineralocorticoids (aldosterone), estrogens and androgens. Lesions arising from the cortex include adenomas, carcinomas and cortical hyperplasia.

A definitive diagnosis of most adrenal lesions can be made by correlating clinical, laboratory and appropriate imaging techniques. Adrenal lesions may manifest a decreased, increased or normal hormonal function. Either the cortex or medulla may be the site of abnormal function. Adrenal cortical hyperfunction includes entities such as Cushing's syndrome, the adrenogenital syndrome and primary aldosteronism. Adrenal medullary hyperfunction is associated with pheochromocytomas. Adrenal cortical hypofunction results in Addison's disease, which may be acute or chronic. Adrenal enlargement with nonfunctioning benign or malignant masses includes stromal lesions such as lipomas, fibromas, neurofibromas, myomas, angiomas or lymphangiomas. Similarly, neuroblastomas, ganglioneuroblastomas and ganglioneuromas usually do not significantly alter adrenal hormone production.

ADRENAL IMAGING

Diagnostic radiology plays an important role in localizing and defining the extent and multiplicity of adrenal lesions. The specific imaging modality chosen is generally dictated by the initial clinical and laboratory data. Some conditions require several complementary imaging procedures before a diagnosis is made. Invasive procedures should be avoided as much as possible.

Various imaging modalities available for the evaluation of adrenal lesions in children are excretory urography, nephrotomography, ultrasonography, computerized axial tomography, adrenal radionuclide scintigraphy and retroperitoneal pneumography. In the evaluation of adrenal lesions in children, excretory urography, ultrasonography and computerized axial tomography are the most frequent initial procedures and these will be discussed in some detail. The sequential diagnostic approach to each clinical syndrome will then be outlined.

Excretory Urography

The excretory urographic examination starts with a frontal film of the abdomen. Oblique or lateral views may then be used. A low KVP technique with a short exposure time should be utilized to prevent motion artifacts and optimally visualize and localize calcification. (A differential diagnosis of suprarenal calcification in children is given in Table 7–1.) Two milliliters per kg of body weight of a water-soluble contrast material is administered intravenously using a dorsal vein of the foot. During continuous injection, a full abdominal film is taken after half of the total dose of contrast material has been injected. The inferior vena cava can usually be visualized and analyzed for compression or displacement by an adrenal mass. A second film is taken immediately following the injection during the total-body opacification phase. This film is frequently helpful in the evaluation of cystic or necrotic adrenal lesions. The remainder of the study is tailored to demonstrate the relationship of the mass to the kidneys.

Ultrasonography

With commercially available gray-scale instrumentation, pediatric patients are studied using a 3.5- or 5.0-MHz focused transducer, depending on their size and body habitus. Conventional transverse and longitudinal scans are performed first with the patient in a supine position, especially when a mass is palpable.

TABLE 7–1.—ADRENAL CALCIFICATION

1. Hemorrhage, e.g., birth trauma (common)
2. Infection, e.g., tuberculosis
3. Waterhouse-Friderichsen syndrome
4. Wolman's syndrome   (extensive bilateral calcification)
5. Adrenal cyst   (unilateral calcification)
6. Adrenal tumors (neuroblastomas, ganglioneuromas, cortical carcinomas and pheochromocytomas)

However, the adrenal glands are frequently best visualized in scans performed with the patient in a decubitus position. The right adrenal gland is more easily visualized since the liver acts as a sonographic window. Although the left adrenal gland can occasionally be imaged using axial scans, coronal scans are usually needed, using the kidney as the sonic window.

The best ultrasonic criterion of an adrenal abnormality is a change in shape. The normal triangular, crescentic or linear shape becomes lentiform or round in appearance. Normally, there may be slight differences in gray-scale texture between the 2 adrenal glands. With existing instrumentation, 1.5- to 2.0-cm lesions have been detected. If calcification is present, it can be localized.

Computerized Axial Tomography

Computerized tomography is most useful in patients with abundant retroperitoneal fat and has not been routinely used in the evaluation of adrenal lesions in children. However, it may be useful in evaluating adrenal lesions in older children. The faster scanners are preferable since there are fewer artifacts related to biological motion. Computerized tomography in younger children is less helpful since suspended respiration is necessary and retroperitoneal fat is minimal.

Radionuclide scintigraphy of the adrenal glands is potentially capable of detecting functional abnormalities prior to the development of significant morphological changes. However, despite the promise in this area, adrenal scintiscanning has not yet become widely used since the labeled precursors are not readily available.

More invasive procedures, such as selective adrenal arteriography and venography, are performed if the diagnosis cannot be made using noninvasive techniques. Arteriography is of value in hypervascular lesions, such as pheochromocytomas, and, rarely, adrenal hemangiomas and carcinomas. This procedure is usually performed after a mass is identified and localized by noninvasive procedures. Adrenal venography and selective venous sampling are valuable in small functioning adrenal lesions that have not been localized by ultrasonography and excretory urography. This is particularly true in aldosteronomas and occasionally in adrenal hyperplasia.

CLINICAL SYNDROMES

Cushing's Syndrome

Excessive secretion of cortisol and other steroids with androgenic activity results in Cushing's syndrome. In adults, Cushing's syndrome is most commonly the result of adrenal hyperplasia. Since the adrenal glands may not be significantly enlarged, ultrasonography and computerized tomography have limited usefulness. In children, however, Cushing's syndrome is caused by adrenal cortical carcinoma in as many as 80% of cases. Since these tumors tend to be large, ultrasonography and excretory urography are usually effective in localizing the lesion. Computerized tomography could be used in older children if ultrasonography is nondiagnostic. Radionuclide scintigraphy and venous sampling may be needed in a small percentage of patients.

Adrenogenital Syndrome

The adrenogenital syndrome can be divided into 2 forms based on the underlying etiology. The congenital form, which is an autosomal recessive disease, is almost always secondary to adrenal hyperplasia. In this form, enzymatic defects result in cortisol deficiency and secondary overproduction of pituitary corticotropin, which in turn results in overproduction of androgens. This syndrome causes pseudohermaphroditism in females and an enlarged penis and precocious puberty in males.

The 2d form of the adrenogenital syndrome is seen in infants and children above 3 months of age, usually secondary to an adrenal neoplasm such as adenoma or carcinoma. In these patients, roentgenographic and ultrasonographic evaluation of the adrenal glands is of prime importance. Other roentgenographic manifestations of this disease are an accelerated bone age, advanced pneumatization of the mastoids and paranasal sinuses, and thickening of the diploic space in the skull. A contrast study of the urogenital sinus in females usually shows the failure of separation of the urethra and vagina.

Primary Aldosteronism

Conn's syndrome is rare in children and is usually caused by cortical adenomas. The initial symptoms include hypertension, headaches, renal potassium loss and sodium retention. The adenomas tend to be small, and although ultrasonography or computerized tomography may detect larger tumors, it is frequently necessary to use adrenal venography and selective venous sampling to make the proper diagnosis.

Adrenocortical Insufficiency

A deficiency in the production of cortisol or aldosterone may result from a variety of congenital and acquired lesions of the hypothalamus, pituitary gland or adrenal cortex.

Acute adrenal insufficiency is a potentially lethal disease and is usually encountered following surgery, infection, hemorrhage or other kinds of stress. Chronic adrenal insufficiency (Addison's disease) is usually the result of a destructive lesion of the adrenal gland and is seen in older children. Formerly, tuberculosis was the most common cause of adrenal insufficiency in children, but now idiopathic atrophy of the gland is the most common cause. Imaging modalities rarely play an important role in this entity.

Pheochromocytomas

Pheochromocytomas originate from chromaffin elements and are usually seen in adults. However, about 10% of these tumors occur in children. In children, unlike adults, males are more commonly affected. The most common location is the adrenal medulla. Extra-adrenal pheochromocytomas are located in the para-aortic and thoracic sympathetic chains, the organ of Zuckerkandl, the carotid bodies or the urinary bladder. Thirty-two percent of affected children have multiple tumors and about 5–10% of pheochromocytomas are malignant. The major initial symptoms are sustained hypertension, headache, weight loss, nausea, vomiting and visual disturbances. About 10% of pheochromocytomas are asymptomatic. Angiographically, these asymptomatic tumors resemble functioning pheochromocytomas. There is a reported familial incidence of pheochromocytomas. Pheochromocytomas might be associated with other tumors (multiple endocrine adenomatosis), cyanotic congenital heart disease and neurofibromatosis (5% of the cases). Ultrasonography, computerized tomography in older children and angiography are of particular importance in localizing the tumor.

Neuroblastomas

Neuroblastomas are the most common solid tumors of infancy and childhood and account for about half of the neonatal malignant tumors. The etiology of neuroblastomas is unknown. Recent immunological data, which show a common tumor-specific antigen, suggest viral causes. Some neuroblastomas are hereditary; these tend to present in early life and are more likely to be multiple. Seventy-five percent of neuroblastomas arise in the abdomen, and 40% of these are adrenal in origin. Neuroblastomas may also occur in the thorax (15%), pelvis (4%) and neck (4%). Those of unknown origin account for 2%. More differentiated forms of neuroblastic tumors, e.g., ganglioneuroblastomas and ganglioneuromas, are less common. Benign ganglioneuromas arise most commonly in the thorax and least commonly in the adrenal gland.

Most neuroblastomas present in the first five years of life, with a peak age of 1 to 1½ years. Clinically, neuroblastomas most commonly present as an abdominal mass, usually found by the mother or pediatrician on a routine examination. Sudden enlargement of the mass may be the result of hemorrhage. Other symptoms include gastrointestinal malfunction, pain, anemia and weight loss. In our experience, urinary symptoms and hypertension are uncommon findings. Sometimes patients have fever and joint pain simulating symptoms of rheumatic fever and juvenile rheumatoid arthritis.

Seventy percent of patients have an abdominal mass that can be seen on plain films of the abdomen, with 50% demonstrating flocculent calcifications. Excretory urography and ultrasonography play an important role in the diagnosis as well as the staging of the disease. In older children, computerized tomography may be helpful in staging, especially in the mediastinum and abdomen.

Staging is defined as follows:

Stage I: Tumor limited to organ of origin
Stage II: Regional spread that does not cross the midline
Stage III: Tumor extends across the midline
Stage IV: Distant metastases
Stage IV-S: Patients have small primary tumors and metastases limited to the liver, skin or bone marrow without radiographic evidence of bone metastasis

Spontaneous regression of neuroblastomas has been reported. Regression consists of complete disappearance of the disease or, in some cases, maturation to a ganglioneuroma. The majority of such patients are infants with Stage II or IV-S disease. Patients with thoracic and pelvic neuroblastomas have higher survival rates than those with abdominal neuroblastomas.

Surgical removal of the tumor is the primary therapy. Survival is best in children under one year of age and in those with Stage I disease. Unfortunately, most patients have more advanced disease at the time of diagnosis. Immunotherapy may have a significant value in the future. Chemotherapy and radiotherapy appear to add very little to the overall cure rate of the disease.

Nonfunctioning Adrenal Lesions

Most nonfunctioning adrenal lesions cause enlargement of the gland, and therefore excretory urography, ultrasonography and computerized tomography are diagnostically useful.

Adrenal cysts are rare lesions that usually present as an abdominal mass and are detected on plain films of the abdomen. Fifteen percent of the cysts are bilateral and 15% show peripheral calcification. Adrenal cysts may be parasitic, epithelial, endothelial or pseudocysts. Lymphangiectatic cysts (endothelial) and pseudocysts (hemorrhagic cysts) are the most common. Adrenal abscesses may also simulate a cystic mass.

Adrenal tumors rarely have stromal origin, and they include neurofibromas, myomas, fibromas, lipomas, hemangiomas and teratomas. Adrenal adenomas and carcinomas are rare and they usually are functioning tumors. Nonfunctioning adrenocortical tumors occur mainly in males.

REFERENCES

Alfidi, R. J., et al.: Arteriography of adrenal neoplasms, A.J.R. 106:637, 1969.

Anderson, B. G., et al.: Adrenal imaging with radioiodocholesterol in the diagnosis of adrenal disorders, Adv. Intern. Med. 19:327, 1974.

Arenson, E. B., et al.: Neuroblastoma in father and son, J.A.M.A. 235:727, 1976.

Arey, J. B.: Tumors of the Adrenal, in Williams, D. I. (ed.): *Urology in Childhood*, vol. 15 (suppl.), *Encyclopedia of Urology* (New York: Springer-Verlag New York, Inc., 1974).

Bearman, S., et al.: B-Scan ultrasound in the evaluation of pediatric abdominal masses, Radiology 108:111, 1973.

Beckmann, C. F., et al.: Angiography of nonfunctioning pheochromocytomas of the adrenal gland, Radiology 124:53, 1977.

Beierwaltes, W. H., et al.: Adrenal imaging agents: Rationale, synthesis, formulation, and metabolism, Semin. Nucl. Med. 8:5, 1978.

Bernardino, M. E., et al.: Gray-scale ultrasonography of adrenal neoplasms, A.J.R. 130:741, 1978.

Birnholz, J. C.: Ultrasound imaging of adrenal mass lesions, Radiology 109:163, 1973.

Boldt, D. W., et al.: Computed tomography of abdominal mass lesions in children, Radiology 124:371, 1977.

Bookstein, J. J., et al.: The role of abdominal radiography in hypertension secondary to renal or adrenal disease, Med. Clin. North Am. 59:169, 1975.

Brascho, D. J.: Clinical applications of diagnostic ultrasound in abdominal malignancy, South. Med. J. 65:1331, 1972.

Brodeur, G. M., et al.: Histochemical demonstration of an increase in acetylcholinesterase in established lines of human and mouse neuroblastomas by nerve growth factor, Cytobios 16:133, 1976.

Brownlie, K., et al.: Computer-assisted tomography of normal suprarenal glands, J. Comput. Assist. Tomogr. 2:1, 1978.

Castellino, R. A., et al.: Lymphographic demonstration of a retroperitoneal lymphangioma, Radiology 115:355, 1975.

Costello, P., et al.: Problems in the diagnosis of adrenal tumors, Radiology 125:335, 1977.

Darling, D. B., et al.: The roentgenographic manifestations of Cushing's syndrome in infancy, Radiology 96:503, 1970.

Davidson, J. K., et al.: Adrenal venography and ultrasound in the investigation of the adrenal gland: An analysis of 58 cases, Br. J. Radiol. 48:435, 1975.

DiGeorge, A. M.: Disorders of the Adrenal Glands, in Nelson, W. E. (ed.): *Textbook of Pediatrics* (Philadelphia: W. B. Saunders Co., 1975).

Duckett, J. W., et al.: Neuroblastoma, Urol. Clin. North Am. 4:285, 1977.

Dunnick, N. R., et al.: Arteriographic manifestations of ganglioneuromas, Radiology 115:323, 1975.

Dunnick, N. R., et al.: Computed tomography in adrenal tumors, A.J.R. 132:43, 1979.

Eklof, O.: Large asymptomatic adrenal haematomas in the neonate, Acta Radiol. Diagn. 11:481, 1971.

Evans, A. E., et al.: Factors influencing survival of children with nonmetastatic neuroblastoma, Cancer 38:661, 1976.

Evans, A. E., et al.: Spontaneous regression of neuroblastoma, Natl. Cancer. Inst. Monogr. 44:49, 1976.

Fritzsche, P., et al.: Vascular specificity in differentiating adrenal carcinoma from renal cell carcinoma, Radiology 125:113, 1977.

Gabriele, O. F., et al.: Bilateral neonatal adrenal hemorrhage, A.J.R. 91:656, 1964.

Ghorashi, B., et al.: Gray-scale sonographic appearance of an adrenal mass: A case report, J. Clin. Ultrasound 4:121, 1976.

Goldberg, B. B., et al.: Ultrasonic evaluation of masses in pediatric patients, A.J.R. 116:677, 1972.

Goldberg, B. B., et al.: Ultrasonography: An aid in the diagnosis of masses in pediatric patients, Pediatrics 56:421, 1975.

Gosink, B. B.: The inferior vena cava: Mass effects, A.J.R. 130:533, 1978.

Grossman, H., et al.: Ultrasonography in children, Pediatrics 54:480, 1974.

Hartman, G. W., et al.: The role of nephrotomography in the diagnosis of adrenal tumors, Radiology 86:1030, 1966.

Hasch, E.: Ultrasound in the investigation of disease of the kidney and urinary tract in children, Acta Paediatr. Scand. 63:42, 1974.

Hassenbusch, S., et al.: Prognostic factors in neuroblastic tumors, J. Pediatr. Surg. 11:287, 1976.

Helson, L., et al.: A rationale for the treatment of metastatic neuroblastoma, J. Natl. Cancer Inst. 57:727, 1976.

Holm, H. H.: Ultrasonic scanning in the diagnosis of space-occupying lesions of the upper abdomen, Br. J. Radiol. 44: 24, 1971.

Holm, H. H., et al.: Errors and pitfalls in ultrasonic scanning of the abdomen, Br. J. Radiol. 45:835, 1972.

Hunig, R.: Ultrasonic diagnosis in pediatrics: The state of the art of ultrasonic diagnosis in pediatrics today: Part I, Pediatr. Radiol. 4:108, 1976.

Kasper, T. E., et al.: Urologic abdominal masses in infants and children, J. Urol. 116:629, 1976.

Keating, J. W., et al.: Remote effects of neuroblastoma, A.J.R. 131:299, 1978.

Kehlet, H., et al.: Comparative study of ultrasound, [131]I-19-iodocholesterol scintigraphy, and aortography in localizing adrenal lesions, Br. Med. J. 2:665, 1976.

Korobkin, M., et al.: Computed tomography in the diagnosis of adrenal disease, A.J.R. 132:231, 1979.

Kurlander, G. J.: Roentgenology of the congenital adrenogenital syndrome, A.J.R. 95:189, 1965.

Lalli, A. F.: Retroperitoneal fibrosis and inapparent obstructive uropathy, Radiology 122:339, 1977.

Lang, E. K.: The roentgenographic diagnosis of suprarenal masses, Radiology 87:35, 1966.

Leonidas, J. C., et al.: Cystic retroperitoneal lymphangioma in infants and children, Radiology 127:203, 1978.

Lieberman, L. M., et al.: Diagnosis of adrenal disease by visualization of human adrenal glands with [131]I-19-iodocholesterol, N. Engl. J. Med. 285:1387, 1971.

Madayag, M., et al.: Renal and suprarenal pseudotumors caused by variations of the spleen, Radiology 105:43, 1972.

Meaney, T. F., et al.: Selective arteriography as a localizing and provocative test in the diagnosis of pheochromocytoma, Radiology 87:309, 1966.

Meyers, M. A.: Characteristic radiographic shapes of pheochromocytomas and adrenocortical adenomas, Radiology 87:889, 1966.

Mineau, D. E., et al.: Ultrasound diagnosis of neonatal adrenal hemorrhage, A.J.R. 132:443, 1979.

Mittelstaedt, C. A., et al.: The sonographic diagnosis of neonatal adrenal hemorrhage, Radiology 131:453, 1979.

Mitty, H. A., et al.: Adrenal venography: Clinical roentgenographic correlation in 80 patients, A.J.R. 119:564, 1973.

Mitty, H. A., et al.: Non-tumorous adrenal hyperfunction: Problems in angiographic-clinical correlation, Radiology 122:89, 1977.

Montagne, J-P., et al.: Computed tomography of the normal adrenal glands, A.J.R. 130:963, 1978.

Morgan, H. E., et al.: Bilateral adrenal enlargement in Addison's disease caused by tuberculosis, Radiology 115:357, 1975.

Older, R. A.: Radiologic approach to adrenal lesions, Urol. Clin. North Am. 4:305, 1977.

Oliff, M., et al.: Retroperitoneal iliac fossa pyogenic abscess, Radiology 126:647, 1978.

Pickering, R. S., et al.: Excretory urographic localization of adrenal cortical tumors and pheochromocytomas, Radiology 114:345, 1975.

Pitts, W. R., et al.: A review of 100 renal and perinephric sonograms with anatomic diagnoses, J. Urol. 114:21, 1975.

Pond, G. D., et al.: Echography: A new approach to the diagnosis of adrenal hemorrhage of the newborn, J. Can. Assoc. Radiol. 27:40, 1976.

Rao, A. K. R., et al.: Normal pancreas and splenic variants simulating suprarenal and renal tumors, A.J.R. 126:530, 1976.

Reuter, S. R., et al.: Adrenal venography, Radiology 89:805, 1967.

Reynes, C. J., et al.: Computed tomography of adrenal glands, Radiol. Clin. North Am. 17:91, 1979.

Rose, J., et al.: Prolonged jaundice as presenting sign of massive adrenal hemorrhage in newborn, Radiology 98: 263, 1971.

Rothberg, M., et al.: Adrenal hemangiomas: Angiographic appearance of a rare tumor, Radiology 126:341, 1978.

Sample, W. F.: A new technique for the evaluation of the

adrenal gland with gray-scale ultrasonography, Radiology 124:463, 1977.

Sample, W. F.: Techniques for improved delineation of normal anatomy of the upper abdomen and high retroperitoneum with gray-scale ultrasound, Radiology 124:197, 1977.

Sample, W. F.: Adrenal ultrasonography, Radiology 127:461, 1978.

Sample, W. F., et al.: Gray-scale ultrasonography: Techniques in pancreatic scanning, Appl. Radiol. Nucl. Med. 4:63, 1975.

Sample, W. F., et al.: Computed tomography and gray-scale ultrasonography of the adrenal gland: A comparative study, Radiology 128:719, 1978.

Scheible, W., et al.: Percutaneous aspiration of adrenal cysts, A.J.R. 128:1013, 1977.

Seabold, J. E., et al.: Adrenal imaging with [131]I-19-iodocholesterol in the diagnostic evaluation of patients with aldosteronism, J. Clin. Endocrinol. Metab. 42:41, 1976.

Seeger, R. C., et al.: Morphology, growth, chromosomal pattern, and fibrinolytic activity of 2 new human neuroblastoma cell lines, Can. Res. 37:1364, 1977.

Sheedy, P. F., et al.: Computed tomography of the body: Initial clinical trial with the EMI prototype, A.J.R. 127:23, 1976.

Stackpole, R. H., et al.: Pheochromocytoma in children, J. Pediatr. 63:315, 1963.

Stewart, D. R., et al.: Carcinoma of the adrenal gland in children, J. Pediatr. Surg. 9:59, 1974.

Thaler, M. M.: Jaundice in the newborn: Algorithmic diagnosis of conjugated and unconjugated hyperbilirubinemia, J.A.M.A. 237:58, 1977.

Thrall, J. H., et al.: Adrenal scintigraphy, Semin. Nucl. Med. 8:23, 1978.

Velick, W. F., et al.: Pheochromocytoma with reversible renal artery stenosis, A.J.R. 131:1069, 1978.

Von Micsky, L., et al.: Optimal diagnosis of renal masses in children by combining and correlating diagnostic features of sonography and radiography, A.J.R. 120:438, 1974.

Wahner, H. W., et al.: Adrenal scanning: Usefulness in adrenal hyperfunction, Clin. Nucl. Med. 2:253, 1977.

Walls, W. J., et al.: B-Scan diagnostic ultrasound in the pediatric patient, A.J.R. 120:431, 1974.

Walls, W. J., et al.: The ultrasonic demonstration of inferior vena caval compression: A guide to pancreatic head enlargement with emphasis on neoplasm, Radiology 123:165, 1977.

Whalen, J. P., et al.: Vector principle in the differential diagnosis of abdominal masses: The left upper quadrant, A.J.R. 113:104, 1971.

Yeh, H.-C., et al.: Ultrasonography of adrenal masses: Unusual manifestations, Radiology 127:475, 1978.

Yeh, H.-C., et al.: Ultrasonography of adrenal masses: Usual features, Radiology 127:467, 1978.

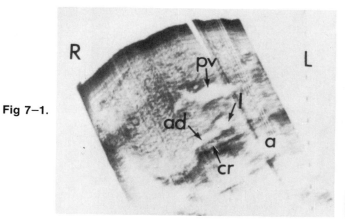

Fig 7-1.

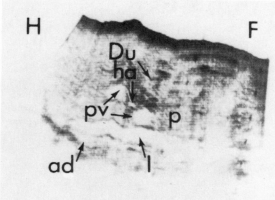

Fig 7-2.

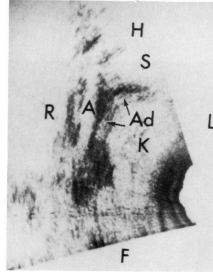

Fig 7-3.

Figs 7-1 to 7-3.—Normal neonatal adrenal glands. A flexible approach must be used in ultrasonic examination of adrenal glands in neonate. On the right, liver can be utilized as acoustic window and transverse scans easily performed with patient in supine position through intercostal spaces (Fig 7-1). Relatively prominent adrenal gland will be seen wedged between medial border of deep right lobe of liver and crus of diaphragm. Inferior vena cava will easily be seen to lie anterior. A 3-dimensional view of right adrenal gland is obtained by performing longitudinal scans either through inferior vena cava or perpendicular to crus of diaphragm (Fig 7-2). Rather linear-appearing adrenal gland will then be seen either lying posterior to inferior vena cava or anterior to crus of diaphragm.

On left side, air within stomach usually prevents more anterior approaches in supine position. As a result, coronal scans performed with patient in right-side-down decubitus position are utilized to visualize adrenal gland (Fig 7-3). Kidney and spleen are utilized as acoustic windows and more curvilinear or triangular-shaped adrenal gland can be seen wedged between kidney, aorta and spleen. R = right; L = left; pv = portal vein; ad = adrenal gland; cr = crus of diaphragm; I = inferior vena cava; a = aorta; Du = duodenum; ha = hepatic artery; p = pancreas; K = kidney; S = spleen; H = head; F = feet.

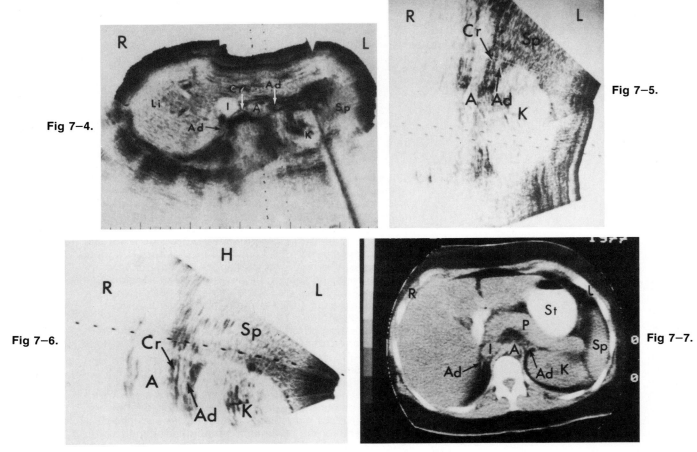

Fig 7–4.

Fig 7–5.

Fig 7–6.

Fig 7–7.

Figs 7–4 to 7–7.—Normal adrenal gland of older child. In the older child, occasionally left lobe of liver extends far enough beyond midline to allow visualization of both adrenal glands in transverse scans performed with patient in supine position (Fig 7–4). Similarly, as in neonate, longitudinal techniques are performed on right to get additional 3-dimensional view of right adrenal gland. In many children, however, gas in stomach prevents visualization in supine position and similar coronal approach is utilized as described for neonate (Figs 7–5 and 7–6). In older children, the crus of diaphragm can be distinguished from adrenal gland, allowing additional anatomical detail. With careful sector scanning in the appropriate intercostal space the relative acoustical texture of spleen, kidney and adrenal gland can be compared.

In many older children, substantial retroperitoneal fat is present, in which case computed tomography is probably superior for demonstration of adrenal glands (Fig 7–7). R = right; L = left; Li = liver; Cr = crus of diaphragm; Ad = adrenal gland; I = inferior vena cava; A = aorta; K = kidney; Sp = spleen; H = head; P = pancreas; St = stomach.

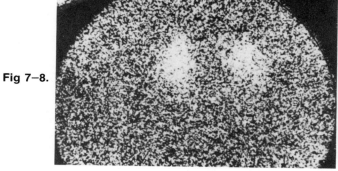

Fig 7–8.

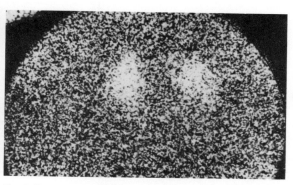

Fig 7–9.

Figs 7–8 and 7–9.—Normal adrenal imaging in nuclear medicine. Adrenal scintiscan is done by labeling cholesterol with ^{131}I. Patients are given Lugol's solution to prevent thyroid uptake of ^{131}I. This technique is quite valuable in identifying functioning adrenal lesions. Patients are also scanned 2 weeks after administration of radiopharmaceu-tical. It would be helpful to administer ^{99m}Tc renal parenchymal imaging agent to localize the adrenal area. This normal study shows equal uptake by both adrenal glands 30 minutes (Fig 7–8) and 10 days (Fig 7–9) following administration of labeled cholesterol.

Fig 7–11.

Fig 7–10.

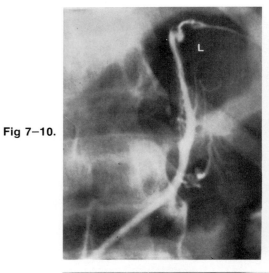

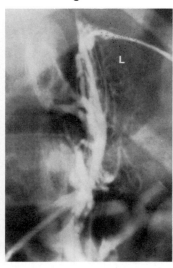

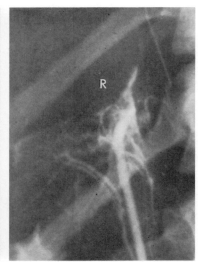

Fig 7–12.

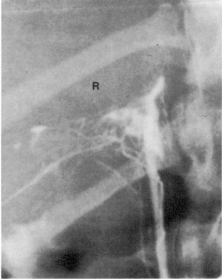

Fig 7–13.

Figs 7–10 to 7–13.—Normal adrenal venogram. Small adrenal lesions are probably best diagnosed by adrenal venography. Furthermore, venous sampling would be helpful in the diagnosis of functioning adrenal lesions. Left gland (Figs 7–10 and 7–11) has more elongated shape and is located superior and medial to left kidney. Right gland (Figs 7–12 and 7–13) has more triangular shape and is located superior to kidney. L = left; R = right.

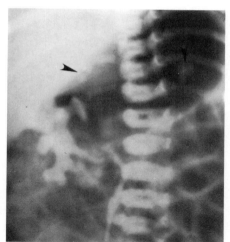

Fig 7–14.

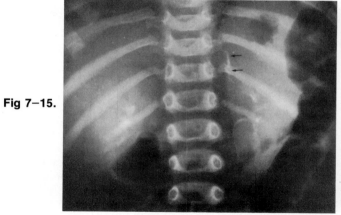

Fig 7–15.

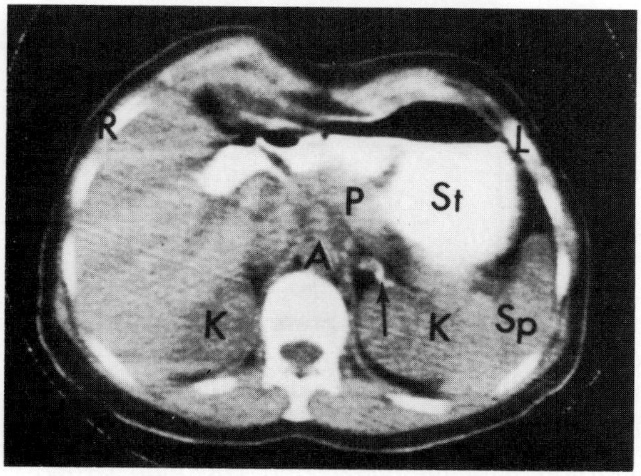

Fig 7–16.

Figs 7–14 to 7–16.—Adrenal calcification. Adrenal calcification may be bilateral (Fig 7–14) or unilateral (Figs 7–15 and 7–16). Differential diagnosis of adrenal calcification is given in Table 7–1. R = right; L = left; P = pancreas; St = stomach; A = aorta; K = kidney; Sp = spleen; arrows and arrowheads = calcified adrenal glands.

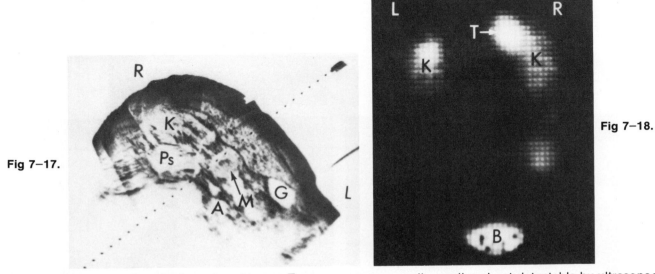

Fig 7–17.

Fig 7–18.

Figs 7–17 and 7–18.—Functioning adrenal tumor. Transverse oblique scan in patient with aldosteronoma (secondary to adenoma) demonstrates large mass in region of adrenal gland (Fig 7–17). Functioning adrenal tumors can be detected with adrenal scintigraphy (Fig 7–18). Aldosterono-mas are usually small and not detectable by ultrasonography. In these patients it would be best to use adrenal scintigraphy or adrenal venography. L = left; R = right; K = kidney; B = bladder; T and M = adrenal mass; A = aorta; G = gallbladder; Ps = psoas muscle.

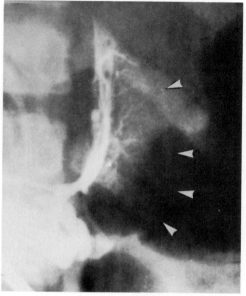

Fig 7–19.—Adrenal hyperplasia. It is very difficult to diagnose adrenal hyperplasia in children using ultrasonography. In these patients, it is usually necessary to perform adrenal venography to demonstrate subtle enlargement of adrenal gland (arrowheads).

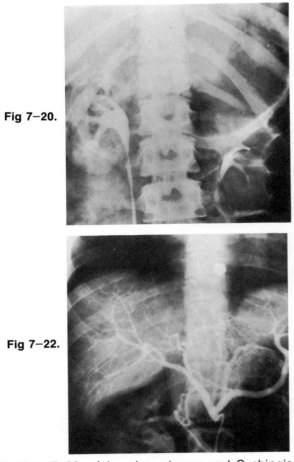

Fig 7–20.

Fig 7–22.

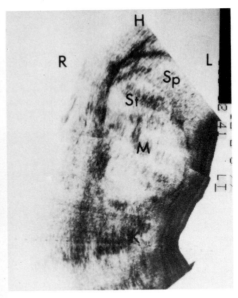

Fig 7–21.

Figs 7–20 to 7–22.—Adrenal carcinoma and Cushing's syndrome. Excretory urography demonstrates displacement of left kidney inferiorly by adrenal mass (Fig 7–20). This large mass is also demonstrated with patient in decubitus position with ultrasonography (Fig 7–21). Angiographically, neovascularity is visible (Fig 7–22). Cushing's syndrome in children is usually due to adrenal carcinoma. H = head; R = right; L = left; Sp = spleen; St = stomach; M = mass; K = kidney.

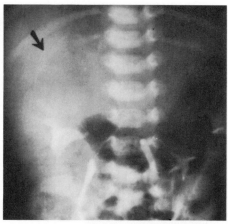

Fig 7–23.—Adrenal cysts. Excretory urography in a neonate demonstrates inferior displacement of kidneys by bilateral hemorrhagic adrenal cysts. Cyst wall is opacified following injection of contrast material during total body opacification phase *(arrow)*.

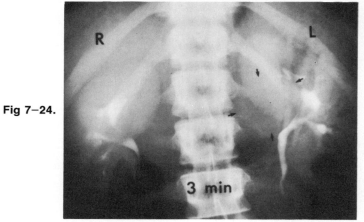

Fig 7–24.

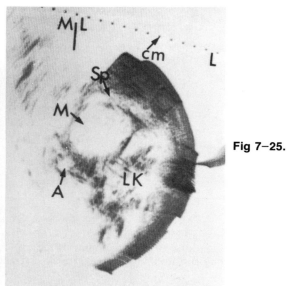

Fig 7–25.

Figs 7–24 to 7–28.—Pheochromocytoma. Excretory urogram (Fig 7–24) shows large mass adjacent to medial and superior pole of left kidney with displacement of renal collecting system *(arrows).* This mass is easily detectable in ultrasonography in supine (Fig 7–25) and decubitus (Fig 7–26) positions. Arteriographically, hypervascular pheochromocytoma can easily be detected (Fig 7–27, *arrows*).

Pheochromocytomas may be bilateral in as many as one third of pediatric patients (Fig 7–28). R = right; L = left; ML = midline; cm = centimeter marker; Sp = spleen; M and T = adrenal pheochromocytoma; LK = left kidney; A = aorta.

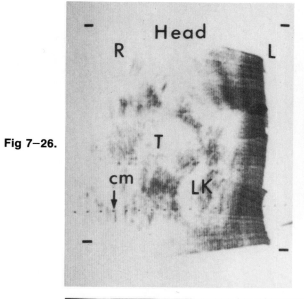

Fig 7–26.

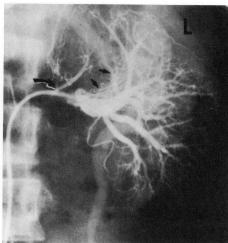

Fig 7–27.

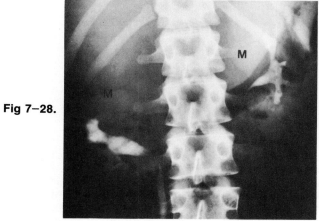

Fig 7–28.

Figs 7–24 to 7–28 (Cont).

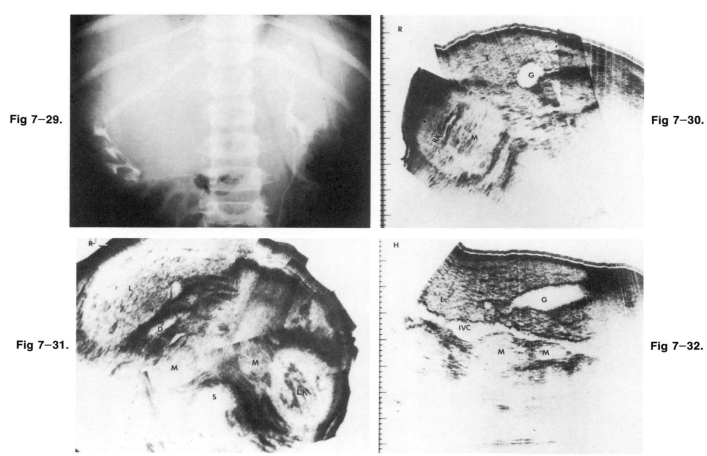

Fig 7–29.

Fig 7–30.

Fig 7–31.

Fig 7–32.

Figs 7–29 to 7–32.—Neuroblastoma. Excretory urogram (Fig 7–29) demonstrates large suprarenal mass displacing the right kidney laterally and inferiorly. Lateral displacement of proximal left ureter is also seen. Transverse scan (Fig 7–30) shows echogenic mass with lateral displacement of right kidney. Contralateral side must always be examined (Fig 7–31) to identify presence or absence of a mass. In this patient, presence of mass adjacent to left kidney indicates at least stage III neuroblastoma. Inferior vena cava should routinely be scanned (Fig 7–32) to detect vascular or tumor thrombosis or displacement of vena cava. RK = right kidney; LK = left kidney; M = mass; S = spine; G = gallbladder; H = head; R = right; L = liver; D = duodenum; IVC = inferior vena cava.

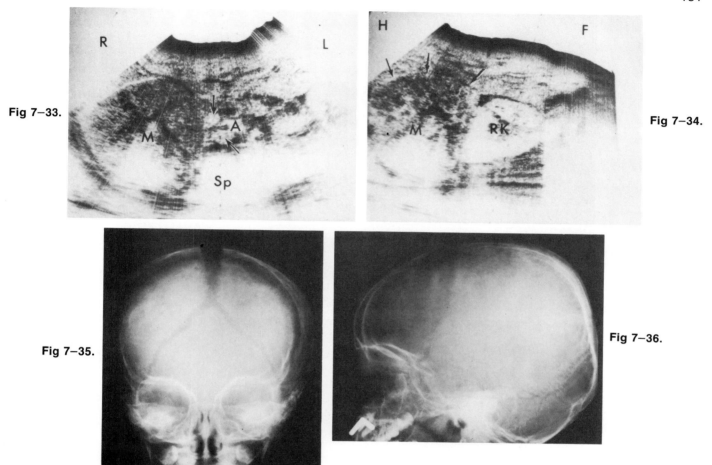

Fig 7–33.

Fig 7–34.

Fig 7–35.

Fig 7–36.

Figs 7–33 to 7–36.—Neuroblastoma with distant metastases. Transverse scan (Fig 7–33) of patient with neuroblastoma demonstrates markedly echogenic mass with metastases to adjacent nodes *(arrows)*. Notice different echographic pattern of mass and adenopathy. This neuroblastoma is demonstrated in longitudinal scan as well (Fig 7–34, *arrows*), displacing the kidney inferiorly. High echogenicity of mass is secondary to small calcifications. Frontal and lateral views of skull on same patient (Figs 7–35 and 7–36) demonstrate metastases to meninges with widening of sutures secondary to erosion by tumor. This is stage IV neuroblastoma. R = right; L = left; H = head; M = mass; A = aorta; RK = right kidney; F = feet; Sp = spine.

Fig 7–37.

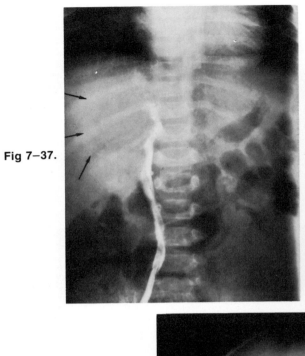

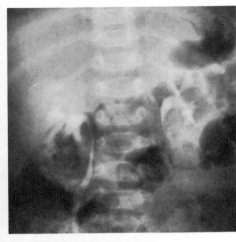

Fig 7–38.

Fig 7–39.

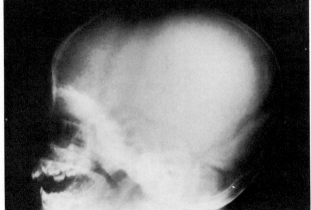

Figs 7–37 to 7–39.—Neuroblastoma with distant metastases. Injection of contrast material in dorsal vein of foot demonstrates good visualization of inferior vena cava (Fig 7–37) and necrotic neuroblastoma in region of adrenal gland *(arrows)*. Later film (Fig 7–38) shows displacement and rotation of upper pole of right kidney inferiorly and laterally. Lateral view of skull in same patient (Fig 7–39) shows metastases to meninges with widening of sutures. This again indicates stage IV neuroblastoma.

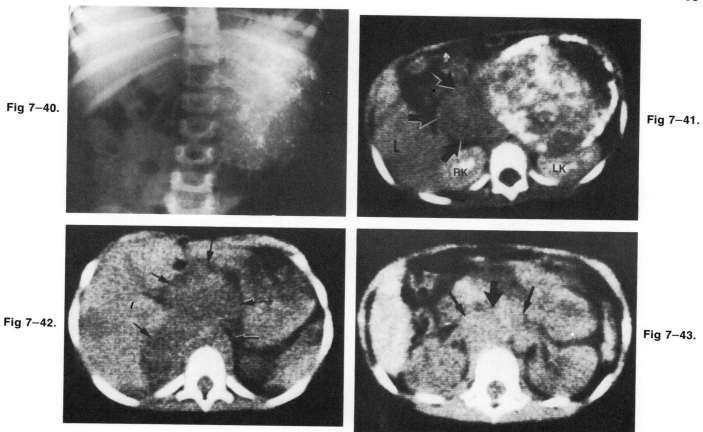

Fig 7–40.

Fig 7–41.

Fig 7–42.

Fig 7–43.

Figs 7–40 to 7–43.—Neuroblastoma. Plain film of abdomen (Fig 7–40) shows large mass with punctate calcification that is highly suggestive of a neuroblastoma. Computed tomographic scan on same patient (Fig 7–41) demonstrates calcified as well as noncalcified *(arrows)* portion of the mass. Right kidney appears normal; left kidney is displaced and compressed by large neuroblastoma. Six months following surgical removal of tumor, patient presented with abdominal pain and computed tomographic scan demonstrated recurrence of lesion in prevertebral region, extending into right suprarenal fossa (Figs 7–42 and 7–43, *arrows*). L = liver; RK = right kidney; LK = left kidney.

8

The Liver and Spleen

DURING THE 3D WEEK OF GESTATION, an epithelial outgrowth of the distal foregut (hepatic diverticulum) penetrates and proliferates within the septum transversum, intimately mixing with the vascular network of the umbilical and vitelline veins giving rise to the hepatic parenchyma. The supporting connective tissue of the liver is derived from the septum transversum itself. The developing liver splits the ventral mesentery into 2 parts: the falciform ligament (which connects the liver to the anterior abdominal wall) and the lesser omentum (which connects the liver to the stomach and 1st portion of the duodenum).

The falciform ligament has been described as dividing the liver into right and left lobes. However, from a functional point of view it is best to consider the named lobes of the liver (right, left, quadrate and caudate) according to their vascular supply, i.e., right and left portal veins and hepatic arteries, as there is no intercommunication between them. Classically, the right branch of the portal vein (and hepatic artery) supplies the right lobe and its respective half of the caudate lobe. The left branch of the portal vein (and hepatic artery) supplies the left lobe, quadrate lobe and its respective half of the caudate lobe. The biliary ducts are intimately associated with the portal vein radicals.

Initially the umbilical and vitelline veins are paired. The right and proximal portions of the left umbilical veins regress early in fetal life. The left umbilical vein resides within the falciform ligament and becomes the ligamentum teres. The most caudal portion of the left vitelline vein forms the ductus venosus. The hepatic veins are formed from the cranial portion of the vitelline plexus. The caudal anastomosis between the right and left vitelline veins forms the portal, splenic and superior mesenteric veins.

At birth the liver occupies a major portion of the abdomen. With growth, the proportionate size of the liver decreases. The size and configuration of the liver at any given age are extremely variable. Although the roentgenographic examination of the liver plays a minor role in the investigation of hepatic diseases in childhood, hepatomegaly or abnormalities manifested by increased or decreased density of the liver may be seen on the plain film of the abdomen. A generalized increase in liver density may be seen in hemachromatosis secondary to increased iron storage, such as thalassemia major, following splenectomy or multiple blood transfusions. A generalized decrease in liver density secondary to fatty infiltration may be seen in children with cystic fibrosis, Reye's syndrome, severe malnutrition and hepatitis. Hepatic (and/or splenic) calcifications have numerous causes, as listed in Table 8–1. Statistically, calcifications less than 1 cm in diameter are granulomas and are not clinically significant.

Ultrasonography has become the major diagnostic modality used for screening and evaluation of pediatric hepatic diseases. Parenchymal hepatic disease, whether focal or generalized, can alter the normal homogeneous acoustical properties of the liver and allow a finite differential diagnosis. If the liver is sec-

TABLE 8–1—CALCIFICATION IN THE LIVER AND SPLEEN OF CHILDREN

Hepatic
Primary tuberculosis, histoplasmosis
Chronic granulomatous disease of childhood
Hepatoblastoma
Hepatoma
Hemangioma
Portal vein phlebolith
Metastatic neuroblastoma
Echinococcal cyst
Abscess, hematoma
Toxoplasmosis, cytomegalovirus, herpes simplex virus
Biliary
Lithiasis
Lymph nodes
Spleen
Phleboliths in a normal spleen or in a hemangioma
Infarction or hematoma
Cysts
Tuberculosis, histoplasmosis
Toxoplasmosis, cytomegalovirus

ondarily involved or affected by adjacent structures, such as the extrahepatic biliary system, pancreas or any mass lesion (intraperitoneal or retroperitoneal), this may also be evaluated. Assessment of the biliary and portal venous systems constitutes a routine part of each examination.

Nuclear scintigraphy is a valuable adjunctive procedure in diagnosing certain pediatric hepatic, biliary or splenic diseases. The current agent of choice for hepatic and splenic imaging is ^{99m}Tc-sulfur colloid. The common finding on the liver scan is a nonspecific photon-deficient area (filling defect). This abnormality may be caused by neoplastic (benign or malignant), inflammatory or traumatic lesions of the liver. Sometimes it is difficult to differentiate filling defects caused by a normal gallbladder or porta hepatis from pathologic processes. Colloidal liver scanning represents a morphologic (Kupffer cells) imaging modality rather than a functional evaluation of the liver. In contrast, functional evaluation of the liver is ascertained with compounds such as rose Bengal sodium I 131 (used for diagnosis of choledochal cysts). Recent reports using ^{99m}TC-HIDA (Technetium-99m labeled N-substituted iminodiacetic acid derivative) are extremely promising in evaluating some hepatobiliary diseases such as cholecystitis.

An alternative scanning agent is gallium. If this is used in conjunction with ^{99m}Tc-sulfur colloid, a more specific differential diagnosis can be suggested. Inflammatory processes and most neoplasms will be "cold" on sulfur colloid liver scans and "hot" on gallium scans.

CONGENITAL AND HEREDITARY DISORDERS OF THE LIVER

Anomalies of Hepatic Lobes

Considerable variation is seen in the size and relative proportion of the various hepatic lobes. Riedel's lobe is a tongue-like projection of the right lobe of the liver that may extend to the right iliac fossa simulating hepatomegaly on abdominal roentgenograms. This is the most common anomaly of the liver and is more often seen in females. Another anomaly is atrophy of the left hepatic lobe secondary to obstruction of the left portal vein, left hepatic artery or left hepatic duct.

Congenital Cystic Diseases of the Liver

There are 2 types of congenital (nonparasitic) cystic disease of the liver: (1) solitary cysts and (2) polycystic disease. The former is rare and usually clinically asymptomatic. Therefore, the cysts are generally diagnosed as incidental findings. These cysts are characteristically single, large and unilocular. The latter is an embryological maldevelopment analogous to and associated with (in 50% of patients) polycystic disease of the kidneys. These cysts are characteristically multiple, variable in size and unilocular. Of differential diagnostic importance, the intervening hepatic parenchyma is normal. Congenital hepatic fibrosis is a complex disorder that may present in infancy through early adult life and is manifested by hepatosplenomegaly, portal hypertension and gastrointestinal bleeding from varices or recurrent cholangitis. There is both a familial and a sporadic form of the disease. It may be associated with renal or hepatic cystic disease and biliary ectasia. Identical-appearing cysts, such as those seen in polycystic disease, may be seen in congenital hepatic fibrosis, but are differentiated by the intervening abnormally fibrotic hepatic parenchyma.

Wilson's Disease

Wilson's disease is a rare, familial disease secondary to a deficiency of ceruloplasmin that results in increased copper deposition in the tissues. It is also characterized by cirrhosis with portal hypertension, basal ganglia degeneration and pigmentation of the cornea (Kayser-Fleischer rings).

Other congenital anomalies that involve the liver, such as biliary atresia, choledochal cysts and Caroli's disease, are described in chapter 9.

INFLAMMATORY DISORDERS OF THE LIVER

Cholestasis and Cholestatic Jaundice

Cholestasis means that bile stagnates in the collecting ducts, with an inadequate amount reaching the duodenum. If cholestasis is prolonged, cirrhosis ensues. There are 2 forms of cholestasis: (1) an intrahepatic form, secondary to biliary atresia, acute hepatitis or sclerosing cholangitis and (2) an extrahepatic form, secondary to an obstruction, a stone or a choledochal cyst.

Acute Hepatitis

In the evaluation of a jaundiced patient, the most important role of diagnostic radiology is to differentiate between surgical and nonsurgical diseases. As a rule, generalized hepatic diseases are medically treated, with certain biliary diseases amenable to surgical correction. Hepatitis may be of the infectious or serum type. If infectious, viruses are by far the most common cause, such as virus A (more common in children), virus B, rubella, cytomegalovirus, herpes simplex and toxoplasmosis. Serum hepatitis in children is usually secondary to complications of hyperalimentation.

Chronic Hepatitis

Chronic hepatitis is defined as hepatitis that persists for more than 6 months. There are 2 types: (1) chronic active hepatitis, which is progressive and the precursor of cirrhosis, and (2) chronic persistent hepatitis, which is nonprogressive and benign.

Sclerosing Cholangitis

Sclerosing cholangitis is a rare disease characterized by extensive narrowing and fibrosis of the bile ducts. It may be an isolated primary disorder or it may be associated with inflammatory bowel disease such as ulcerative colitis or Crohn's disease.

Liver Abscess

PYOGENIC LIVER ABSCESSES.—Fifty percent of patients with pyogenic hepatic abscesses have a predisposing cause, such as umbilical sepsis, appendicitis, cholecystitis, ulcerative colitis or Crohn's disease. The responsible organisms may result in gas gangrene of the liver.

AMEBIC LIVER ABSCESSES.—A liver abscess secondary to *Entamoeba histolytica*, while endemic in tropical areas, is only occasionally seen in this country. It may also cause hepatitis or a suppurative abscess.

Hydatid Disease of the Liver

There are 2 types of hydatid disease of the liver: (1) *Echinococcus granulosus*, the more common form, involves the liver 70% of the time. It may show 3 different types of calcification: curvilinear calcification of the wall, multiple small calcifications within the cyst itself and small irregular calcifications secondary to hemorrhage. (2) *E. multilocularis*, the rarer form (alveolar form), causes hepatic necrosis. Roentgenographic findings are typical and show calcifications surrounding central lucencies.

Granulomas of the Liver

Tuberculosis involving the liver is usually secondary to tuberculosis elsewhere in the body. Sarcoidosis, brucellosis, syphilis, histoplasmosis and chronic granulomatous disease of childhood are other causes of hepatic granulomas.

CIRRHOSIS OF THE LIVER IN CHILDREN

Various severe hepatic diseases may result in cirrhosis of the liver. Numerous causes in children include (1) hepatitis, which causes postnecrotic cirrhosis; (2) biliary cirrhosis, either primary, which is a disease of older women, or secondary to an obstruction, such as extrahepatic biliary atresia or a choledochal cyst; (3) vascular obstruction such as the Budd-Chiari syndrome, congestive heart failure, constrictive pericarditis, veno-occlusive disease of Jamaican children; (4) hereditary hepatic diseases, such as polycystic disease of the liver, congenital hepatic fibrosis, hereditary hemorrhagic telangiectasia; (5) metabolic disorders, such as Wilson's disease, galactosemia, fructose intolerance, glycogen storage disease, tyrosinosis, Fanconi's syndrome, hepatic porphyria, hemosiderosis, hemochromatosis, and α_1-antitrypsin deficiency; (6) serum hepatitis, secondary to therapeutic complications (hyperalimentation) of inflammatory bowel diseases; (7) nutritional liver diseases, such as kwashiorkor; and (8) other causes, including cystic fibrosis, sickle cell disease and schistosomiasis.

PRIMARY VASCULAR DISORDERS OF THE LIVER

Variations in the Arterial Supply of the Liver

The most common anomalies involve the right and left hepatic arteries. Normally, the hepatic artery arises from the celiac axis and branches into a right and left hepatic artery. The right (or, rarely, the common hepatic artery) may arise from the superior mesenteric artery. This is termed a replaced right (common) hepatic artery. Occasionally, an accessory right hepatic artery will arise from the superior mesenteric artery in addition to the one from the celiac axis. The left hepatic artery may similarly be "replaced" and arise from the left gastric artery. Alternatively, an accessory left hepatic artery may arise from the left gastric artery with a normally located left hepatic artery.

Hepatic Aneurysms

Hepatic artery aneurysms are rare and almost always involve the extrahepatic branches. They may be associated with the mucocutaneous lymph node syndrome (Kawasaki's disease), syphilis, polyarteritis nodosa or arteriosclerosis and may be mycotic or idiopathic in origin. Hepatic artery stenosis or occlusion may be secondary to fibromuscular hyperplasia, compression by an adjacent mass or surgery.

Hematobilia

Hemorrhage into the biliary tract is uncommon. It may occur with biliary lithiasis, hepatic infection or following trauma or liver biopsy.

Disorders of the Hepatic Veins

The hepatic veins are valveless and carry blood from the liver into the inferior vena cava via 3 major branches. The veins of the caudate lobe enter the inferior vena cava separately caudad to the main right and left hepatic veins.

The Budd-Chiari syndrome is an obstruction of the hepatic veins at any site from the small lobular veins to the intrahepatic inferior vena cava. The patients present with ascites, hepatomegaly and abdominal pain. The cause is variable and includes entities such as polycythemia, oral contraceptive drugs and obstruction by tumors or inflammatory processes.

Portal Hypertension

There are 2 types of portal hypertension: extrahepatic and intrahepatic. The majority of children with the extrahepatic type of portal hypertension have upper gastrointestinal bleeding but no intrinsic liver disease. They have had occlusion of the portal vein in infancy or childhood, with subsequent development of collateral channels (so-called cavernous transformation of the portal vein). Most of them have had an insidious onset of abdominal distention or splenomegaly since infancy without documented evidence of neonatal sepsis or omphalitis. However, infection with resulting thrombosis and occlusion of the portal vein is believed to be the major cause. Developmental abnormalities of the portal vein, such as hypoplasia or atresia, although uncommon, must be considered in the differential diagnosis.

A minority of children develop the intrahepatic type

of portal hypertension and present with symptoms secondary to hepatic cirrhosis. The multiple causes have been described above.

Roentgenographic signs of portal hypertension include splenomegaly, esophageal varices and azygos vein dilatation. Prior to ultrasonography, differentiation between the intrahepatic and extrahepatic types needed more invasive techniques, such as endoscopic retrograde cholangiopancreatography (ERCP), transhepatic cholangiography, celiac arteriography or, possibly, splenoportography. However, ultrasonography can often make this differentiation and obviate more invasive techniques in many patients, or indicate which invasive techniques may be necessary for the proper diagnosis.

TUMORS OF THE LIVER

In children, neoplasms involving the liver are usually metastatic, particularly from neuroblastomas or Hodgkin's disease.

Primary neoplasms, benign or malignant, can arise from the liver parenchyma, the bile ducts, the blood vessels or the connective tissues. Benign tumors of the liver are rare and usually are not clinically significant, with the exception of hemangiomas in infants and adenomas in older children and adults.

Hemangiomas may be capillary (hemangioendothelioma) or cavernous and are the most common benign tumors of the liver. They should be considered as simple vascular hamartomas rather than true neoplasms and may be associated with extrahepatic hemangiomas in some instances. In infancy, they may present as an abdominal mass and might be associated with anemia, ascites, jaundice and high-output congestive heart failure secondary to arterial venous shunts within the tumor. These lesions can be solitary, and best treated surgically, or multicentric, in which case they may either regress spontaneously or may require irradiation for treatment.

Adenomas are rare, solitary, circumscribed neoplasms composed of hepatic cells. They contain no bile ducts or portal triads. Adenomas should be differentiated from adenomatous hyperplastic nodules associated with hepatic damage. Focal nodular hyperplasia of the liver is a rare tumor, the exact nature of which is not known, but probably it is not a true neoplasm.

Carcinoma of the Liver

The majority of primary tumors in infants and children are malignant. There are 2 distinct forms of carcinoma of the liver: hepatoblastoma and hepatoma. They both present, in most patients, as an abdominal mass in an otherwise well child. Systemic manifestations of the tumor, such as precocious puberty or virilization, may occasionally be the initial clinical symptom. Hepatoblastomas are more common in the pediatric age group. They occur almost entirely during the first 3 years of life and may be present at birth. Hepatomas tend to occur after 5 or 6 years of age and may complicate other hepatic diseases, such as neonatal hepatitis, glycogen storage disease or biliary cirrhosis (hepatoblastomas appear to bear no relationship to preexisting hepatic disease). Metastasis from hepatoblastomas or hepatomas occur principally in the lungs, liver, abdominal lymph nodes and bones.

THE SPLEEN

The spleen is a complex lymphatic organ anatomically located in the left upper quadrant; it is derived from a mass of mesenchymal cells between the layers of the dorsal mesogastrium. The spleen acquires its characteristic shape early in the fetal period. As the stomach rotates, the left surface of the mesogastrium fuses with the peritoneum over the left kidney. This fusion anatomically explains the dorsal attachment of the lienorenal ligament, and the course of the splenic artery, passing to the left behind the peritoneum to enter this ligament. There is significant individual variation in the size, shape and position of the spleen. If the spleen is not located in the left upper quadrant (wandering spleen), it may present as an abdominal mass or may undergo torsion, causing acute abdominal pain. Although radiographic findings are not specific, preoperative diagnosis may be suggested on the basis of combined roentgenographic, ultrasonographic and scintigraphic studies.

The spleen is relatively large at birth and proportionately decreases with growth. Abnormalities of the spleen are usually manifested as an increase in size. The multiple causes are listed below:

1. Acute and chronic bacteremias: syphilis, tuberculosis, bacterial endocarditis
2. Malaria
3. Hemolytic anemias
4. Congestive splenomegaly
5. Reticuloendotheliosis
6. Leukemia
7. Rheumatoid arthritis
8. Amyloid disease
9. Osteopetrosis
10. Splenic cysts: true cysts (lined with secreting membrane); and pseudocysts: hemorrhagic or inflammatory, cystic lymphangiomatosis

Occasionally, the spleen may be abnormally small, such as that seen in sickle cell disease.

Accessory spleens are common in childhood. The absence of the spleen (asplenia) is a rare anomaly and almost always is associated with Ivemark's syndrome. Associated findings include viscerosymmetry and congenital heart disease. In 75% of these patients the left lobe of the liver is larger than the right. Incomplete rotation of the bowel and stomach is seen. Multiple cyanotic congenital heart lesions can be associated. Common anomalies include defect of septation (97%), particularly atrioventricular canal; conus-truncus abnormalities (97%), such as pulmonic stenosis and pulmonary atresia; cardiac malposition; and transposition of the great vessels. Polysplenia may be considered an abortive form of asplenia. In these patients, however, there are multiple splenic tissues and the congenital anomalies of the heart and great vessels are less severe.

REFERENCES

Abrams, R. M., et al.: Angiographic features of cavernous hemangioma of liver, Radiology 92:308, 1969.

Aksoy, M., et al.: Osseous changes in Wilson's disease, Radiology 102:505, 1972.

Alfidi, R. J., et al.: Computed tomography of the liver, A.J.R. 127:69, 1976.

Allen, R. P., et al.: Epidermoid cysts of the spleen in children, A.J.R. 86:534, 1961.

Alpert, E., et al.: α-Fetoprotein in human hepatoma: Improved detection in serum, and quantitative studies using a new sensitive technique, Gastroenterology 61:137, 1971.

Astley, R., et al.: Miliary calcification of the liver, Br. J. Radiol. 22:723, 1949.

Ayers, A. B., et al.: Hepatic haematoma in polyarteritis nodosa, Br. J. Radiol. 49:184, 1976.

Babcock, D. S., et al.: Ultrasound diagnosis of hydatid disease (echinococcosis) in 2 cases. A.J.R. 131:895, 1978.

Baker, D. H., et al.: Congenital absence of the intrahepatic bile ducts, A.J.R. 91:875, 1964.

Baltaxe, H. A., et al.: The angiographic appearance of hydatid disease, Radiology 97:599, 1970.

Bass, E. M., et al.: Caroli's disease: An ultrasonic diagnosis, Br. J. Radiol. 50:366, 1977.

Baum, J. K., et al.: Possible association between benign hepatomas and oral contraceptives, Lancet 2:926, 1973.

Behan, M., et al.: The echographic characteristics of fatty tissues and tumors, Radiology 129:143, 1978.

Bekerman, C., et al.: Other Malignancies in Which Gallium-67 Is Useful: Hepatoma, Melanoma and Leukemia, in Hoffer, P., et al. (eds.): Gallium-67 Imaging (New York: John Wiley & Sons, Inc., 1978).

Bhimji, S. D., et al.: Ultrasound diagnosis of splenic cysts, Radiology 122:787, 1977.

Biello, D. R., et al.: Computed tomography and radionuclide imaging of the liver: A comparative evaluation, Radiology 127:159, 1978.

Birnholz, J. C.: Sonic differentiation of cysts and homogenous solid masses, Radiology 108:699, 1973.

Boley, S. J., et al.: Congenital hepatic fibrosis causing portal hypertension in children, Pediatr. Surg. 54:356, 1963.

Bonakdarpour, A.: Echinococcus disease, A.J.R. 99:660, 1967.

Bookstein, J. J., et al.: Histological-venographic correlates in portal hypertension, Radiology 116:565, 1975.

Brasch, R. C., et al.: Computed body tomography in children: Evaluation of 45 patients, A.J.R. 131:21, 1978.

Brasch, R. C., et al.: Computed tomographic scanning in children: Comparison of radiation doses and resolving power of commercial CT scanners, A.J.R. 131:95, 1978.

Brennan, R., et al.: Liver metastases discovered during high-dose excretory urography, Radiology 127:373, 1978.

Bryan, P. J., et al.: Correlation of computed tomography, gray-scale ultrasonography, and radionuclide imaging of the liver in detecting space-occupying processes, Radiology 124:387, 1977.

Campbell, H. E., et al.: Aneurysm of hemiazygos vein associated with portal hypertension, A.J.R. 83:1024, 1960.

Carlsen, E. N.: Liver, gallbladder, and spleen, Radiol. Clin. North Am. 13:543, 1975.

Casarella, W. J., et al.: Focal nodular hyperplasia and liver cell adenoma: Radiologic and pathologic differentiation, A.J.R. 131:393, 1978.

Castaneda-Zuniga, W. R., et al.: Angiography of the liver in lymphoma, Radiology 122:679, 1977.

Cavaluzzi, J. A., et al.: Hepatic venography and wedge hepatic vein pressure measurements in diffuse liver disease, A.J.R. 129:441, 1977.

Chafetz, N., et al.: Portal and hepatic veins: Accuracy of margin echoes for distinguishing intrahepatic vessels, Radiology 130:725, 1979.

Chafetz, N., et al.: The heterogeneous liver scan: Ultrasound correlation, Radiology 130:201, 1979.

Chuan, V. P., et al.: The paradoxical halo sign in hepatic pseudotumor, Radiology 123:315, 1977.

Clatworthy, H. W., et al.: Liver tumors in infancy and childhood, Ann. Surg. 154:475, 1961.

Cook, A., et al.: Radiographic findings in the mucocutaneous lymph node syndrome, A.J.R. 132:107, 1979.

Coutsoftides, T., et al.: Nonparasitic cysts of the liver, Surg. Gynecol. Obstet. 138:906, 1974.

Cutler, B., et al.: Primary sclerosing cholangitis and obliterative cholangitis, Am. J. Surg. 117:502, 1969.

Dardik, H., et al.: Congenital hepatic cysts causing jaundice, Ann. Surg. 159:585, 1964.

Desser, P. L., et al.: Nonparasitic liver cysts in children, J. Pediatr. 49:297, 1956.

Deutsch, V., et al.: Angiography in the diagnosis of subphrenic abscess, Clin. Radiol. 25:133, 1974.

Eade, M. N., et al.: Liver disease in Crohn's colitis: A study of 21 consecutive patients having colectomy, Ann. Intern. Med. 74:518, 1971.

Elias, E., et al.: Endoscopic retrograde cholangiopancreatography in the diagnosis of jaundice associated with ulcerative colitis, Gastroenterology 67:907, 1974.

Feist, J. H., et al.: Extra- and intrasplenic artery aneurysms in portal hypertension, Radiology 125:331, 1977.

Finley, A., et al.: Pediatric gastroenterology 1/1/69 – 12/31/75: A review: II. The liver and biliary tract, Am. J. Dig. Dis. 22:155, 1977.

Fleming, M. P., et al.: Percutaneous transhepatic cholangiography: The differential diagnosis of bile duct pathology, A.J.R. 116:327, 1972.

Freeman, M. H., et al.: Focal splenic defects, Radiology 121:689, 1976.

Geslien, G. E., et al.: Gallium scanning in acute hepatic amebic abscess, J. Nucl. Med. 15:561, 1974.

Gilby, E. D., et al.: Ultrasound monitoring of hepatic metastases during chemotherapy, Br. Med. J. 1:371, 1975.

Gooneratne, N. S., et al.: "Hot spot": On hepatic scintigraphy and radionuclide venacavography, A.J.R. 129:447, 1977.

Gordon, D. H., et al.: Wandering spleen: The radiological and clinical spectrum, Radiology 125:39, 1977.

Gracey, L.: Tuberculous abscess of the liver, Br. J. Surg. 52:442, 1965.

Green, B., et al.: Gray-scale ultrasound evaluation of hepatic neoplasms: Patterns and correlations, Radiology 124:203, 1977.

Griscom, N. T., et al.: The visibly fatty liver, Radiology 117:385, 1975.

Grossman, H., et al.: Ultrasonography in children, Pediatrics 54:480, 1974.

Hamlyn, A. N., et al.: Portal hypertension with varices in unusual sites, Lancet 2:1531, 1974.

Hays, D. M., et al.: Diagnosis of biliary atresia: Relative accuracy of percutaneous liver biopsy, open liver biopsy, and operative cholangiography, J. Pediatr. 71:598, 1967.

Heck, L. L., et al.: The appearance of intrahepatic biliary duct dilatation on the liver scan, Radiology 99:135, 1971.

Hillman, B. J., et al.: Ultrasonic appearance of the falciform ligament, A.J.R. 132:205, 1979.

Holder, L. E., et al.: Liver size determination in pediatrics using sonographic and scintigraphic techniques, Radiology 117:349, 1975.

Hungerford, G. D., et al.: Pseudo-metastases in the liver: A presentation of the Budd-Chiari syndrome, Radiology 120:627, 1976.

James, O., et al.: [67]Gallium scanning in the diagnosis of liver disease, Gut 15:414, 1974.

Jensen, P. S.: Hemochromatosis: A disease often silent but not invisible, A.J.R. 126:343, 1976.

Johnson, J. D.: Medical intelligence: Current concepts: Neonatal nonhemolytic jaundice, N. Engl. J. Med. 292: 194, 1975.

Jones, C. A., et al.: Choledochal cyst with associated cholelithiasis diagnosed by infusion cholangiography and tomography, Br. J. Radiol. 46:711, 1973.

Kamin, P. D., et al.: Ultrasound manifestations of hepatocellular carcinoma, Radiology 131:459, 1979.

Karras, B. G., et al.: Hepatic calcifications, Acta Radiol. Diagn. 57:458, 1962.

Katzen, B. T., et al.: Pseudomass of the liver due to pleural effusion and inversion of the diaphragm, A.J.R. 131:1077, 1978.

King, D. L.: Ultrasonography of echinococcal cysts, J. Clin. Ultrasound 1:64, 1973.

Kutzen, B. M., et al.: Splenosis simulating an intramural gastric mass, Radiology 126:45, 1978.

Lipchik, E. O., et al.: Angiographic and scintillographic identification of Riedel's lobe of the liver, Radiology 88: 48, 1967.

MacCarty, R. L., et al.: Retrospective comparison of radionuclide scans and computed tomography of the liver and pancreas, A.J.R. 129:23, 1977.

MacCarty, R. L., et al.: Hepatic imaging by computed tomography, Radiol. Clin. North Am. 17:137, 1979.

Madden, J. J., et al.: Multiple biliary papillomatosis, Cancer 34:1216, 1974.

Maguire, R., et al.: Angiographic abnormalities in partial Budd-Chiari syndrome, Radiology 122:629, 1977.

Malini, S., et al.: Ultrasonography in obstructive jaundice, Radiology 123:429, 1977.

Marquis, J. R., et al.: Rupture of the spleen in a newborn infant, Radiology 119:177, 1976.

Matthews, A. W., et al.: The use of combined ultrasonic and isotope scanning in the diagnosis of amoebic liver disease, Gut 14:50, 1973.

McDonald, P.: Hepatic tumours in childhood, Clin. Radiol. 18:74, 1967.

McLoughlin, M. J., et al.: Angiography and colloid scanning of benign mass lesions of the liver, Clin. Radiol. 23:377, 1972.

McLoughlin, M. J., et al.: Angiographic findings in multiple bile-duct hamartomas of the liver, Radiology 116:41, 1975.

Melki, G.: Ultrasonic patterns of tumors of the liver, J. Clin. Ultrasound 1:306, 1973.

Meyer, P., et al.: Hepatoblastoma associated with an oral contraceptive, Lancet 2:1387, 1974.

Mikkelsen, W. P.: Extrahepatic portal hypertension in children, Am. J. Surg. 111:333, 1966.

Miller, J. H., et al.: The radiologic investigation of hepatic tumors in childhood, Radiology 124:451, 1977.

Miller, J. H., et al.: Radiography of glycogen storage diseases, A.J.R. 132:379, 1979.

Moss, A. A., et al.: Angiographic appearance of benign and malignant hepatic tumors in infants and children, A.J.R. 113:61, 1971.

Nahum, H., et al.: The study of the gallbladder and biliary ducts, Prog. Pediatr. Radiol. 2:65, 1969.

Odievre, M., et al.: Anomalies of the intrahepatic portal venous system in congenital hepatic fibrosis, Radiology 122: 427, 1977.

Parulekar, S. G.: Ligaments and fissures of the liver: Sonographic anatomy, Radiology 130:409, 1979.

Piepsz, A., et al.: A real clinical indication for selective spleen scintigraphy with ^{99m}Tc-labeled red blood cells, Radiology 123:407, 1977.

Prando, A., et al.: Ultrasonic pseudolesions of the liver, Radiology 130:403, 1979.

Raghavendra, B. N., et al.: Bone changes in intrahepatic biliary atresia, Br. J. Radiol. 49:179, 1976.

Robins, J. M., et al.: Regressing aneurysms in periarteritis nodosa, Radiology 104:39, 1972.

Rosch, J., et al.: Extrahepatic portal obstruction in childhood and its angiographic diagnosis, A.J.R. 112:143, 1971.

Rosch, J., et al.: "Vascular" benign liver cyst in children: Report of 2 cases, Radiology 126:747, 1978.

Rosenfield, N., et al.: Choledochal cysts: Roentgenographic techniques, Radiology 114:113, 1975.

Rosewarne, M. D.: Cystic dilatation of the intrahepatic bile ducts, Br. J. Radiol. 45:825, 1972.

Rubin, B. E., et al.: Selective hepatic artery embolization to control massive hepatic hemorrhage after trauma, A.J.R. 129:253, 1977.

Sanders, R. C., et al.: Normal and abnormal upper abdominal venous structures as seen by ultrasound, A.J.R. 128: 657, 1977.

Scherer, U., et al.: Diagnostic accuracy of CT in circumscript liver disease, A.J.R. 130:711, 1978.

Scheuer, P. J.: Primary biliary cirrhosis, Proc. R. Soc. Med. 60:1257, 1967.

Schmidt, A. G.: Plain film roentgen diagnosis of amebic hepatic abscess, A.J.R. 107:47, 1969.

Shackelford, B. D., et al.: Neonatal hepatic calcifications secondary to transplacental infection, Radiology 122:753, 1977.

Sherlock, S.: Hepatic adenomas and oral contraceptives, Gut 16:753, 1975.

Six, R., et al.: A spectrum of renal tubular ectasia and hepatic fibrosis, Radiology 117:117, 1975.

Slovis, T. L., et al.: Hemangiomas of the liver in infants: Review of diagnosis, treatment and course, A.J.R. 123:791, 1975.

Smith, W. L., et al.: Radiodense liver in transfusion hemochromatosis, A.J.R. 128:316, 1977.

Sniderman, K. W., et al.: Hepatic schistosomiasis: A case with intrahepatic shunting and extrahepatic portal vein occlusion, A.J.R. 130:565, 1978.

Spiegel, R. M., et al.: Ultrasonography of primary cysts of the liver, A.J.R. 131:235, 1978.

Stanley, P., et al.: Hepatic cavernous hemangiomas and hemangioendotheliomas in infancy, A.J.R. 129:317, 1977.

Stephens, D. H., et al.: Computed tomography of the liver, A.J.R. 128:579, 1977.

Strack, P. R., et al.: An integrated procedure for the rapid diagnosis of biliary obstruction, portal hypertension and liver disease of uncertain etiology, N. Engl. J. Med. 285:1225, 1971.

Sullivan, D. C., et al.: The use of ultrasound to enhance the diagnostic utility of the equivocal liver scintigraphy, Radiology 128:727, 1978.

Taylor, K. J. W., et al.: A clinical evaluation of grey-scale ultrasonography, Br. J. Radiol. 49:244, 1976.

Taylor, K. J. W., et al.: Gray-scale ultrasound and isotope scanning: Complementary techniques for imaging the liver, A.J.R. 128:277, 1977.

Tewfik, H., et al.: Infantile hepatic hemangioendothelioma: A surviving case, Radiology 123:723, 1977.

Thaler, M. M., et al.: Congenital fibrosis and polycystic disease of the liver and kidneys, Am. J. Dis. Child. 126:374, 1973.

Thompson, E. N., et al.: The aetiology of portal vein thrombosis with particular reference to the role of infection and exchange transfusion, Q. J. Med. 33:465, 1964.

Thompson, W. M., et al.: Plain film roentgenographic findings in alveolar hydatid disease-*Echinococcus multilocularis*, A.J.R. 116:345, 1972.

Tuttle, R. J., et al.: Splenic cystic lymphangiomatosis: An unusual cause of massive splenomegaly, Radiology 126:47, 1978.

Unite, I., et al.: Congenital hepatic fibrosis associated with renal tubular ectasia, Radiology 109:565, 1973.

Vermess, M., et al.: Computed tomographic demonstration of hepatic tumor with the aid of intravenous iodinated fat emulsion, Radiology 125:711, 1977.

Vicary, R. R., et al.: Ultrasound and jaundice, Gut 18:161, 1977.

Wastie, M. L., et al.: Roentgenologic findings in recurrent pyogenic cholangitis, A.J.R. 119:71, 1973.

Weaver, R. M., et al.: Gray-scale ultrasonographic evaluation of hepatic cystic disease, A.J.R. 130:849, 1978.

Westcott, J. L., et al.: Portal vein visualization during intravenous cholangiography, Radiology 120:427, 1976.

Whitley, N. O., et al.: Angiographic and echographic findings in avascular focal nodular hyperplasia of the liver, A.J.R. 130:777, 1978.

Wistow, B. W., et al.: Experimental and clinical trials of new ^{99m}Tc-labeled hepatobiliary agents, Radiology 128:793, 1978.

Wooten, W. B., et al.: Computed tomography of necrotic hepatic metastases, A.J.R. 131:839, 1978.

Wooten, W. B., et al.: Ultrasonography of necrotic hepatic metastases, Radiology 128:447, 1978.

Young, A. E.: The clinical presentation of pyogenic liver abscess, Br. J. Surg. 63:216, 1976.

Yousefzadeh, D. K., et al.: The radiographic signs of fatty liver, Radiology 131:351, 1979.

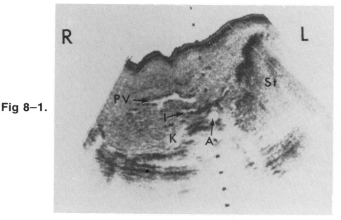

Fig 8–1.

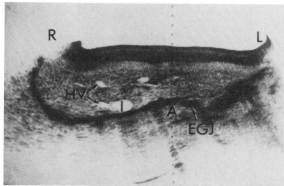

Fig 8–2.

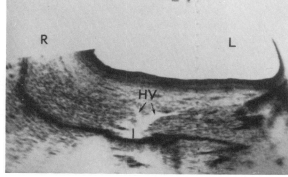

Fig 8–3.

Figs 8–1 to 8–3.—Normal neonatal liver. Neonatal liver should be examined with high-resolution transducers (5 MHz) and scans obtained in both transverse and longitudinal planes with patient in supine position. In transverse planes (Figs 8–1 to 8–3), liver architecture will vary depending on level of scan as well as specific anatomy of individual patient. In general, major segments of right and left portal vein and the intrahepatic course of the inferior vena cava can be seen. In addition, hepatic veins can be seen throughout the liver as well as their convergence and entry into inferior vena cava in very high scans. Hepatic veins are distinguished by relative absence of echogenic margins and their convergence toward inferior vena cava from the confluence of portal venous system with superior mesenteric and splenic veins. Remainder of liver texture is relatively homogeneous with medium echogenicity. Occasionally, high-level circular echoes can be visualized highlighting liver; these represent fibrofatty tissue associated with 2d- and 3d-order branches of portal triad structures. Usually, right and left portal branches, as well as 3 main hepatic vein branches, can be identified. R = right; L = left; PV = portal vein; I = inferior vena cava; A = aorta; K = kidney; St = stomach; EGJ = esophagogastric junction; HV = hepatic vein.

Fig 8–4.

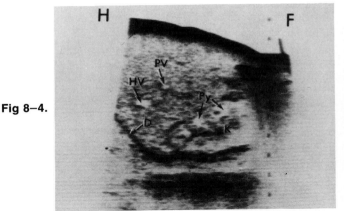

Fig 8–5.

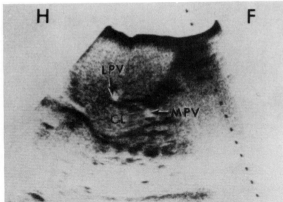

Fig 8–6.

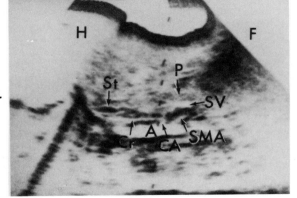

Figs 8–4 to 8–6.—Normal neonatal liver. Longitudinal scans are equally important in evaluating neonatal liver. Frequently, it is easiest to simply roll patient from supine to decubitus position while scanning. Rapid scanning will negate need for respiratory suspension; however, scans frequently are best obtained at end-expiration when significant pause occurs. In the most lateral longitudinal scans (Fig 8–4) branches of both right portal vein and right hepatic veins are evident. Kidney will usually lie inferior to liver with homogeneous texture of liver more echogenic than normal kidney. Longitudinal scans in the plane of inferior vena cava, demonstrate the confluence of left portal vein, right portal vein and main portal vein, which courses posteriorly and inferiorly just anterior to inferior vena cava. At this point, it separates head of the pancreas inferiorly from caudate lobe of liver superiorly (Fig 8–5). In midline scans in plane of aorta (Fig 8–6) smaller branches of left portal vein may interrupt normal homogeneous texture of liver. Deep to liver, significant detail in high retroperitoneum is appreciated, including such structures as stomach, crus of diaphragm, body of pancreas, branches of aorta and portal venous system.

In general, texture of liver on longitudinal scans is very homogeneous, except for the punctate sonolucent vessels. However, a band of increased echogenicity may be noted in midportion of liver a variable distance from skin surface, depending on actual focal pattern of transducer. With newer instrumentation, correction for this beam intensity profile artifact has been made. H = head; F = feet; HV = hepatic vein; PV = portal vein; D = diaphragm; Py = pyramids; K = kidney; LPV = left portal vein; MPV = main portal vein; CL = caudate lobe of liver; St = stomach; P = pancreas; SV = splenic vein; Cr = crus of diaphragm; A = aorta; CA = celiac artery; SMA = superior mesenteric artery.

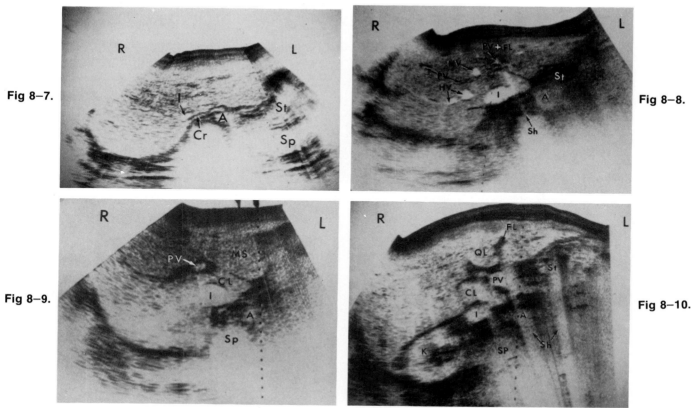

Figs 8–7 to 8–10. —Normal liver in older child. In older child, transverse scans of normal liver will demonstrate similar anatomical detail. However, lobular nature of liver is frequently better appreciated. This leads to some inherent variations of liver that must not be interpreted as abnormal. Careful attention to normal liver acoustical texture will usually prevent sonographer from mistaking normal lobulation for pathological process. Left portal vein tends to course anteriorly through the liver and ends in dense echogenic focus representing fibrofatty tissue surrounding ligamentum teres and falciform ligament. This branch divides left lobe of liver into its medial and lateral segments. Right and left branches of portal vein pass around quadrate lobe of liver, which may also have prominent lobular appearance. Caudate lobe of liver is identified by right portal vein anteriorly and inferior vena cava posteriorly. True surgical distinction between left and right lobe of liver can be estimated by a line passing from gallbladder fossa to inferior vena cava. Another normal variant is shadowing effect of dense falciform ligament and ligamentum teres. This should not be mistaken for either air or stones in the biliary tree. R = right; L = left; I = inferior vena cava; Cr = crus of diaphragm; A = aorta; St = stomach; Sp = spleen (Fig 8–7) and spine (Figs 8–9 and 8–10); PV = portal vein; FL = falciform ligament; HV = hepatic vein; Sh = shadowing; CL = caudate lobe of liver; MS = medial segment of left lobe of liver; QL = quadrate lobe; K = kidney.

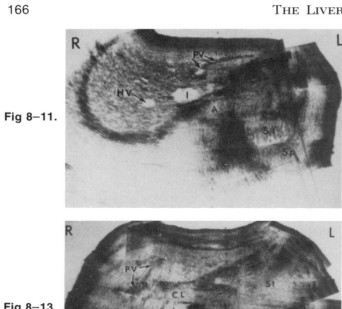

Fig 8–11.

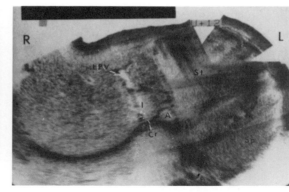

Fig 8–12.

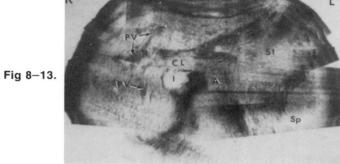

Fig 8–13.

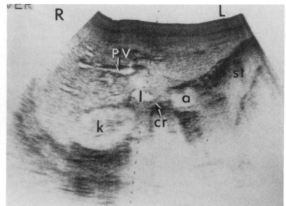

Fig 8–14.

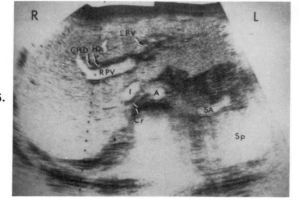

Fig 8–15.

Figs 8–11 to 8–15.—Normal liver in older child. On transverse scans of liver in older children, a variety of branching patterns of portal system can be appreciated. Variable prominence of left and right lobe branches is seen. Also, anatomical location of branching confluence varies from patient to patient, depending on relative size of left and right lobes. In addition, fibrofatty tissue surrounding smaller branches may extend to periphery of liver; beam width artifact associated with these high-level echoes may actually simulate a mass separate from liver. The more bizarre branching patterns of portal venous system can lead to unexplained defects on liver-spleen scans that frequently are accurately identified on ultrasonography. In older children, small tubular or round sonolucent regions anterior to right portal vein can be identified. These represent 1st-order branches of biliary and hepatic arterial systems and do not necessarily imply biliary dilatation. Although no normal measurements for pediatric age group have been obtained, any tubular structure in this region over 4 mm in diameter is usually dilated bile duct in the adult. R = right; L = left; HV = hepatic vein; PV = portal vein; I = inferior vena cava; A = aorta; St = stomach; Sp = spleen; LPV = left portal vein; Cr = crus of diaphragm; CL = caudate lobe; CHD = common hepatic duct; HA = hepatic artery; RPV = right portal vein; SA = splenic artery; k = kidney.

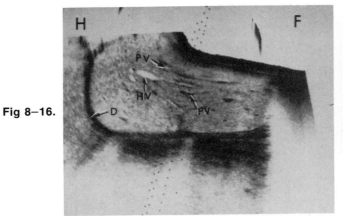

Fig 8–16.

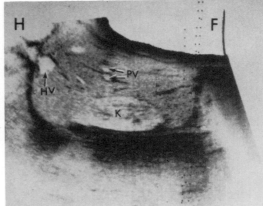

Fig 8–17.

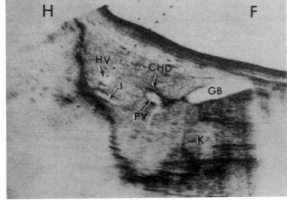

Fig 8–18.

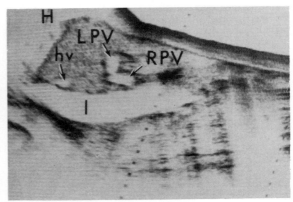

Fig 8–19.

Figs 8–16 to 8–19.—Normal liver in older child. On longitudinal sonograms of liver in older child, reproducible sequence of portal venous anatomy exists. On the most lateral scans (Fig 8–16) 2d-order branches of portal and hepatic venous systems can be seen. These may take the form of very thin tubular sonolucent areas but usually are tubular echogenic bands representing fibrofatty tissue around the portal triads. As one scans more medially (Fig 8–17), the 2 major branches of right portal vein can ordinarily be identified. This usually occurs in sagittal plane of the kidney. The 2 branches of right portal vein then unite to form main right portal vein (Fig 8–18). This single portal branch can be identified for several scans more medially. At this point the common hepatic duct may be seen passing anterior to right portal vein. Usually in this region the echogenic fissure that leads to gallbladder is also seen. More medially (Fig 8–19), ordinarily in plane of inferior vena cava, confluence of left and right portal veins can be visualized. Similarly, confluence of hepatic veins can be visualized adjacent to diaphragm, giving appearance of cystic mass. However, usually enhancement phenomenon causing increased echogenicity deep to cyst will not be observed. In addition, correlation with transverse scans will identify this as hepatic vein confluence. H = head; F = feet; PV = portal vein; HV = hepatic vein; D = diaphragm; K = kidney; CHD = common hepatic duct; GB = gallbladder; LPV = left portal vein; RPV = right portal vein; I = inferior vena cava.

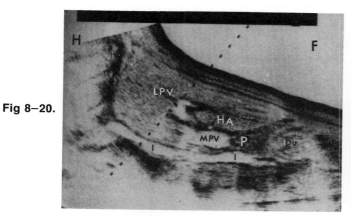

Fig 8–20.

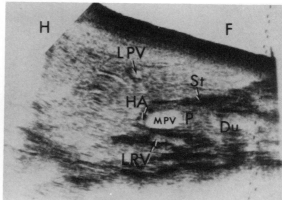

Fig 8–21.

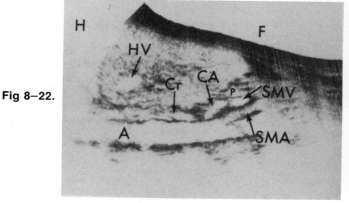

Fig 8–22.

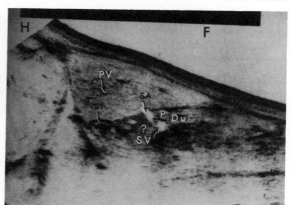

Fig 8–23.

Figs 8–20 to 8–23.—Normal liver in older child. The reproducible anatomical sequence of portal venous system continues into midline longitudinal scans. In region of inferior vena cava (Fig 8–20) main portal vein passes inferiorly and posteriorly, almost touching inferior vena cava, whereas left portal vein courses anteriorly into left lobe of liver. At this point, main portal vein separates caudate lobe of liver from pancreas. Scans progressing sequentially to left demonstrate 2d-order branching of left portal vein as well as the branching pattern of hepatic venous system (Figs 8–21 and 8–22). If left lobe of liver extends across midline, it acts as acoustic window for substantial detail to high retroperitoneum in left upper quadrant (Fig 8–23). Frequently, portions of stomach, pancreas, splenic vasculature and 4th portion of duodenum can be identified. H = head; F = feet; LPV = left portal vein; HA = hepatic artery; MPV = main portal vein; P = pancreas; Du = duodenum; I = inferior vena cava; St = stomach; LRV = left renal vein; HV = hepatic vein; Cr = crus of diaphragm; A = aorta; CA = celiac artery; SMV = superior mesenteric vein; SMA = superior mesenteric artery; SA = splenic artery; SV = splenic vein; PV = portal vein.

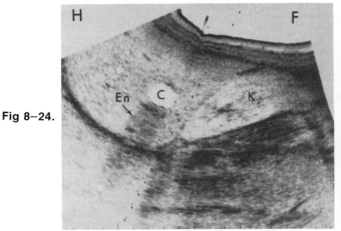

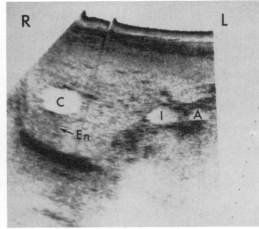

Fig 8–24.

Fig 8–25.

Figs 8–24 and 8–25.—Simple cysts of the liver. Simple cystic disease of the liver is being discovered more frequently now as an ancillary finding with ultrasonography and computed body tomography. On ultrasonograms, classic findings of simple fluid collection are encountered. The mass tends to be completely echo free, with exception of some ringdown artifact on near-transducer side in anteriorly located cysts. Sharp posterior margins are evident, usually with strong echo boundary. In addition, lack of attenuation focusing effect of fluid leads to enhanced echoes, deep to the fluid region. Although simple cystic structures tend to be round, lateral margins are less well defined due to refractive changes of sound beam. In fact, if transducer is moved in linear fashion, refractive shadow effects can be observed. When simple fluid collection is identified, it must be carefully located anatomically to avoid confusion with hepatic vein confluence. In addition, careful search for irregularities of wall should be made since some abscesses, hemorrhagic tumors and cystic metastases can have a very similar appearance. H = head; F = feet; C = cyst; K = kidney; En = enhancement; I = inferior vena cava; A = aorta; R = right; L = left.

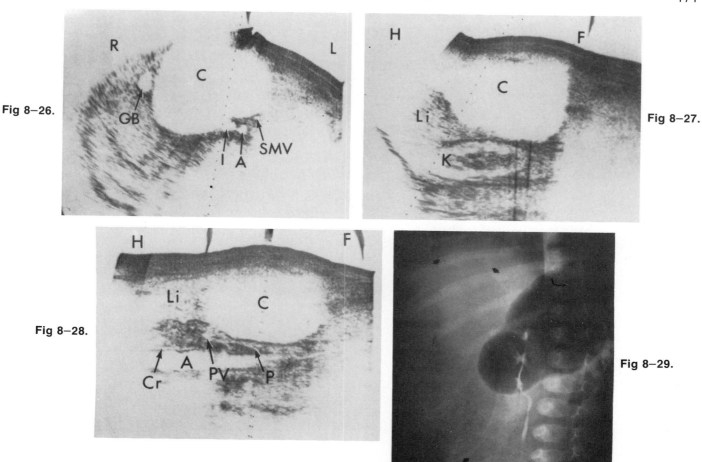

Fig 8–26.

Fig 8–27.

Fig 8–28.

Fig 8–29.

Figs 8–26 to 8–29.—Simple cysts of the liver. Simple cysts of the liver may be quite large, either inherently or secondary to hemorrhage, and present as abdominal masses. Sonographically their cystic character is obvious but they cannot always be distinguished from other cystic masses such as choledochal cysts, mesenteric cysts or pancreatic pseudocysts. Confusion often exists if the cyst is located between left and right lobes of liver or if it hangs exophytically from lower aspect of liver. Careful scanning and multiple planes (Figs 8–26 to 8–28) will usually separate cystic mass from kidney, gallbladder and pancreas. However, further evaluation of biliary system and gastrointestinal tract is frequently needed to determine the organ of origin of these masses. Occasionally, liver surrounds majority of cyst, correctly identifying its hepatic origin. Total-body opacification studies (Fig 8–29) may identify cystic nature of mass *(arrows)* but are less specific in determining anatomical organ of origin. R = right; L = left; GB = gallbladder; C = cyst; I = inferior vena cava; A = aorta; SMV = superior mesenteric vein; K = kidney; Li = liver; H = head; F = feet; Cr = crus of diaphragm; PV = portal vein; P = pancreas.

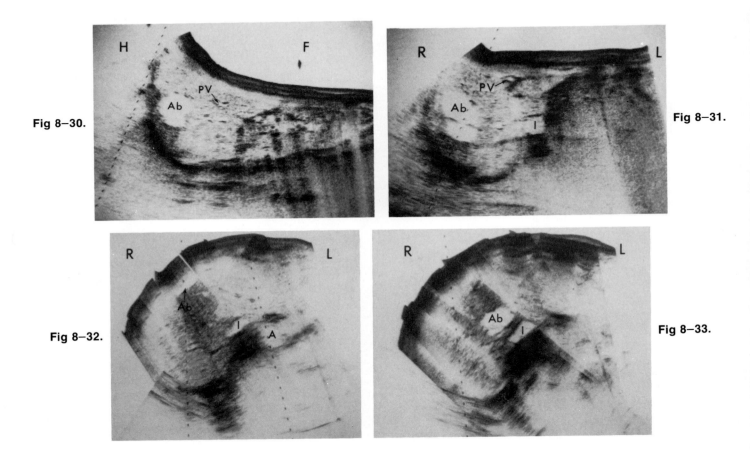

Fig 8–30.

Fig 8–31.

Fig 8–32.

Fig 8–33.

Figs 8–30 to 8–33.—Liver abscesses. Sonographic features of liver abscesses are in part similar to any fluid collection. They may be relatively echo free and demonstrate enhancement phenomenon. In addition, there may be refractive shadowing at margins. Nevertheless, careful scanning will usually show more ellipsoid or irregular shape and frequently some septations. There may also be dependent echoes representing thicker debris. Careful anatomical localization is also necessary to ensure against misdiagnosing the normal hepatic vein confluence. If abscesses contain air, there may be strong echogenic foci within them, with or without shadowing. Abscesses may be predominantly air-containing, in which case, particularly if they are at periphery of liver, they may be mistaken for loops of bowel. In this situation, if clinical suspicion is high, and extraluminal air is not detected on plain films, computed tomography can be of great value. H = head; F = feet; Ab = abscess; PV = portal vein; I = inferior vena cava; R = right; L = left; A = aorta.

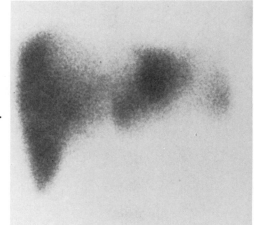

Fig 8–34.

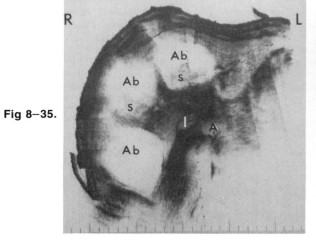

Fig 8–35.

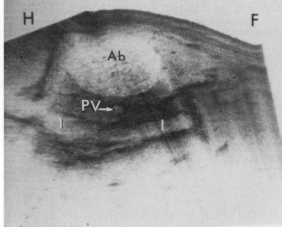

Fig 8–36.

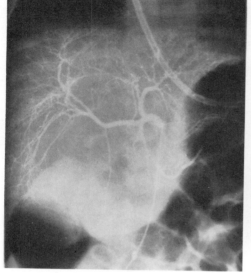

Fig 8–37.

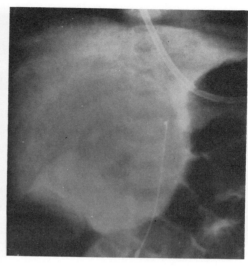

Fig 8–38.

Figs 8–34 to 8–38.—Amebic abscess. Amebic abscess has no distinguishing ultrasonic features from pyogenic abscess. Although nuclear scintiscans (Fig 8–34) are an excellent screening modality for focal lesions of liver, unless multiple isotope techniques are used, a useful differential diagnosis is often not possible due to its nonspecificity. On ultrasonograms, amebic abscesses have a variety of appearances, from sonolucent irregular walled masses to moderately echogenic masses (Figs 8–35 and 8–36). Furthermore, an abscess cavity will change with time, usually with partial clearing of internal debris. If abscess has more solid appearance (see Fig 8–36) the ultrasonographer must rely on criteria other than the absence of internal echoes to ascertain that this is basically fluid-containing mass. In some cases, enhancement is maintained; however, an additional important finding is evidence of refractive changes. Shadows at margin of lesion are related to velocity changes occurring across solid tissue-fluid interface. This usually indicates that an echogenic mass such as this either has a capsule or, indeed, contains isolated components.

Angiographically, amebic abscess is not different from other types of abscesses. In arterial phase (Fig 8–37), stretching of intrahepatic branches is seen, and in later phase (Fig 8–38) relative lucency of the abscess is noted. R = right; L = left; Ab = abscess; S = sediment; I = inferior vena cava; A = aorta; H = head; F = feet; PV = portal vein.

Fig 8–39.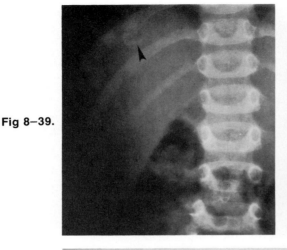

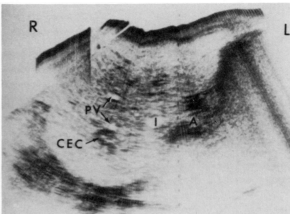 **Fig 8–40.**

Fig 8–41.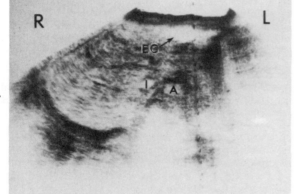

Figs 8–39 to 8–41.—Echinococcal cysts. Echinococcal cystic disease may or may not have a specific pattern on ultrasonography. Calcifications, which are frequently associated, may be seen on plain films (Fig 8–39, *arrowhead*) or recognized on ultrasonograms (Fig 8–40) by strong echogenicity usually associated with some shadowing. However, ultrasonography has capability of visualizing noncalcified lesions, which may have appearance similar to pyogenic abscesses characterized by irregularly marginated fluid collections (Fig 8–41). More specific pattern can occasionally be seen (not demonstrated in this case) whereby complex mass with multiple internal rings or septations suggests daughter cysts. R = right; L = left; PV = portal vein; CEC = calcified echinococcal cyst; I = inferior vena cava; A = aorta; EC = echinococcal cyst.

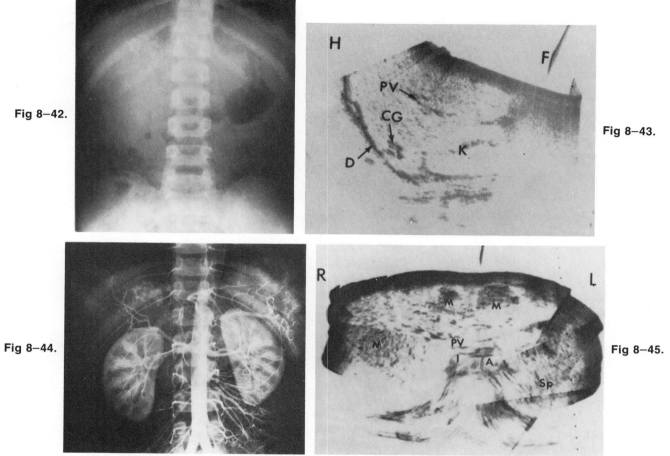

Fig 8–42.

Fig 8–43.

Fig 8–44.

Fig 8–45.

Figs 8–42 to 8–45. —Hepatic granulomas. Most calcifications in the liver that are less than 1 cm are benign and require no additional investigation (Fig 8–42). However, these calcifications may be easily localized to liver by ultrasonography (Fig 8–43). Rarely, angiography is necessary for evaluation of this kind of calcification, which usually is the result of benign granuloma (Fig 8–44). Calcified granulomas of the liver may be numerous and appear as multiple echogenic masses with acoustical shadowing, as in this patient with tuberculosis involving the liver (Fig 8–45). H = head; F = feet; R = right; L = left; PV = portal vein; CG = calcified granuloma; K = kidney; D = diaphragm; M = masses secondary to calcified granulomas; I = inferior vena cava; A = aorta; Sp = spleen.

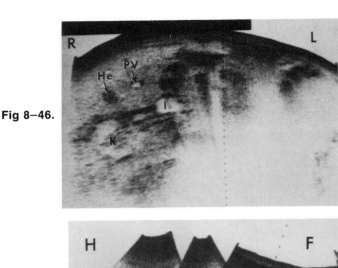

Fig 8—46.

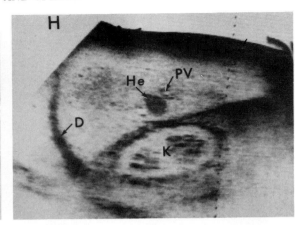

Fig 8—47.

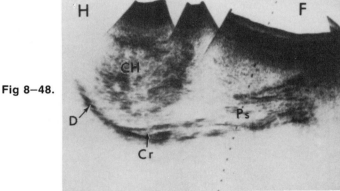

Fig 8—48.

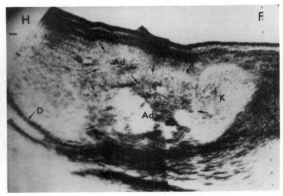

Fig 8—49.

Figs 8—46 to 8—49. — Benign lesions of liver. Small hepatic hemangiomas may be incidentally found on ultrasonography as they have been for years on hepatic angiography (Figs 8–46 and 8–47). These frequently constitute a very well-circumscribed echogenic mass that tends to be round. The echogenic pattern is similar to fibrofatty tissue around portal triad structures; therefore, such a mass must be identified well in periphery of liver, or nearby portal triads must be distinctly separated from mass.

Larger cavernous hemangiomas have less specific pattern, with variable degrees of random echogenicity mixed with smaller fluid components (Fig 8–48). Usually additional diagnostic studies such as computed tomography or angiography are necessary for diagnosis.

Although hepatic adenomas induced by birth control pills are more common in adults, with earlier use of contraceptives they are occasionally seen in the older pediatric population. These adenomas develop most commonly in right lobe of liver and frequently are exophytic (Fig 8–49). Acoustical texture, however, is not specific, with mixed pattern of solid and fluid components. However, one may occasionally see an echographic pattern suggesting capsule (*arrows* in Fig 8–49). R = right; L = left; He = hemangioma; PV = portal vein; K = kidney; I = inferior vena cava; H = head; F = feet; D = diaphragm; CH = cavernous hemangioma; Cr = crus of diaphragm; Ps = psoas muscle; Ad = adenoma.

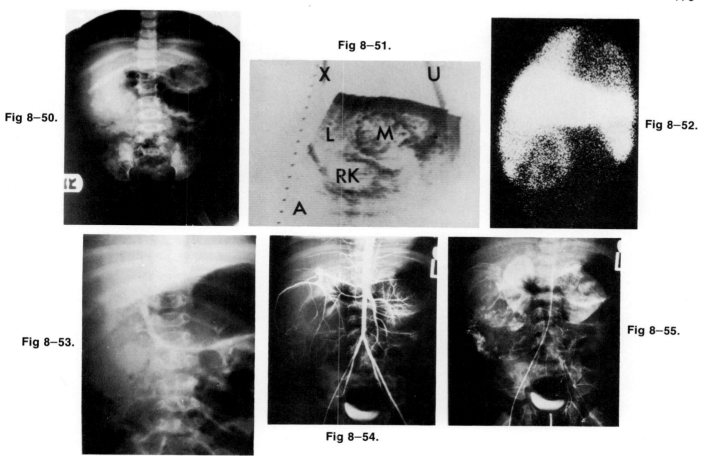

Figs 8–50 to 8–55.—Cavernous hemangioma of infancy. Children with this lesion usually present in congestive heart failure. Lesions may be large and show areas of faint calcification (Fig 8–50). Ultrasonography demonstrates an intrahepatic mass that is echogenic, particularly if calcifications are present (Fig 8–51). An easy and accurate way to make the diagnosis is a liver scintiscan with a flow study followed by static views (Fig 8–52). Excretory urography may demonstrate lesion in total-body opacification phase (Fig 8–53). Angiography (Figs 8–54 and 8–55) is diagnostic with characteristic pooling and puddling of contrast material and no evidence of neovascularity. M = mass; L = liver; RK = right kidney; U = umbilicus; X = xiphoid; A = posterior part of patient.

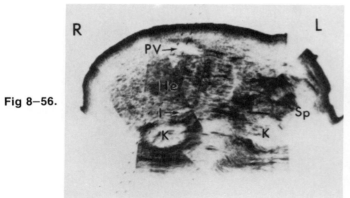

Fig 8–56.

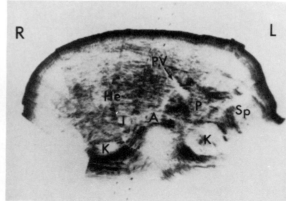

Fig 8–57.

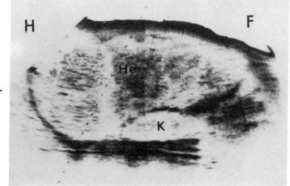

Fig 8–58.

Figs 8–56 to 8–58.—Hepatoma. Hepatoma has a variety of ultrasonic patterns and in some instances may be very difficult to detect. When texture change occurs, it may be an area of increased echogenicity (Figs 8–56 to 8–58) or decreased echogenicity. Former pattern may be confused with metastatic disease, whereas latter may be confused with metastatic disease or lymphoma. R = right; L = left; PV = portal vein; He = hepatoma; I = inferior vena cava; K = kidney; Sp = spleen; P = pancreas; A = aorta; H = head; F = feet.

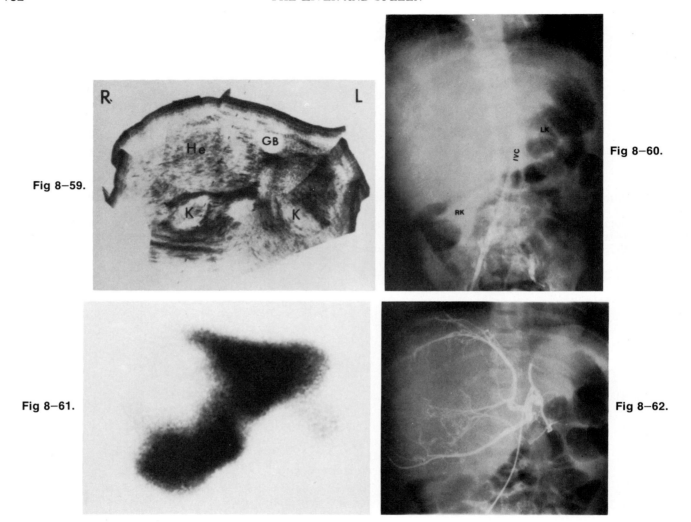

Fig 8–59.

Fig 8–60.

Fig 8–61.

Fig 8–62.

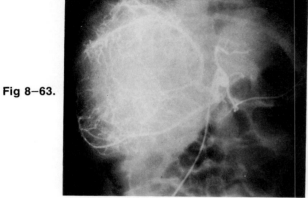

Fig 8–63.

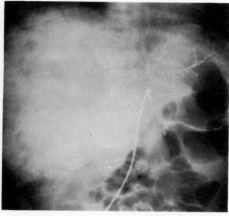

Fig 8–64.

Figs 8–59 to 8–64. — Hepatoblastoma. This lesion is identified as solid mass on ultrasonography (Fig 8–59). It is important to identify uninvolved portion of liver. During excretory urography an inferior venacavogram should be obtained in suspected abdominal masses. The total body opacification phase may identify the origin of mass, as in this patient (Fig 8–60) where origin is clearly from liver as shown by inhomogeneous hepatogram. Technetium-99m-sulfur colloid scan (Fig 8–61) is also excellent method for detection of space-occupying lesions of liver. Angiography (Figs 8–62 to 8–64) is necessary in most patients, specifically to demonstrate uninvolved portion of liver and to demonstrate vascular anatomy. L = left; R = right; He = hepatoblastoma; GB = gallbladder; K = kidney; RK = right kidney; IVC = inferior vena cava; LK = left kidney.

Fig 8–65.

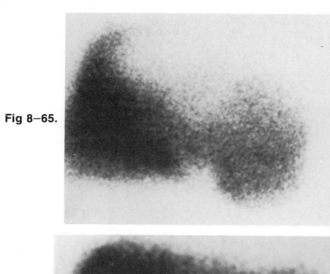

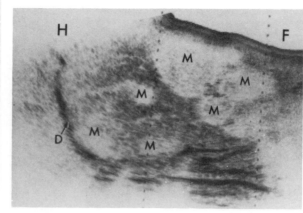

Fig 8–66.

Fig 8–67.

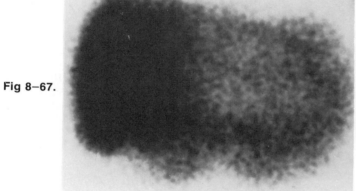

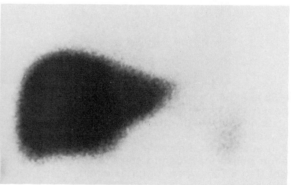

Fig 8–68.

Figs 8–65 to 8–68.—Undifferentiated sarcoma of liver. This large, rare lesion is identified in the ^{99m}Tc-sulfur colloid scan (Fig 8–65) as space-occupying lesion of liver. Ultrasonographically, mass appears solid, involving major portion of liver (Fig 8–66). One month following therapy (Fig 8–67), lesion is much smaller. Eight months later, liver appears almost normal (Fig 8–68). H = head; F = feet; D = diaphragm; M = mass.

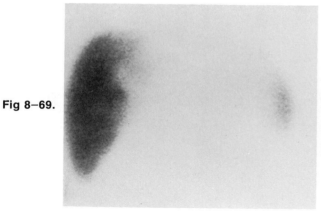

Fig 8–69.

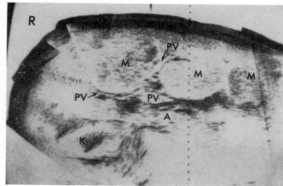

Fig 8–70.

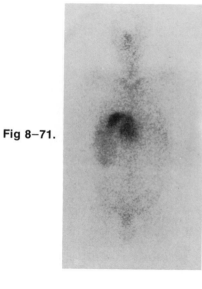

Fig 8–71.

Figs 8–69 to 8–71.—Lymphoma of the liver. In over 60% of cases Hodgkin's disease may involve the liver as diffuse or focal process. Latter may be detected on ^{99m}Tc-sulfur colloid scans (Fig 8–69) as focal-type defects. Similarly, on ultrasonograms (Fig 8–70) focal abnormalities and texture changes may be appreciated. These are usually sonolucent but, rarely, can be sonodense. Latter occurs particularly after treatment with chemotherapy. The abnormalities on scintigram and sonogram may be nonspecific and seen in other entities. Occasionally a gallium scan will aid in differential diagnosis (Fig 8–71). R = right; PV = portal vein; M = mass; A = aorta; K = kidney.

Fig 8–72.

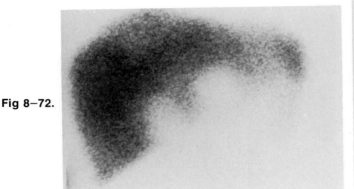

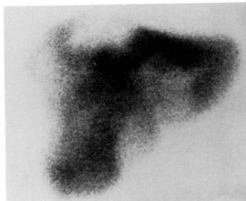

Fig 8–73.

Fig 8–74.

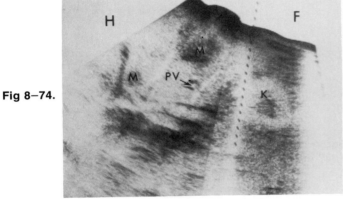

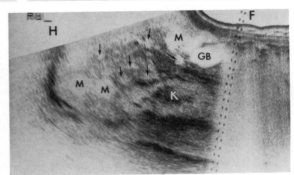

Fig 8–75.

Figs 8–72 to 8–75.—Liver metastases. Liver metastases may appear as nonspecific single (Fig 8–72) or multiple (Fig 8–73) defects on ^{99m}Tc-sulfur colloid scan. Many times these defects, in conjunction with clinical history, need no further evaluation. In other instances, additional imaging modality is necessary to determine whether they are cystic or solid abnormalities. Ultrasonography or computed tomography can serve this function, and former is preferred in children to diminish radiation. Ultrasonography may also be used effectively as screening procedure for metastatic disease.

A variety of acoustical texture has been seen with metastatic disease, including focal echogenic (Fig 8–74) and nonechogenic types (Fig 8–75, *arrows*). For any given tumor, both patterns may be visualized in same liver. In addition, there appears to be no real specificity to any one of the patterns to particular tumor type. In addition to focal patterns, one may visualize a rather bizarre diffuse type of abnormality to liver texture that may mimic other entities, such as hepatoma or diffuse benign diseases of liver. H = head; F = feet; M = mass; PV = portal vein; K = kidney; GB = gallbladder.

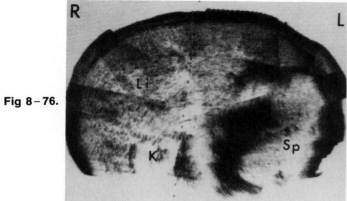

Fig 8–76.

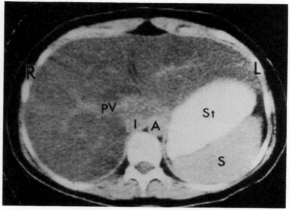

Fig 8–77.

Figs 8–76 and 8–77.—Fatty infiltration of liver in cystic fibrosis. One cause of hepatic cirrhosis is cystic fibrosis, which might be seen as markedly echogenic liver on ultrasonography (Fig 8–76) and is easily detectable as fatty infiltration of liver in computerized axial tomography (Fig 8–77). R = right; L = left; Li = liver; Sp and S = spleen; St = stomach; A = aorta; I = inferior vena cava; PV = portal vein; K = kidney.

Fig 8–79.

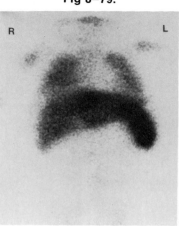

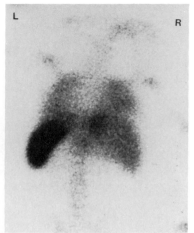

Fig 8–80.

Fig 8–78.

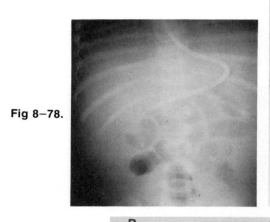

Fig 8–81.

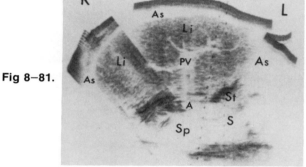

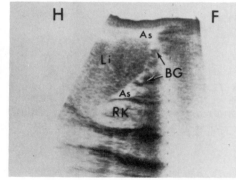

Fig 8–82.

Figs 8–78 to 8–82. — Cirrhosis of liver. Cirrhosis of liver may be detected by primary or secondary signs on a number of imaging modalities. On plain films of abdomen (Fig 8–78), ascites may be suspected by a generalized ground-glass appearance as well as the midline position of the bowel. Similarly, on ⁹⁹ᵐTc-sulfur colloid scans, liver may be noted to be medially displaced from the body wall, suggesting ascites. In addition, there may be splenomegaly and disproportionate increased distribution of isotope in spine and possibly in lung (Figs 8–79 and 8–80). On ultrasonograms (Figs 8–81 and 8–82), ascites can readily be detected. In addition, in cases of cirrhosis, diffuse abnormality to liver texture is noted with generalized increased echogenicity and frequently associated increased attenuation of sound. In cases of portal hypertension, portal vein may also be enlarged. R = right; L = left; As = ascites; Li = liver; PV = portal vein; A = aorta; St = stomach; Sp = spine; S = spleen; RK = right kidney; BG = bowel gas.

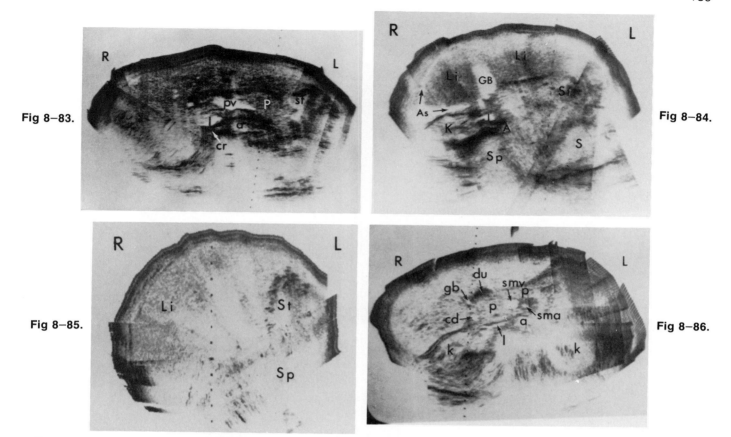

Figs 8–83.

Fig 8–84.

Fig 8–85.

Fig 8–86.

Figs 8–83 to 8–86. — Diffuse diseases of the liver. In a variety of diffuse diseases of the liver, generalized change in texture pattern may occur on ultrasonograms. With acute hepatitis (Fig 8–83), liver may show increased or decreased echogenicity. With diffuse fatty infiltration or fibrosis (Figs 8–84 and 8–85), liver may show increasing echogenicity and ultimately appear as highly attenuative solid mass with or without associated ascites. Finally, diffuse metastatic disease to liver (Fig 8–86) may result in generalized decreased or increased echogenicity. R = right; L = left; pv = portal vein; P = pancreas; I = inferior vena cava; a = aorta; cr = crus of diaphragm; St = stomach; Li = liver; GB = gallbladder; As = ascites; K = kidney; Sp = spine (Fig 8–84) and spleen (Fig 8–85); S = spleen; cd = common duct; du = duodenum; smv = superior mesenteric vein; sma = superior mesenteric artery.

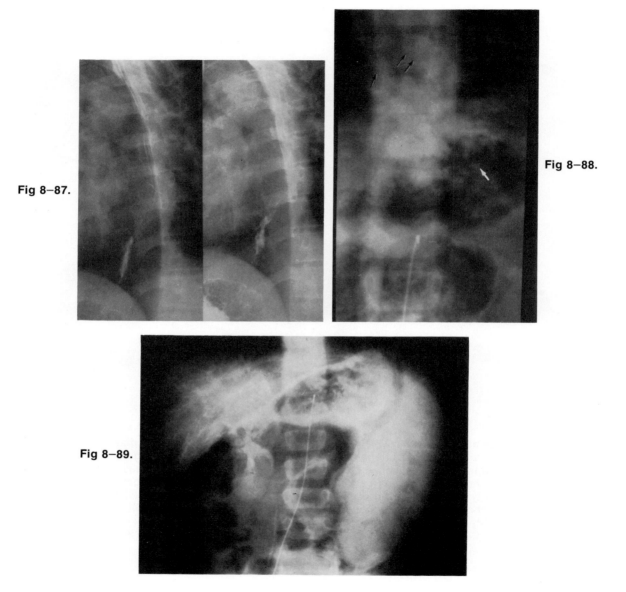

Fig 8–87.

Fig 8–88.

Fig 8–89.

Figs 8–87 to 8–89.—Hepatic cirrhosis and portal hypertension. In addition to the sonographic abnormalities in cirrhosis and secondary portal hypertension, esophageal varices are seen on an esophagogram (Fig 8–87) as nodular filling defects involving distal portion of esophagus. These dilated veins are visible in late phase of a celiac or superior mesenteric arteriogram (Fig 8–88, *arrows*). Associated splenomegaly is easily detected in late phase of arteriogram (Fig 8–89), as well as with nuclear scintigraphy and ultrasonography.

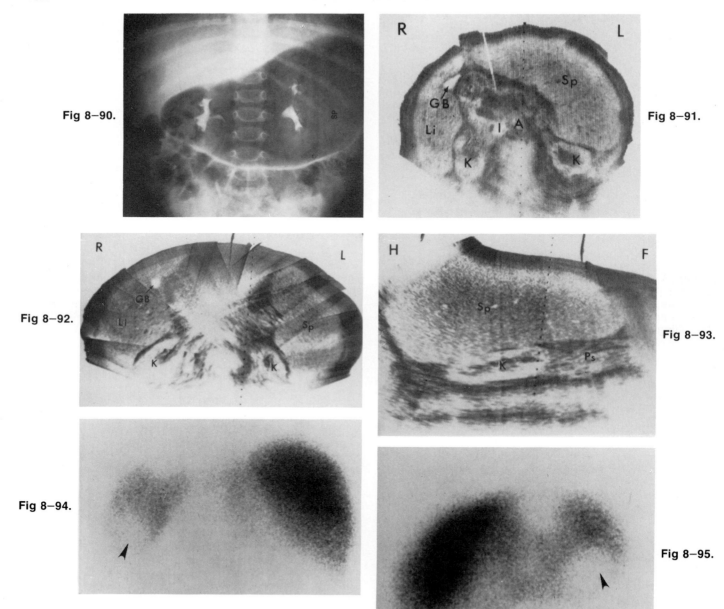

Fig 8–90.

Fig 8–91.

Fig 8–92.

Fig 8–93.

Fig 8–94.

Fig 8–95.

Figs 8–90 to 8–95. — Spleen. Abnormalities of the spleen can be detected on a variety of imaging modalities. On plain film of abdomen or during other contrast studies, such as excretory urogram (Fig 8–90), splenomegaly can be readily appreciated. Similarly, on ultrasonograms an increased size of spleen is usually demonstrated by abnormal anterior extension of the spleen or loss of normally concave medial margin of spleen (Figs 8–91 and 8–92). Additional assessment of spleen size is obtained with longitudinal scans (Fig 8–93) and, if multiple scans are obtained using planimeter type of volume determination, actual splenic volume can be calculated. Ultrasonograms may demonstrate punctate areas of increased echogenicity consistent with calcification or show focal texture abnormalities. There has been no reliable acoustical texture pattern to distinguish benign from malignant splenomegaly.

Technetium-99m-sulfur colloid scan is also excellent way to determine splenic size. In addition, focal areas of abnormality can be appreciated in frontal (Fig 8–94, *arrowhead*) or oblique projections (Fig 8–95, *arrowhead*). R = right; L = left; H = head; F = feet; Li = liver; GB = gallbladder; Sp and sp = spleen; A = aorta; I = inferior vena cava; K = kidney; Ps = psoas muscle.

9

Gallbladder and Biliary System

WHEN AN EMBRYO IS 2.5 mm (4th week of gestation), a bud forms along the ventral margin of the primitive foregut, bifurcates and grows laterally into the adjacent mesenchymal tissue, inducing formation of the liver, gallbladder and biliary system. The superior division initiates formation of the liver and intrahepatic biliary ducts; the inferior division initiates formation of the gallbladder and extrahepatic biliary ducts. The portal vein as well as the hepatic veins, hepatocytes and Kupffer cells develop prior to the intrahepatic biliary ducts, with the latter developing along the framework provided by the portal vein and its branches. This close anatomical relationship of the intrahepatic biliary ducts and the portal vein and its branches is helpful in the ultrasonographic demonstration of intrahepatic biliary dilatation.

GALLBLADDER

The gallbladder is a relatively thick-walled sac lying in its fossa and attached to the undersurface of the right lobe of the liver. The fundus of the gallbladder is located anteriorly and approximates the superior aspect of the intraperitoneal portion of the hepatic flexure of the colon. The body, infundibulum (Hartmann's pouch) and neck of the gallbladder course superiorly, medially and posteriorly to join the cystic duct just superior, lateral and anterior to the junction of the 1st and 2d portions of the duodenum. The common hepatic duct joins the cystic duct to become the common bile duct, which descends in the free edge of the lesser omentum behind the duodenal cap, then continues medial to the proximal 2d portion of the duodenum, and inserts into the ampulla of Vater.

Anomalous positions of the gallbladder are rare. If ectopic, however, it may be suprahepatic, retrohepatic, within the falciform ligament or abdominal wall or completely within the liver parenchyma. This latter anomaly may present problems clinically or diagnostically in differentiating acute cholecystitis from a liver abscess. Ultrasonography may be of help in this situation as a search for the gallbladder in either a normal or an abnormal position can be made.

If the gallbladder is attached to the liver by only a small pedicle of tissue, it can be somewhat mobile and may herniate into the lesser sac through the foramen of Winslow. Rarely, the gallbladder may be located in the left side of the abdomen. This anomalous position is almost always associated with situs inversus.

Developmental anomalies of the gallbladder include septation, duplication and agenesis. Rarely, the gallbladder may contain heterotopic pancreatic or gastric tissue.

Abnormalities in Size

In newborns the gallbladder is proportionately small and located deep in the hepatic tissue. However, it grows rapidly and reaches its proportionate adult size by 2 years of age.

Abnormalities in the size of the gallbladder may be observed in association with other diseases. This is a subjective finding as there is extreme variation in the size of the gallbladder with the time of day, and whether or not the patient has eaten.

Cholecystomegaly may be seen in diabetic patients and following surgical vagotomy. Hydrops of the gallbladder has been reported in septicemia, mucocutaneous lymph node syndrome (Kawasaki's disease) and leptospirosis.

The gallbladder is small in infants with extrahepatic biliary atresia. A small, contracted and poorly functioning gallbladder may be seen in patients with cystic fibrosis. Thirty percent of patients with cystic fibrosis have some form of gallbladder abnormality (nonvisualization, size, cholelithiasis, etc.), but the importance of these findings is not yet known.

Cholelithiasis

Cholelithiasis is infrequent in children and, if present, should arouse suspicion of an underlying abnormality such as a blood dyscrasia (hemolytic anemia), cystic fibrosis or various abnormalities of the terminal ileum (such as Crohn's disease) which disturb the enterohepatic circulation of bile salts. Roentgenograms of the abdomen are helpful in children since approximately 50% of gallstones are calcified and therefore visible.

Cholecystitis

Acute cholecystitis is initially a chemical inflammation that may be followed by bacterial infection, necrosis or, rarely, rupture of the gallbladder. In the majority of older children, this condition is the result of obstruction of the cystic duct by a small stone. In younger children, the cause is usually not known or may be related to septicemia. In the early stages of the disease, the gallbladder wall is swollen by edema and hemorrhage. This is used as a diagnostic criterion in ultrasonography. As the time-course is prolonged, this acute edema subsides and the wall returns to normal size.

Chronic cholecystitis is the result of chronic or recurrent inflammation of the gallbladder and may be associated with cholelithiasis. Ultrasonography can again be of aid as the stone(s) is easily demonstrated by this modality.

BILIARY SYSTEM

Biliary Atresia

Biliary atresia is one of the most common serious conditions in infants. It is not a congenital developmental defect; rather, it represents a progressive obliterative inflammatory process that may involve the extrahepatic and intrahepatic ducts to varying degrees. Thus, neonatal hepatitis, extrahepatic and intrahepatic biliary atresia, and biliary hypoplasia are probably different manifestations of the same disease process. The close embryologic relationship between the biliary system and duodenal development accounts for the association of biliary malformations in children with duodenal atresia. Patients with extrahepatic biliary atresia have a small gallbladder and absent hepatic ducts.

Choledochal Cysts

A choledochal cyst is a congenital cystic dilatation of any segment of the extrahepatic biliary ducts, usually involving the major portion of the common bile duct. Dilatation of the intrahepatic bile ducts may also be associated. It is more common in females and the Japanese. The majority of patients are diagnosed prior to 10 years of age. The pathogenesis of this disease, although not well understood, is probably related to anomalous insertion of the common bile duct into the proximal portion of the pancreatic duct. This anomalous insertion allows reflux of pancreatic enzymes into the biliary ducts, causing inflammation and subsequent fibrosis, which leads to segmental narrowing and proximal dilatation. Neonates and infants present with symptoms of obstructive jaundice, but older children present with the typical triad of jaundice, abdominal pain and a palpable abdominal mass.

Choledochal cysts can be divided into 2 major types; in turn, each type may be subdivided. Type 1 is concentric dilatation of the common bile duct; this accounts for the majority of choledochal cysts (about 90%). Type 2 is eccentric dilatation of the common bile duct (bile duct diverticulum). Type 1A is concentric dilatation of the common bile duct without intrahepatic biliary dilatation and type 1B is concentric dilatation of the common bile duct with intrahepatic biliary dilatation. Type 2A is eccentric dilatation of the common bile duct without intrahepatic biliary dilatation, and type 2B is eccentric dilatation of the common bile duct with intrahepatic biliary dilatation.

Choledochoceles

A choledochocele is a bulbous dilatation of the most distal portion of the common bile duct (analogous to a ureterocele) and may cause jaundice, intermittent abdominal pain and emesis. Pathogenesis of a choledochocele is unknown but probably differs from that described for choledochal cysts. There is no definite association of anomalous insertion of the common bile duct into the pancreatic duct. The differential diagnosis includes a duplication cyst of the duodenum and an intraluminal diverticulum. These lesions may be differentiated as follows: a choledochocele will appear as a filling defect on an upper gastrointestinal examination but opacifies on intravenous cholangiogram. An intraluminal diverticulum fills with barium on an upper gastrointestinal series but does not opacify on an intravenous cholangiogram. Duplication of cysts of the duodenum do not fill with contrast material on upper gastrointestinal series or intravenous cholangiograms.

Biliary Dilatation

ECTASIA. — There are two forms of ductal ectasia. The first is more common and shows intrahepatic biliary dilatation with associated periportal fibrosis. This entity is properly termed congenital hepatic fibrosis with biliary ectasia. The disease has a poor prognosis, with cirrhosis usually present at birth. Patients die at a young age of complications from portal hypertension secondary to the hepatic cirrhosis.

The second form, Caroli's disease, is less common and shows segmental intrahepatic biliary dilatation without associated periportal fibrosis. Although Caroli's disease may present in infancy, it is usually not diagnosed until adult life. Patients usually are not jaundiced. Intrahepatic biliary calculi may form within the dilated segments and cause biliary obstruction.

STRICTURES. — Bile duct strictures are most commonly acquired and are only rarely congenital. The majority of acquired strictures are secondary to previous operations. The rare congenital form may cause partial biliary obstruction.

OTHER CAUSES OF DILATATION. — Other, less common, causes of biliary dilatation include the Mirizzi syndrome and tumors, particularly rhabdomyosarcomas. The Mirizzi syndrome is an obstruction of the common hepatic duct by impacted stones in the cystic duct. These impacted stones cause pressure necrosis and inflammation of the common hepatic duct.

Sarcoma botryoides (rhabdomyosarcoma) is a rare malignant tumor of the bile ducts that occurs exclusively in children. Since the tumor is slow growing, at the time of diagnosis there is massive dilatation of the ducts containing the tumor, but the ducts proximal to it are only slightly dilated. Patients have symptoms of obstructive jaundice.

Other abnormalities related to the biliary system that are only rarely seen in childhood are cholangitis and congenital tracheobiliary fistula. Acute cholangitis is a rare cause of fever, abdominal distress and a palpable mass in a child. Cholangitis secondary to ascariasis occurs in endemic areas. Suppurative cholangitis is usually secondary to partial obstruction of the bile ducts. Primary sclerosing cholangitis is of unknown cause and may be associated with ulcerative colitis.

Congenital tracheobiliary fistula is rare and causes

symptoms from birth. Patients have respiratory distress and cough, with productive yellow or green sputum. The anomalous bronchus originates near the carina and inserts into the left hepatic duct. This rare anomaly is probably the result of either a union between an anomalous bronchial bud with an anomalous bile duct or the connection of a foregut duplication with a hepatic diverticulum.

REFERENCES

Babbitt, D. P., et al.: Choledochal cyst: A concept of etiology, A.J.R. 119:57, 1973.

Balthazar, E. J., et al.: The Mirizzi syndrome, inflammatory stricture of the common hepatic duct, Am. J. Gastroenterol. 64:144, 1975.

Bass, E. M., et al.: Choledochal cysts: A clinical and radiological evaluation of 21 cases, Pediatr. Radiol. 5:81, 1976.

Behan, M., et al.: Sonography of the common bile duct: Value of the right anterior oblique view, A.J.R. 130:701, 1978.

Belsito, A. A., et al.: Measurement of biliary tract size and drainage time, Radiology 122:65, 1977.

Bergman, A. B., et al.: Ultrasonographic evaluation of pericholecystic abscesses, A.J.R. 132:201, 1979.

Black, E. B., et al.: New cholangiographic sign of common bile duct obstruction: Initial opacification of intrahepatic ducts, A.J.R. 130:61, 1978.

Bloom, A. A., et al.: Diabetic cholecystomegaly, J.A.M.A. 208:357, 1969.

Burgener, F. A., et al.: Contraction of the canine gallbladder in different degrees of common bile duct obstruction, Radiology 116:49, 1975.

Burhenne, H. J.: Problem areas in the biliary tract, Curr. Probl. Radiol. 5:(#5)3, 1975.

Callen, P. W., et al.: The left portal vein: A possible source of confusion on ultrasonograms, Radiology 130:205, 1979.

Campbell, D. P., et al.: The differential diagnosis of neonatal hepatitis and biliary atresia, J. Pediatr. Surg. 9:699, 1974.

Caroli, J.: Diseases of the intrahepatic biliary tree, Clin. Gastroenterol. 2:147, 1973.

Chiavarini, R. L., et al.: The wandering gallbladder, Radiology 115:47, 1975.

Clemett, A. R., et al.: The roentgen features of the Mirizzi syndrome, A.J.R. 94:480, 1965.

Conrad, M. R., et al.: Sonographic "parallel channel" sign of biliary tree enlargement in mild to moderate obstructive jaundice, A.J.R. 130:279, 1978.

Cooperberg, P. L.: High-resolution real-time ultrasound in the evaluation of the normal and obstructed biliary tract, Radiology 129:477, 1978.

Crade, M., et al.: Surgical and pathologic correlation of cholecystosonography and cholecystography, A.J.R. 131:227, 1978.

Cremin, B. J., et al.: Biliary ascariasis in children, A.J.R. 126: 352, 1976.

Cynn, W. S., et al.: Infusion hepatotomography for evaluation of obstructive jaundice, A.J.R. 132:187, 1979.

Danks, D. M., et al.: Extrahepatic biliary atresia: Further comments on potentially operable cases, J. Pediatr. Surg. 3:584, 1968.

Danzi, J. T., et al.: Primary sclerosing cholangitis, Am. J. Gastroenterol. 65:109, 1976.

DeLorimier, A. A.: Surgical management of neonatal jaundice, N. Engl. J. Med. 288:1284, 1973.

Dodds, W. J., et al.: Upright spot filming of the gallbladder using pneumatic compression, A.J.R. 128:334, 1977.

Dusol, M., et al.: Congenital hepatic fibrosis with dilation of intrahepatic bile ducts: A therapeutic approach, Gastroenterology 71:839, 1976.

Felson, B. (ed.): The gallbladder and biliary tract: I. Methodology, Semin. Roentgenol. 11:141, 1976.

Felson, B. (ed.): The gallbladder and biliary tract: II. Diseases, Semin. Roentgenol. 11:231, 1976.

Ferrucci, J. T., et al.: Refinements in Chiba needle transhepatic cholangiography, A.J.R. 129:11, 1977.

Filly, R. A., et al.: Choledochal cyst: Report of a case with specific ultrasonographic findings, J. Clin. Ultrasound 4:7, 1976.

Fisher, M. M., et al.: Congenital diaphragm of the common hepatic duct, Gastroenterology 54:605, 1968.

Fonkalsrud, E. W., et al.: Choledochal cysts in infancy and childhood, Surg. Gynecol. Obstet. 121:733, 1965.

Franken, E. A., et al.: Percutaneous cholangiography in infants, A.J.R. 130:1057, 1978.

Ghahremani, G. G., et al.: The cholecysto-colic relationships: A roentgenanatomic study of the colonic manifestations of gallbladder disorders, A.J.R. 125:21, 1975.

Gillis, D. A., et al.: Prolonged biliary obstruction and massive gastrointestinal bleeding secondary to choledochal cyst, Surgery 52:391, 1962.

Goldberg, B. B.: Ultrasonic cholangiography: Gray-scale B-scan evaluation of the common bile duct, Radiology 118:401, 1976.

Goldberg, B. B., et al.: Ultrasonic and radiographic cholecystography, Radiology 111:405, 1974.

Hammerman, H. J., et al.: Biliary matrix: Matrix stones as a cause of biliary obstruction, Radiology 124:31, 1977.

Handler, S. J.: Ultrasound of gallbladder: Wall thickening and its relation to cholecystitis, A.J.R. 132:581, 1979.

Harbin, W. P., et al.: Nonvisualized gallbladder by cholecystosonography, A.J.R. 132:727, 1979.

Harley, W. D., et al.: Gas in the bile ducts (pneumobilia) in emphysematous cholecystitis, A.J.R. 131:661, 1978.

Harned, R. K, et al.: Cholelithiasis in children, Radiology 117:391, 1975.

Harned, R. K., et al.: Preliminary abdominal films in oral cholecystography: Are they necessary? A.J.R. 130:477, 1978.

Hatfield, P. M., et al.: Anatomic variation in the gallbladder and bile ducts, Semin. Roentgenol. 11:157, 1976.

Hatfield, P. M., et al.: Congenital diseases of the gallbladder and bile ducts, Semin. Roentgenol. 11:235, 1976.

Haughton, V., et al.: Agenesis of the gallbladder: Is preoperative diagnosis possible? Radiology 106:305, 1973.

Havrilla, T. R., et al.: Computed tomography of the gallbladder, A.J.R. 130:1059, 1978.

Hays, D. M., et al.: Botryoid sarcoma (rhabdomyosarcoma) of the bile ducts, Am. J. Dis. Child. 110:595, 1965.

Hays, D. M., et al.: Diagnosis of biliary atresia: Relative accuracy of percutaneous liver biopsy, open liver biopsy, and operative cholangiography, J. Pediatr. 71:598, 1967.

Isenberg, J. N., et al.: Clinical observations of the biliary system in cystic fibrosis, Am. J. Gastroenterol. 65:134, 1976.

Jander, H. P., et al.: Emergency embolization in blunt hepatic trauma, A.J.R. 129:249, 1977.

Kimura, K., et al.: Congenital cystic dilatation of the common bile duct: Relationship to anomalous pancreaticobiliary ductal union, A.J.R. 128:571, 1977.

Kittredge, R. D., et al.: Percutaneous transhepatic cholangiography, A.J.R. 125:35, 1975.

Lee, T. G., et al.: Ultrasound diagnosis of common bile duct dilatation, Radiology 124:793, 1977.

L'Heureux, P. R., et al.: Gallbladder disease in cystic fibrosis, A.J.R. 128:953, 1977.

Leopold, G. R.: Ultrasonography of jaundice, Radiol. Clin. North Am. 17:127, 1979.

Leopold, G. R., et al.: Gray-scale ultrasonic cholecystography: A comparison with conventional radiographic techniques, Radiology 121:445, 1976.

Lilly, J. R.: The surgery of biliary hypoplasia, J. Pediatr. Surg. 11:815, 1976.

Loeb, P. M., et al.: The effect of fasting on gallbladder opacification during oral cholecystography: A controlled study in normal volunteers, Radiology 126:395, 1978.

Longmire, W. P.: Congenital biliary hypoplasia, Ann. Surg. 159:335, 1964.

Malini, S., et al.: Ultrasonography in obstructive jaundice, Radiology 123:429, 1977.

Mall, J. C., et al.: Caroli's disease associated with congenital hepatic fibrosis and renal tubular ectasia, Gastroenterology 66:1029, 1974.

Meyers, C., et al.: Diverticulum of the hepatic duct: A rare anomaly, Radiology 119:38, 1976.

Mojab, K., et al.: Mycotic aneurysm of the hepatic artery causing obstructive jaundice, A.J.R. 128:143, 1977.

Morin, M. E., et al.: Demonstration of dilated biliary ducts by total-body opacification: Differentiation of surgical from nonsurgical jaundice, Radiology 121:307, 1976.

Morin, M. E., et al.: Visualization of the gallbladder wall at excretory urography: Implications for infusion tomography of the gallbladder, Radiology 125:35, 1977.

Mujahed, Z., et al.: Communicating cavernous ectasia of the intrahepatic ducts (Caroli's disease), A.J.R. 113:21, 1971.

Ounjian, Z. J., et al.: Stratification in the gallbladder on intravenous cholangiography: The value of delayed or 24-hour radiographs, Radiology 121:591, 1976.

Perlmutter, G. S., et al.: Ultrasonic evaluation of the common bile duct, J. Clin. Ultrasound 4:107, 1976.

Phillips, J. C., et al.: The incidence of cholelithiasis in sickle cell disease, A.J.R. 113:27, 1971.

Pizzolato, N. F., et al.: A new contrast agent for oral cholecystography: Iopronic (Oravue), A.J.R. 130:845, 1978.

Poley, J. R., et al.: Lipoprotein-X and the double ^{131}I-rose Bengal test in the diagnosis of prolonged infantile jaundice, J. Pediatr. Surg. 7:660, 1972.

Reid, M. H.: Visualization of the bile ducts using focused ultrasound, Radiology 118:155, 1976.

Robinson, A. E., et al.: Cholecystitis and hydrops of the gallbladder in the newborn, Radiology 122:749, 1977.

Rohrmann, C. A., et al.: Endoscopic retrograde intrahepatic cholangiogram: Radiographic findings in intrahepatic disease, A.J.R. 128:45, 1977.

Rosenfield, N., et al.: Choledochal cysts: Roentgenographic techniques, Radiology 114:113, 1975.

Rosenthall, L., et al.: Diagnosis of hepatobiliary disease by ^{99m}Tc-HIDA cholescintigraphy, Radiology 126:467, 1978.

Rovsing, H., et al.: Micro-gallbladder and biliary calculi in mucoviscidosis, Acta Radiol. Diagn. 14:588, 1973.

Sample, W. F., et al.: Nuclear imaging, tomographic nuclear imaging, and gray-scale ultrasound in evaluation of the porta hepatis, Radiology 122:773, 1977.

Sample, W. F., et al.: Gray-scale ultrasonography of the jaundiced patient, Radiology 128:719, 1978.

Sane, S. M., et al.: Congenital bronchobiliary fistula, Surgery 69:599, 1971.

Scholz, F. J., et al.: The choledochocele: Correlation of radiological, clinical and pathological findings, Radiology 118:25, 1976.

Shanser, J. D., et al.: Computed tomographic diagnosis of obstructive jaundice in the absence of intrahepatic ductal dilatation, A.J.R. 131:389, 1978.

Smeets, R., et al.: Gallbladder: Common cause of antral pad sign, A.J.R. 132:571, 1979.

Stadalnik, R. C., et al.: Technetium-99m pyridoxylideneglutamate (P.G.) cholescintigraphy, Radiology 121:657, 1976.

Stone, L. B., et al.: Gray-scale ultrasound diagnosis of obstructive biliary disease, A.J.R. 125:47, 1975.

Thaler, M. M.: Jaundice in the newborn: Algorithmic diagnosis of conjugated and unconjugated hyperbilirubinemia, J.A.M.A. 237:58, 1977.

Unite, I., et al.: Congenital hepatic fibrosis associated with renal tubular ectasia, Radiology 109:565, 1973.

Vint, W. A.: Herniation of the gallbladder through the epiploic foramen into the lesser sac: Radiologic diagnosis, Radiology 86:1035, 1966.

Weill, F., et al.: Ultrasonic study of the normal and dilated biliary tree, Radiology 127:221, 1978.

Weinstein, D. P., et al.: Ultrasonography of biliary tract dilatation without jaundice, A.J.R. 132:729, 1979.

Weissmann, H. S., et al.: Rapid and accurate diagnosis of acute cholecystitis with ^{99m}Tc-HIDA cholescintigraphy, A.J.R. 132:523, 1979.

Wright, R. M., et al.: Ascariasis of the biliary system, Arch. Surg. 86:402, 1963.

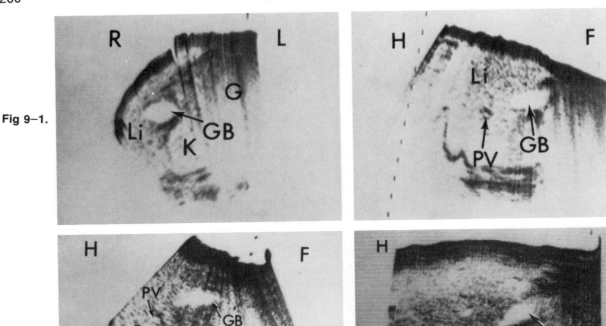

Figs 9–1 to 9–4. — Normal neonatal gallbladder. The normal neonatal gallbladder can readily be examined with ultrasound. Patients should fast for 4–6 hours prior to examination to ensure that gallbladder is not contracted. Transverse scans can initially be done (Fig 9–1) to locate gallbladder in gallbladder fossa. Once alignment of gallbladder is established, longitudinal scans along long axis of gallbladder can be obtained (Fig 9–2). Sometimes it is easiest to find gallbladder initially in longitudinal scans by following portal vein to point where fissure for gallbladder leads inferiorly (Figs 9–3 and 9–4). In neonate, scans must be performed rapidly since voluntary suspension of respiration is not possible. Convenient point to perform a scan is at end of expiration, where pause naturally occurs in breathing cycle. Scanning direction should be perpendicular to walls of gallbladder to prevent irregularities secondary to beam width artifact. R = right; L = left; H = head; F = feet; Li = liver; GB = gallbladder; K = kidney; G = gas; PV = portal vein; D = diaphragm.

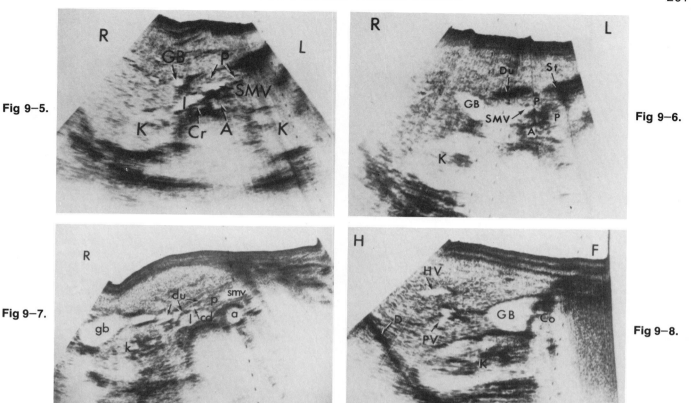

Fig 9–5.

Fig 9–6.

Fig 9–7.

Fig 9–8.

Figs 9–5 to 9–8. — Normal gallbladder in older child. In the older child gallbladder may have a variable location. Most commonly, it is located lateral to duodenal bulb in junctional notch between quadrate and right lobes of liver (Figs 9–5 and 9–6). However, gallbladder may lie more inferiorly in Morison's pouch (Fig 9–7). In this location, it can be confused for abnormality of the kidney. As a result, it is easier to localize gallbladder utilizing longitudinal scans (Fig 9–8). If portal vein is followed medially, eventually fissure for gallbladder leading from portal vein can be seen. This fissure can then be traced distally to gallbladder. Close relationship of gallbladder to both colon and duodenal sweep must also be appreciated (see Fig 9–8), since gas in these structures can mimic gallstones.

Normal gallbladder should be oval, pear- or sausage-shaped and walls should be smooth without any measurable thickness. To assess wall thickness it is important to keep transducer beam perpendicular to plane of wall to prevent beam width artifacts. In addition, one should use transducer with focal point corresponding to gallbladder depth in individual patient. R = right; L = left; H = head; F = feet; GB = gallbladder; P = pancreas; I = inferior vena cava; K = kidney; Cr = crus of diaphragm; A = aorta; SMV = superior mesenteric vein; Du = duodenum; St = stomach; cd = common duct; PV = portal vein; HV = hepatic vein; D = diaphragm; Co = colon.

Fig 9–9.

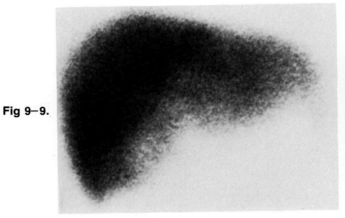

Fig 9–10.

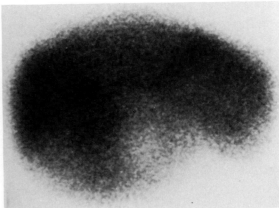

Fig 9–11.

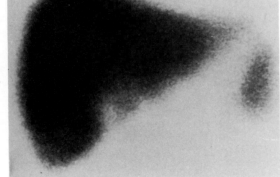

Figs 9–9 to 9–11.—Gallbladder fossa on liver scintigrams. On scintigrams gallbladder fossa has a variable appearance. When in its usual location along inferior margin of liver on anterior views (Figs 9–9 and 9–11) or along anteroinferior margin of liver on lateral or oblique views (Fig 9–10), defect usually causes no problem. However, when this defect is in an unusual position or merges with porta hepatis defect, it may lead to confusion. In this situation ultrasonography is an excellent way of evaluating these marginal defects within the liver.

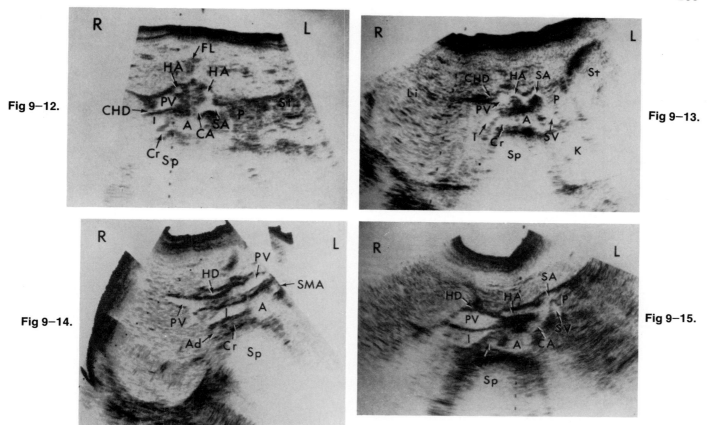

Figs 9–12 to 9–15.—Normal hepatoduodenal ligament. On most ultrasonograms, structures within the free edge of the hepatoduodenal ligament can usually be demonstrated somewhere along their course. Anatomy of this region has become important in the evaluation of various biliary, portal venous, and hepatic arterial diseases. In hepatoduodenal ligament, portal vein tends to be most posterior structure. Hepatic artery resides anteriorly on the left and common hepatic or common bile duct resides anteriorly or laterally on the right (Fig 9–12). If confusion exists as to which particular structure one is observing, especially when only 2 or 3 structures are seen, then course of each structure must be traced to its origin. Hepatic artery can usually be traced back to bifurcation of celiac artery, giving batwing appearance (Fig 9–13). Portal vein, on the other hand, can be traced back to midline, where it is joined initially in liver by left branch of portal vein and eventually by splenic and superior mesenteric veins. Common hepatic duct will usually course posteriorly and medially to lie in its usual location in posterolateral aspect of head of pancreas. Another reliable relationship exists along right branch of portal vein (Fig 9–14). In between 2 main branches of right portal vein and its junction with left portal vein is a long segment anterior to which there should be no large tubes. Occasionally portions of right hepatic duct can be seen (Fig 9–15) but these are rarely more than a few millimeters in diameter in children. Any tubular structure anterior to this segment of right portal vein greater than 4 mm in diameter is most likely dilated hepatic duct. R = right; L = left; HA = hepatic artery; PV = portal vein; CHD = common hepatic duct; Cr = crus of diaphragm; Sp = spine; A = aorta; CA = celiac artery; SA = splenic artery; FL = falciform ligament; P = pancreas; St = stomach; Li = liver; I = inferior vena cava; SV = splenic vein; K = kidney; Ad = adrenal gland; SMA = superior mesenteric artery; HD = hepatic duct.

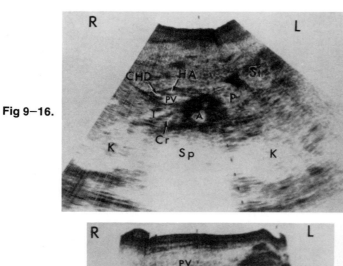

Fig 9–16.

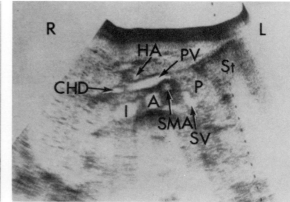

Fig 9–17.

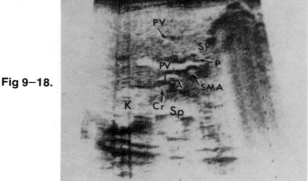

Fig 9–18.

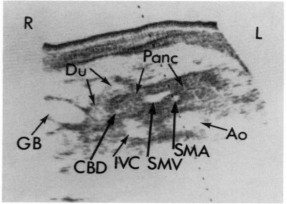

Fig 9–19.

Figs 9–16 to 9–19.—Normal hepatoduodenal ligament. As hepatoduodenal ligament is followed distally, each structure takes a different course (Figs 9–16 to 9–19). Common hepatic duct courses posteriorly to join the cystic duct and become common bile duct, which lies in the posterolateral aspect of head of pancreas (Fig 9–19). Portal vein courses medially and slightly anteriorly. Hepatic artery, on the other hand, courses medially in same coronal plane of abdomen.

R = right; L = left; CHD = common hepatic duct; HA = hepatic artery; PV = portal vein; St = stomach; P and Panc = pancreas; I and IVC = inferior vena cava; A = aorta; Cr = crus of diaphragm; K = kidney; Sp = spine; SMA = superior mesenteric artery; SV = splenic vein; Du = duodenum; GB = gallbladder; SMV = superior mesenteric vein; Ao = aorta; CBD = common bile duct.

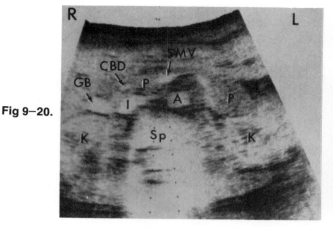

Fig 9-20.

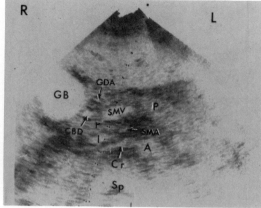

Fig 9-21.

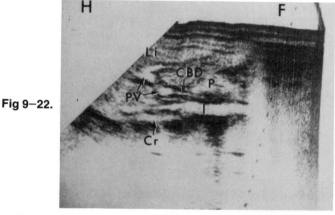

Fig 9-22.

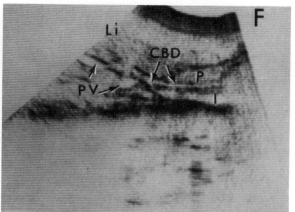

Fig 9-23.

Figs 9-20 to 9-23.—Normal common bile duct. Normal common bile duct is located on posterolateral aspect of head of pancreas (Fig 9-20). Although no normal size criteria have been established for children, size criteria under specific clinical situations have been described for adults. In patients who have intact biliary system without prior biliary surgery and who do not have acute pancreatitis, diameter of the distal common bile duct should not be greater than 6 mm. In patients with previous cholecystectomy, with prior surgery for obstructive jaundice or with concomitant pancreatitis, common bile duct may be as large as 1 cm in diameter. In transverse scans, one may also visualize gastroduodenal artery (Fig 9-21), which should not be con-

fused with common bile duct. The gastroduodenal artery normally courses more anteriorly along lateral aspect of head of pancreas.

Distal common bile duct may best be seen on longitudinal scans as it courses posterior to head of pancreas (Figs 9-22 and 9-23). It can be distinguished from gastroduodenal artery, which passes anterior to head of pancreas. R = right; L = left; GB = gallbladder; CBD = common bile duct; K = kidney; I = inferior vena cava; P = pancreas; Sp = spine; SMV = superior mesenteric vein; A = aorta; SMA = superior mesenteric artery; Cr = crus of diaphragm; PV = portal vein; Li = liver; GDA = gastroduodenal artery; F = feet; H = head.

Fig 9–24.

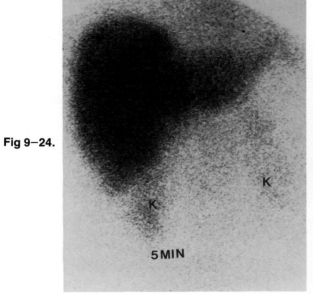

5 MIN

Fig 9–25.

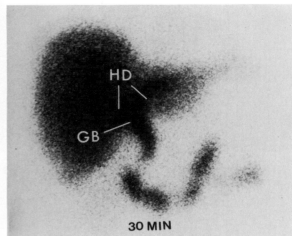

HD

GB

30 MIN

Fig 9–26.

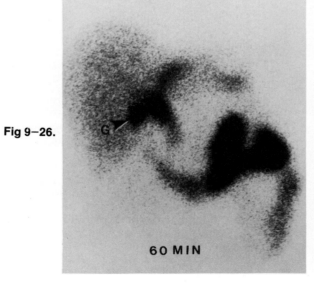

G

60 MIN

Fig 9–27.

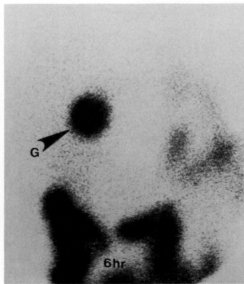

G

6 hr

Figs 9–24 to 9–27.—Normal ^{99m}Tc-HIDA cholescintigraphy. Technetium-99m-dimethylacetanilide iminodiacetic acid (HIDA) cholescintigraphy is an accurate method in evaluation of hepatobiliary tract. Intrahepatic bile ducts, extrahepatic bile ducts and gallbladder can easily be identified. Gallbladder can be visualized, in normal patients, within 1 hour, which indicates patency of cystic duct. Since technetium-labeled agents have a short half-life (6 hours) and are pure gamma emitters, they can be administered in much higher doses compared to sodium rose Bengal I 131. Following intravenous injection of ^{99m}Tc-HIDA, sequential scintigrams provide dynamic representation of hepatobiliary function. Patients fast for 2 hours prior to examination. About 85% of ^{99m}Tc-HIDA is taken up by hepatocytes and excreted unchanged into biliary system; remaining 15% is excreted by kidneys. Normally, this renal excretion is only seen in first 10 minutes. Activity peaks in the liver within 5–10 minutes, and common bile duct, gallbladder and duodenum are usually visualized within first half hour. This agent provides reasonably good visualization of hepatobiliary tract with bilirubin levels up to 7–8 mg %. K = kidney; G = gallbladder; HD = hepatic duct.

Fig 9–29.

Fig 9–28.

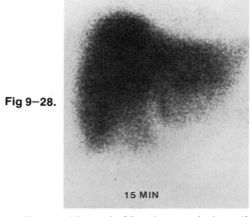

15 MIN

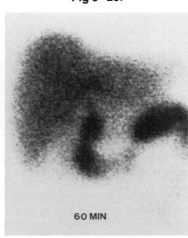

60 MIN

Fig 9–30.

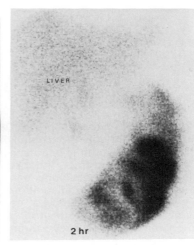

2 hr

Figs 9–28 to 9–30.—Acute cholecystitis. Technetium-99m-HIDA cholescintigraphy has an accuracy of 98% and specificity of 100% in diagnosis of acute cholecystitis. In patients with right upper quadrant pain, nonvisualization of the gallbladder with normal hepatocyte uptake and common bile duct excretion is diagnostic of cholecystitis (Figs 9–28 to 9–30). It is important to be certain that patient has been fasting for at least 2 hours. In patient who has not fasted, gallbladder may normally not fill. However, this study does not differentiate between acute and chronic cholecystitis. To differentiate between these 2 conditions, a second injection of the agent may be given 30 minutes following administration of cholecystokinin. Persistent nonvisualization of gallbladder confirms diagnosis of acute cholecystitis, whereas, if gallbladder visualizes, diagnosis of chronic cholecystitis can be made.

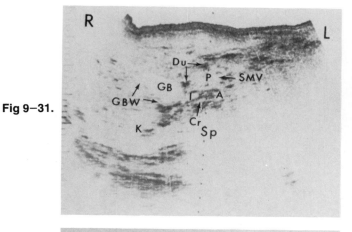

Fig 9–31.

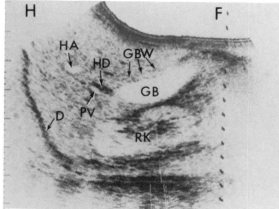

Fig 9–32.

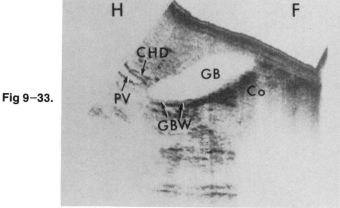

Fig 9–33.

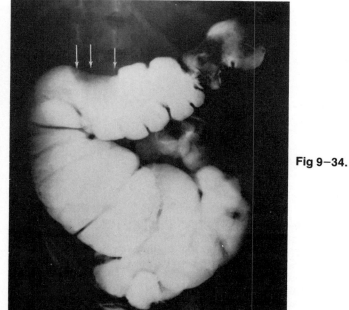

Fig 9–34.

Figs 9–31 to 9–34.—Cholecystitis. Main sonographic finding of cholecystitis is thickened gallbladder wall (Figs 9–31 to 9–33). Acoustic texture of thickened wall should be low-level. Some patients will have substantial fatty tissue between gallbladder and liver that gives appearance of gallbladder wall but will be echogenic. Neck of gallbladder should be carefully evaluated to assess whether a stone is impacted in this region. Shadowing effect of spiral valves of Heister may be seen normally and, therefore, shadowing alone is not sufficient evidence to diagnose lithiasis. One should also assess common hepatic duct to determine whether it is dilated (Fig 9–33). Barium enema (Fig 9–34) may show impression on transverse colon *(arrows)* in patients with cholecystitis. R = right; L = left; H = head; F = feet; GB = gallbladder; GBW = gallbladder wall; Du = duodenum; P = pancreas; SMV = superior mesenteric vein; I = inferior vena cava; A = aorta; Cr = crus of diaphragm; Sp = spine; K = kidney; HD = hepatic duct; PV = portal vein; D = diaphragm; RK = right kidney; CHD = common hepatic duct; Co = colon; HA = hepatic artery.

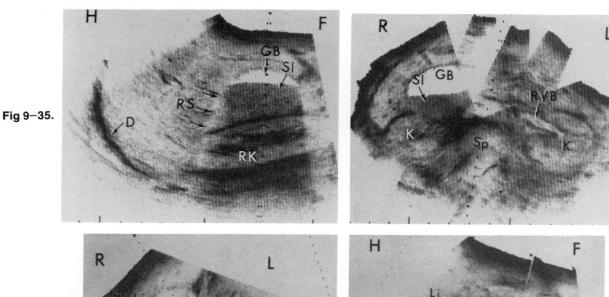

Fig 9–35.

Fig 9–36.

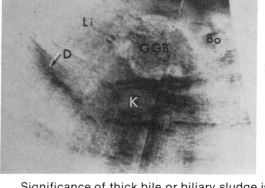

Fig 9–37.

Fig 9–38.

Figs 9–35 to 9–38.—Biliary sludge. Biliary sludge is a term analogous to thick bile manifested by presence of dependent echoes within gallbladder. A number of features distinguish thick bile from gallstones. Dependent echoes should have sharp-layered margin and should not attenuate sound beam (Figs 9–35 and 9–36). In fact, sound is frequently enhanced through gallbladder as it would be in any fluid-containing structure. There may, however, be refractive shadows (see Fig 9–35) at edges of gallbladder secondary to velocity changes in bile. Biliary sludge should have medium- to low-level homogeneous echogenicity. Final requirement, not demonstrated on these scans, is that changes in patient position cause very slow relayering of bile-sludge interface. This is in contrast to stones or biliary sand, which rapidly reestablish dependent echogenic level with changes in position.

Significance of thick bile or biliary sludge is uncertain at present. It is frequently visualized in patients who are on prolonged fasts (1 week) or who have had prolonged obstructive jaundice. This phenomenon has been reproduced experimentally by Doctor Filly at the University of California at San Francisco in dog-animal model. Doctor Filly has also established that this echogenic material can be filtered out with 10-μ filter and under microscope appears to be calcium bilirubinate crystals.

A number of patients will have biliary sludge after only 12- to 24-hour fast. It is unclear whether these patients have lithogenic bile and are prone to gallbladder disease. An example of such a case is demonstrated in Figures 9–37 and 9–38. The patient shown in these figures is same as in Figures 9–35 and 9–36, after a period of several months. On second examination patient was complaining of right

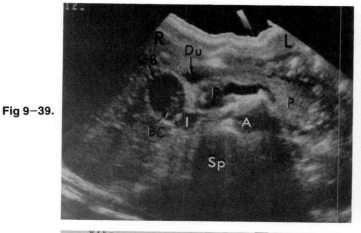

Fig 9-39.

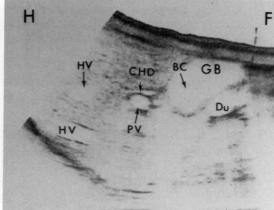

Fig 9-40.

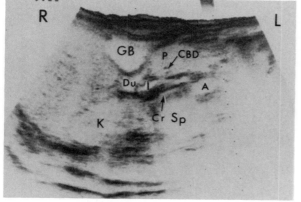

Fig 9-41.

Figs 9-39 to 9-41. — Gallbladder hematoma. In contrast to biliary sludge, hematomas within gallbladder tend to be more irregular, without dependent layering effect. Typical hematoma is demonstrated in Figure 9-39 in patient in whom this complication developed following liver biopsy.

Gallbladder hematoma may follow blunt trauma to abdomen, as demonstrated in Figures 9-40 and 9-41. In this patient, mild thickening of gallbladder wall is seen in association with very subtle echoes from blood clot within gallbladder. Common hepatic duct is also slightly dilated, but this is not abnormal in patient with accompanying pancreatitis (see Fig 9-41). Echogenic pattern of gallbladder hematoma is indistinguishable from that seen with carcinoma or polyps of gallbladder. These entities, however, generally have different clinical history and are very rare in children. R = right; L = left; H = head; F = feet; GB = gallbladder; BC = blood clot; Du = duodenum; I = inferior vena cava; P = pancreas; A = aorta; Sp = spine; HV = hepatic vein; PV = portal vein; CHD = common hepatic duct; CBD = common bile duct; Cr = crus of diaphragm; K = kidney.

---

upper quadrant pain, and ultrasonic findings are typical for acute cholecystitis with irregularity and thickening of gallbladder wall with biliary sludge completely filling the gallbladder (see Figs 9-37 and 9-38). H = head; F = feet; R = right; L = left; D = diaphragm; RS = refractive shadows; RK = right kidney; GB = gallbladder; Sl = sludge; Sp = spine; RVB = renal vascular bundle; K = kidney; Li = liver; GGB = gangrenous gallbladder; I = inferior vena cava; A = aorta; Bo = bowel.

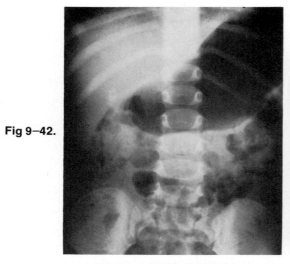

Fig 9-42.

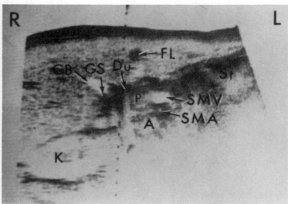

Fig 9-43.

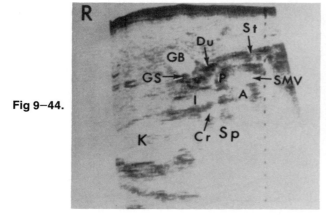

Fig 9-44.

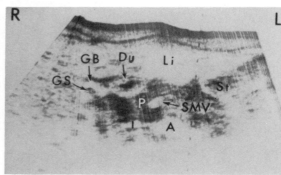

Fig 9-45.

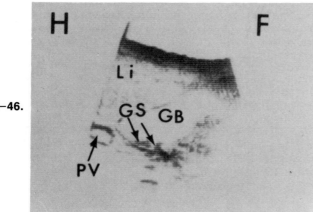

Fig 9-46.

Figs 9–42 to 9–46.—Cholelithiasis. Although gallstones are much more common in adults, they may be present in pediatric age group (Fig 9–42). On ultrasonograms, they are dependent filling defects within gallbladder with rounded or jagged edge and relatively high echogenicity. Stones demonstrated in Figures 9–43 to 9–46 do not demonstrate shadowing. Absence of acoustical shadowing occurs in approximately 15–20% of cases and is related to technical aspects. A number of investigators have demonstrated under experimental conditions in phantoms that gallstones, regardless of their composition, will shadow if they reside within focal point of transducer and are not significantly smaller than the focal width. Since stone may not be at focal point of the transducer, it may not demonstrate shadowing. Frequently, using a transducer that is more highly focused in this region will bring out shadowing effect. Shadowing per se appears to be related to critical-angle phenomena occurring at edge of stone secondary to acoustical velocity changes occurring at this interface. R = right; L = left; H = head; F = feet; GB = gallbladder; GS = gallstone; Du = duodenum; FL = falciform ligament; P = pancreas; A = aorta; K = kidney; SMV = superior mesenteric vein; SMA = superior mesenteric artery; St = stomach; Cr = crus of diaphragm; Sp = spine; Li = liver; PV = portal vein; I = inferior vena cava.

Fig 9–47.

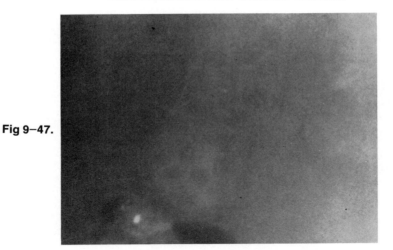

Fig 9–48.

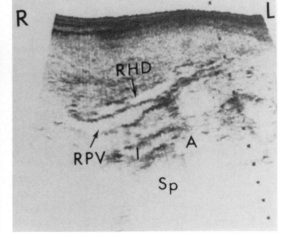

Fig 9–49.

Figs 9–47 to 9–49.—Cholelithiasis. Although oral cholecystography has certainly been the mainstay of diagnosis for cholelithiasis (Fig 9–47), ultrasonography represents excellent screening procedure or backup procedure to a nonvisualization on oral cholecystography. Since ultrasonography does not use radiation, and since cholelithiasis is less common in pediatric age group, it may be procedure of choice as screening imaging modality. Figure 9–48 shows more typical appearance of shadowing gallstones with echogenic rounded or irregular margins. It is always important to evaluate intrahepatic and extrahepatic biliary system for dilatation, even in absence of jaundice, for their enlargement (Fig 9–49) may indicate that gallstones are being overlooked. H = head; F = feet; R = right; L = left; PV = portal vein; D = diaphragm; GB = gallbladder; GS = gallstones; RK = right kidney; Sh = shadow; RPV = right portal vein; RHD = right hepatic duct; I = inferior vena cava; A = aorta; Sp = spine.

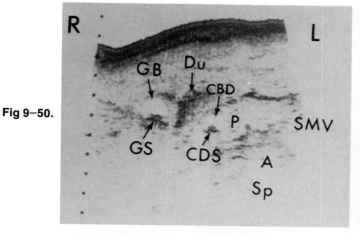

Fig 9–50.

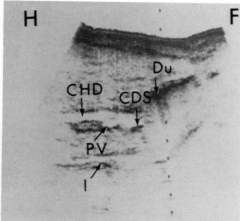

Fig 9–51.

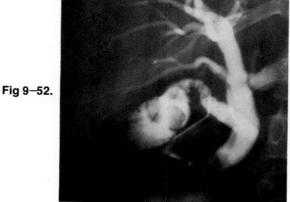

Fig 9–52.

Figs 9–50 to 9–52.—Cholelithiasis and choledocholithiasis. Ultrasound is excellent modality for evaluating jaundice in older child. Stones in gallbladder and extrahepatic biliary system (Figs 9–50 and 9–51) can be demonstrated. This operative cholangiogram (Fig 9–52) provides anatomical correlation. It should be noted that no intrahepatic biliary dilatation is present, and that extrahepatic biliary system has absorbed the increased pressure. This is not uncommon and supports necessity for visualizing both intrahepatic and extrahepatic biliary system to differentiate surgical from medical jaundice. Ultrasound must be considered nondiagnostic if extrahepatic biliary system is not imaged. R = right; L = left; GB = gallbladder; GS = gallstones; Du = duodenum; CBD = common bile duct; CDS = common duct stone; A = aorta; SMV = superior mesenteric vein; Sp = spine; I = inferior vena cava; PV = portal vein; CHD = common hepatic duct; P = pancreas; H = head; F = feet.

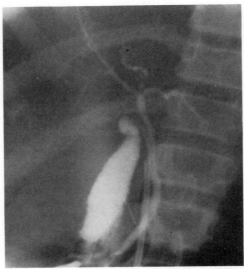

Fig 9–53. — Hypoplasia of biliary tract. It is extremely difficult to demonstrate small size of biliary tract either in ultrasonography or roentgenographically. Even following operative cholangiogram (Fig 9–53), it may be difficult to make
accurate diagnosis of biliary hypoplasia. It is also difficult to
make diagnosis of biliary atresia by available diagnostic
modalities (e.g., contrast cholecystography, ultrasonography and nuclear scintigraphy) with any degree of certainty.

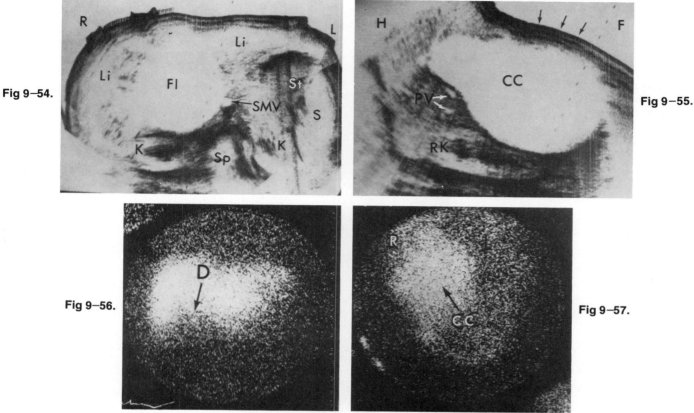

Figs 9–54 to 9–57.—Choledochal cysts. Choledochal cysts may present in pediatric age group as palpable right upper quadrant or midabdominal mass. Ultrasonography is excellent screening modality in such a clinical situation; however, it may be difficult to determine with ultrasound alone the origin of large cystic structure. Differential diagnoses always include choledochal cyst, duplication cysts of duodenum and pancreatic pseudocysts. When mass is extremely large (Figs 9–54 and 9–55, *arrows*) this differentiation may not be possible. One may have to resort to other imaging modalities, such as isotope scans. On ⁹⁹ᵐTc-sulfur colloid scan, defect in portal area will usually be demonstrated (Fig 9–56). With aid of hepatobiliary agent such as rose Bengal or, more recently, the ⁹⁹ᵐTc-HIDA analogues, communication with biliary system can be demonstrated in approximately 60–80% of cases (Fig 9–57). Alternatively, if jaundice is not present intravenous cholangiogram may show similar findings, particularly when delayed films are obtained. Finally, if there is intrahepatic biliary dilatation, percutaneous transhepatic cholangiogram may be procedure of choice. R = right; L = left; H = head; F = feet; Li = liver; Fl = fluid; K = kidney; Sp = spine; SMV = superior mesenteric vein; St = stomach; S = spleen; PV = portal vein; RK = right kidney; CC = choledochal cyst; D = defect on technetium scan.

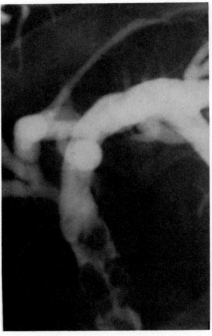

Fig 9–58.—Percutaneous transhepatic cholangiogram. Detailed anatomical evaluation of biliary tract dilatation is best achieved with direct cholangiography performed either percutaneously or intraoperatively. Although rare, biliary tract dilatation may be result of rhabdomyosarcoma, which might be difficult to differentiate from impacted stones. Rhabdomyosarcoma is most common neoplasm of biliary tract in children. Appearance similar to "bunch of grapes" may suggest diagnosis.

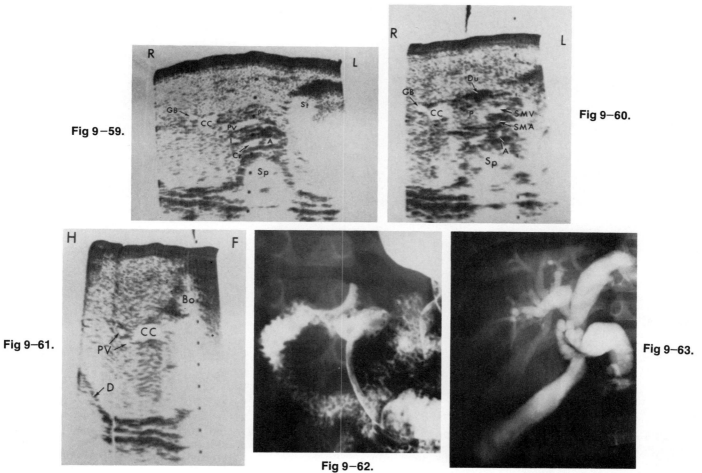

Fig 9–59.

Fig 9–60.

Fig 9–61.

Fig 9–62.

Fig 9–63.

Figs 9–59 to 9–63.—Choledochal-cyst (type 1A). This may present as neonatal jaundice. Ultrasound is an effective way to evaluate these patients by demonstrating cystic mass separate from gallbladder in hepatoduodenal ligament and head of pancreas region (Figs 9–59 to 9–61). Detailed scans must be performed with anatomical identification of gallbladder, duodenum and head of pancreas. This case (Figs 9–59 to 9–63) represents concentric dilatation of common bile duct without dilatation of intrahepatic bile ducts (type 1A). The diagnosis may be suggested indi-rectly on upper gastrointestinal series that shows extrinsic defect on duodenal bulb (Fig 9–62). Operative cholangio-gram, in this case, confirms diagnosis of choledochal cyst (Fig 9–63). R = right; L = left; GB = gallbladder; CC = cho-ledochal cyst; PV = portal vein; P = pancreas; I = inferior vena cava; Cr = crus of diaphragm; A = aorta; St = stom-ach; Sp = spine; Du = duodenum; SMV = superior mes-enteric vein; SMA = superior mesenteric artery; D = dia-phragm; Bo = bowel; H = head; F = feet.

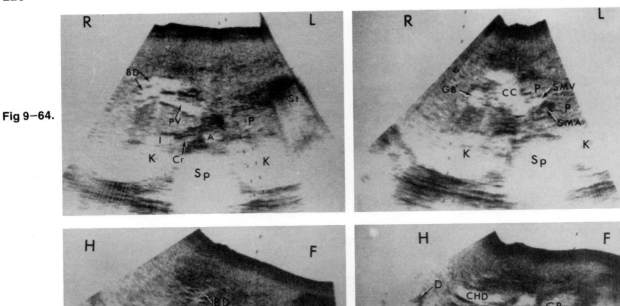

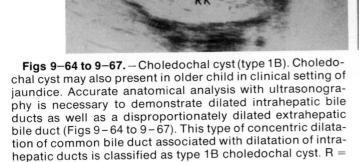

Fig 9–64.

Fig 9–65.

Fig 9–66.

Fig 9–67.

Figs 9–64 to 9–67. – Choledochal cyst (type 1B). Choledochal cyst may also present in older child in clinical setting of jaundice. Accurate anatomical analysis with ultrasonography is necessary to demonstrate dilated intrahepatic bile ducts as well as a disproportionately dilated extrahepatic bile duct (Figs 9–64 to 9–67). This type of concentric dilatation of common bile duct associated with dilatation of intrahepatic ducts is classified as type 1B choledochal cyst. R = right; L = left; BD = bile ducts; PV = portal vein; I = inferior vena cava; Cr = crus of diaphragm; K = kidney; A = aorta; Sp = spine; P = pancreas; St = stomach; GB = gallbladder; CC = choledochal cyst; SMV = superior mesenteric vein; SMA = superior mesenteric artery; D = diaphragm; RK = right kidney; CHD = common hepatic duct; H = head; F = feet.

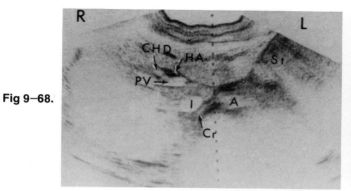

Fig 9–68.

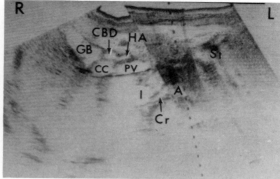

Fig 9–69.

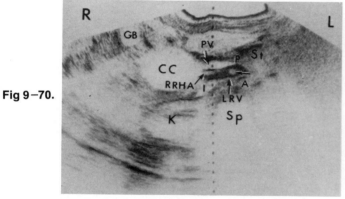

Fig 9–70.

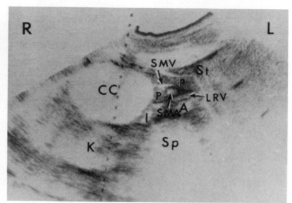

Fig 9–71.

Figs 9–68 to 9–71.—Choledochal cyst (type 2). Eccentric dilatation of common bile duct (CBD) (type 2) is much less common than concentric dilatation of CBD (type 1). Anatomical detail on ultrasound may be sufficient to strongly suggest the diagnosis. In Figures 9–68 to 9–71, progressive caudal scans of abdomen in transverse plane performed with patient in supine position are provided. High in hepatoduodenal ligament, 3 major components are readily identified. As these are followed distally, cystic mass arises in hepatoduodenal ligament separate from gallbladder and appears separate from CBD (eccentric dilatation of CBD). As scans are performed more caudally, this cystic mass moves into lateral aspect of head of pancreas and anatomically is consistent with biliary origin. If this eccentric dilatation of CBD is associated with dilatation of intrahepatic ducts, it is classified as type 2B; conversely, if intrahepatic ducts are normal, it is classified as type 2A. R = right; L = left; CHD = common hepatic duct; PV = portal vein; HA = hepatic artery; I = inferior vena cava; A = aorta; Cr = crus of diaphragm; St = stomach; GB = gallbladder; CC = choledochal cyst; RRHA = replaced right hepatic artery; K = kidney; Sp = spine; LRV = left renal vein; SMA = superior mesenteric artery; P = pancreas; SMA = superior mesenteric artery; SMV = superior mesenteric vein.

Fig 9-72.

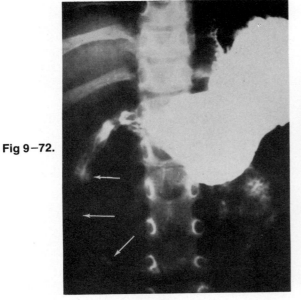

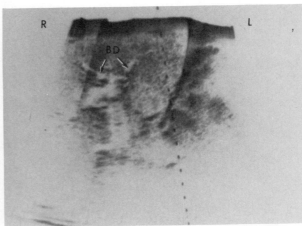

Fig 9-73.

Fig 9-74.

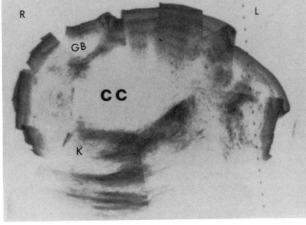

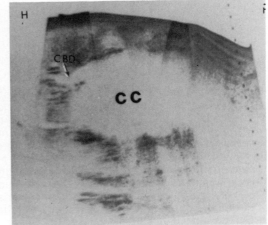

Fig 9-75.

Figs 9-72 to 9-79. — Choledochal cyst. In this example of choledochal cyst, a variety of imaging modalities are illustrated to show how they provide many similar findings. On upper gastrointestinal series (Fig 9-72), mass effect on duodenal sweep is evident *(arrows)*. Actual organ of origin of mass is unclear from this study. Ultrasonograms (Figs 9-73 to 9-75) demonstrate dilated intrahepatic bile ducts as well as large right upper quadrant cystic mass separate from gallbladder and seemingly in communication with common bile duct. Nevertheless, it is unclear without better identification of duodenum or pancreas what exact cause of mass is.

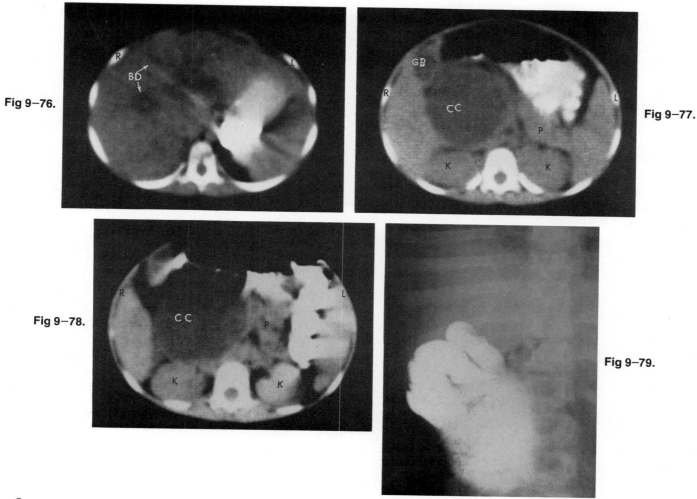

Fig 9–76.

Fig 9–77.

Fig 9–78.

Fig 9–79.

On computed tomograms (Figs 9–76 to 9–78) intrahepatic bile duct dilatation is again documented, as is the large cystic mass separate from gallbladder in right upper quadrant. Pancreas is visualized better and mass does not enhance following intravenous contrast injection. Additional information is provided by location of mass medial to duodenal sweep. Nevertheless, it is still uncertain whether this indeed represents pancreatic or biliary abnormality.

Final confirmation in this case came at surgery during operative cholangiogram (Fig 9–79). Percutaneous transhepatic cholangiogram could have provided same information preoperatively. R = right; L = left; H = head; F = feet; BD = bile ducts; GB = gallbladder; CC = choledochal cyst; K = kidney; CBD = common bile duct; P = pancreas; S = spleen.

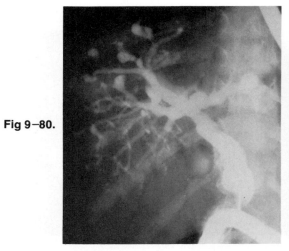

Fig 9–80.

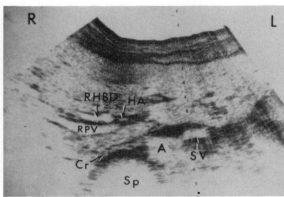

Fig 9–81.

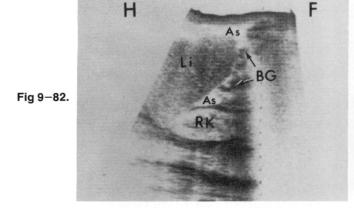

Fig 9–82.

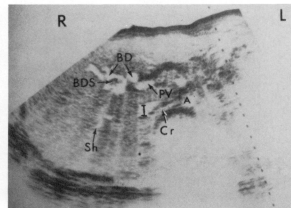

Fig 9–83.

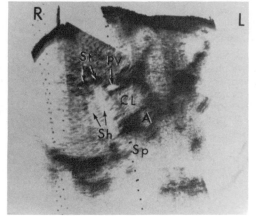

Fig 9–84.

224

Figs 9–80 to 9–84. – Congenital ductal ectasia. Dilatation of intrahepatic bile ducts can be demonstrated by variety of techniques (Figs 9–80 and 9–81). Most accurate method is direct visualization of bile ducts. There are 2 distinct forms of biliary ductal ectasia. More common one is associated with periportal fibrosis and cirrhosis of liver (Fig 9–82). Patients may have ascites and other complications of portal hypertension. In less common form (Caroli's disease) there is no associated periportal fibrosis. Patients do not develop jaundice or abdominal pain when calculi develop (Figs 9–83 and 9–84), with or without resultant cholangitis.

Both forms are commonly associated with renal abnormalities similar to medullary sponge kidney. However, in contrast to polycystic disease of liver, renal involvement in biliary ductal ectasia does not influence prognosis. R = right; L = left; H = head; F = foot; Sp = spine; Cr = crus of diaphragm; A = aorta; SV = splenic vein; RPV = right portal vein; RHBD = right hepatic bile duct; HA = hepatic artery; RK = right kidney; As = ascites; BG = bowel gas; Li = liver; PV = portal vein; I = inferior vena cava; BD = bile ducts; BDS = bile duct stones; Sh = shadowing; CL = caudate lobe of liver; St = stones.

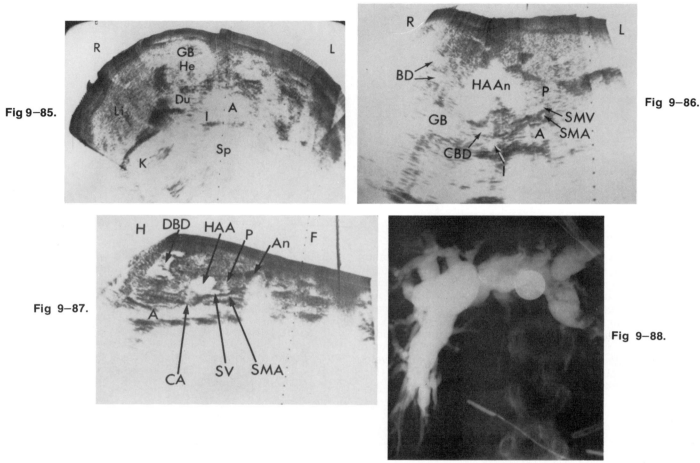

Fig 9–85.

Fig 9–86.

Fig 9–87.

Fig 9–88.

Figs 9–85 to 9–90. — Hepatic artery aneurysm. Although most cases of obstructive jaundice in children are related to abnormalities of biliary system or pancreas, occasionally other organ systems may be responsible. In this rare case of hepatic artery aneurysm, diagnosis was possible after careful anatomical analysis of ultrasonograms (Figs 9–85 to 9–87). On lower transverse scan of abdomen, enlarged gallbladder filled with inhomogeneous echoes consistent with either gangrenous gallbladder, gallbladder tumor or gallbladder hematoma was observed (see Fig 9–85). In higher transverse scan, dilated intrahepatic bile ducts were seen and sausage-shaped fluid mass was identified in anterolateral aspect of head of pancreas separate from common bile duct and gallbladder (see Fig 9–86). Anatomically, this is an appropriate location for hepatic artery; however, one cannot completely rule out choledochal cyst or pancreatic pseudocyst. On midline longitudinal scan, this fluid area can be seen to be in direct communication with celiac artery (see Fig 9–87). Transhepatic cholangiogram confirms dilatation of intrahepatic biliary system and obstruction of common hepatic duct (Fig 9–88).

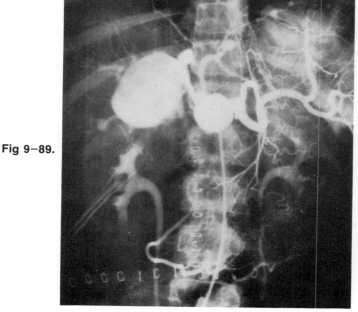

Fig 9–89.

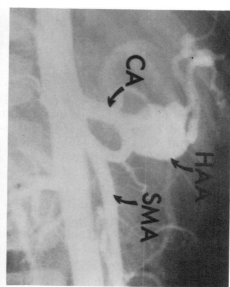

Fig 9–90.

Two films from subsequent angiogram correlate re-markably well anatomically with ultrasonogram and demon-strate not only aneurysm near origin of hepatic artery but multiple aneurysms throughout hepatic arterial system (Figs 9–89 and 9–90). This was a 15-year-old patient with Kawa-saki's disease, aneurysms involving hepatic arterial and cor-onary arterial systems. R = right; L = left; H = head; F = feet; GB He = gallbladder hematoma; Li = liver; Du = duo-denum; K = kidney; Sp = spine; I = inferior vena cava; A = aorta; BD = bile ducts; HAAn and HAA = hepatic artery aneurysm; GB = gallbladder; CBD = common bile duct; SMV = superior mesenteric vein; SMA = superior mesen-teric artery; P = pancreas; DBD = dilated bile ducts; An = antrum of stomach; SV = splenic vein; CA = celiac artery.

10

Pancreas

THE PANCREAS DEVELOPS FROM THE ENDODERMAL CELLS arising from the most caudal portion of the foregut. Two pancreatic buds develop about the 4th week of embryonic life. The dorsal bud develops first and grows rapidly into the dorsal mesentery; the smaller ventral bud develops near the entry of the common bile duct into the duodenum. Each bud has its own duct. When the duodenum grows and rotates to the right, the ventral bud is carried into the dorsal mesentery, where it fuses with the dorsal bud. The ventral bud forms the uncinate process and the inferior part of the head of the pancreas. The dorsal bud forms the remainder of the pancreas. As the pancreatic buds fuse, the ducts anastomose; the main pancreatic duct (Wirsung) is formed by fusion of the short ventral duct with the distal portion of the dorsal duct. The proximal portion of the dorsal duct forms the accessory pancreatic duct (Santorini).

The pancreatic parenchyma originates from endoderm which forms a network of primitive ducts. Acini develop from clusters of cells around the ends of the ducts, and the islets of Langerhans develop between the acini. The acinar cells provide the exocrine function of the pancreas, while the islets of Langerhans provide the endocrine function. The islets of Langerhans are composed of 3 cell types: β, α and δ cells that produce insulin, glucagon and gastrin, respectively.

Evaluation of the pancreas by any imaging modality requires a thorough understanding of its anatomical boundaries. The head of the pancreas lies anterior to the 2d and 3d lumbar vertebrae; the body lies in the region of the 1st lumbar vertebra. The duodenal bulb lies above and anterior, while the 2d portion of the duodenum lies lateral and slightly posterior to the head of the pancreas. The common bile duct (which runs in the free border of the hepatoduodenal ligament) is also closely related to the posterolateral aspect of the pancreatic head. The 3d portion of the duodenum passes below and slightly posterior to the head of the pancreas; the 4th portion lies to the left and anterior to the uncinate process. The transverse colon is anterior to the head of the pancreas, and the roentgenographic splenic flexure of the colon is related to the inferior margin of the body and the anterior surface of the pancreatic tail. The major part of the anterior surface of the pancreas lies adjacent to the posterior wall of the stomach, being separated from it by the potential space of the lesser peritoneal sac. The spleen is posterior and lateral to the tail of the pancreas; the superior pole of the left kidney is posterior to the body of the pancreas; the left adrenal gland lies directly posterior to the junction of the body and tail of the pancreas.

Close attention to the vascular anatomy of the upper abdomen is of particular value in evaluating the pancreas by ultrasonography and computerized axial tomography. The inferior vena cava passes behind the head of the pancreas. The left renal vein courses behind the head, uncinate process and body of the pancreas and over the aorta; the right renal vein passes behind the head of the gland. The splenic vein courses transversely along the posterosuperior aspect of the body and tail of the pancreas; the superior mesenteric vein ascends anterior to the uncinate process and joins the splenic vein to become the portal vein.

The aorta lies behind the body of the pancreas. The celiac axis arises from the anterior aspect of the aorta at the superior border of the body of the pancreas. The splenic and hepatic arteries arise from the celiac axis at this level and course to the left and right, respectively. The superior mesenteric artery arises from the anterior aspect of the aorta below the origin of the celiac axis and, at its origin, lies posterior to the neck of the pancreas coursing inferiorly and ventrally, anterior to the uncinate process and 3d portion of the duodenum.

CONGENITAL ANOMALIES OF THE PANCREAS

The ductal system of the pancreas may show several anatomical variations. In the majority of cases, the duct of Wirsung and common bile duct form a single channel, and the duct of Santorini is present and communicates with the main pancreatic duct. The duct of Santorini forms the main pancreatic duct in about 2–10% of individuals.

Congenital anomalies of the pancreatic tissue are rare, with the exception of 2 entities: annular pancreas and ectopic pancreatic tissue.

Annular Pancreas

Annular pancreas is the most common congenital anomaly of the pancreas, and is characterized by a band of pancreatic tissue completely or incompletely encircling the 2d portion of the duodenum at or just above the ampulla of Vater. Embryologically, an annular pancreas results from failure of the ventral pancreatic bud to rotate dorsally and fuse with the dorsal bud. Embryological development of the pancreas clearly demonstrates that the normal development of the gland is dependent on the normal development of the duodenum. Hence, it is logical to deduce that annular pancreas is secondary to failure of normal development of the duodenum (always associated with intrinsic stenosis or atresia of the duodenum) and

not an isolated finding. Patients present at varying ages, depending on the degree of duodenal obstruction.

Ectopic Pancreas

Aberrant ectopic tissue may be distributed anywhere along the alimentary tract. It is most commonly found as a submucosal lesion in the gastric antrum or duodenal bulb. However, it may occur in the esophagus, jejunum, ileum, spleen, liver, gallbladder or lungs. The majority of patients with ectopic pancreatic tissue are asymptomatic, but occasionally they may have associated abdominal pain, vomiting or pyloric obstruction. It has also been reported in patients with hypoglycemia, jaundice, diabetes, neutropenia and metaphyseal chondrodysplasia. Roentgenographically, the lesion is a small (less than 2.5 cm) filling defect that may show a central umbilication indicating the orifice of the duct draining the ectopic pancreatic tissue. Multiple lesions have been described and are potentially subject to all the pathological processes that involve the pancreas.

Another anomaly, foregut duplication of the pancreas, is a duplication sac lined by gastric epithelium, containing a well-defined ductal system that connects with the pancreas.

Congenital Atresia of the Pancreatic Duct

The distal part of the pancreatic duct is completely occluded, with marked cystic dilatation of the duct proximal to this obstruction. The parenchyma of the gland is atrophic and fibrotic, similar to that seen in cystic fibrosis. However, in cystic fibrosis the clinical onset is after the 2d month of life. Congenital atresia of the pancreatic duct may be related to a less severe form of stenosis of the sphincter of Oddi or pancreatic duct, which have been described as rare causes of childhood pancreatitis.

PANCREATITIS

Primary inflammatory diseases of the pancreas are uncommon in children.

Acute Pancreatitis

Acute pancreatitis is more common than chronic relapsing pancreatitis. Since one third of children with acute pancreatitis have signs suggestive of an acute surgical condition of the abdomen, and surgery may be detrimental to such patients, it is important to make an accurate diagnosis and initiate conservative treatment. Ultrasonography or computerized axial tomography will usually establish or confirm the diagnosis of acute pancreatitis and may also be able to demonstrate the possible etiological factors. Unlike adults, in whom pancreatitis is most often associated with alcoholism or hepatobiliary disease, in children a variety of factors may be responsible. The causes of acute pancreatitis in children may be divided into 7 categories:

1. *Infectious.* Most of these patients have associated acute tonsillitis or otitis media; other causes include bacteremia and generalized peritonitis. Pancreatitis may occur as a complication of mumps 4–5 days following the onset of the parotid enlargement. In rare instances, only the pancreas may be involved.

2. *Obstructive.* In this group of patients, acute pancreatitis is usually the result of obstruction of the pancreatic or biliary ducts. Obstruction of the pancreatic duct may be the result of congenital stenosis or ascariasis. Obstruction of the biliary tract may be the result of lithiasis or congenital stenosis of the sphincter of Oddi. Of the causes mentioned above, the most common is obstruction of the pancreatic duct by the ascaris worm.

3. *Metabolic, toxic or chemical.* Various causes in this category include steroid therapy, immunosuppressive drugs, nutritional disturbances (such as kwashiorkor) and cirrhosis of the liver. Although diabetic coma was a major cause of pancreatitis in the past, excellent medical prevention of diabetic coma has made this an infrequent cause.

4. *Traumatic.* Included in this category are blunt trauma secondary to accidents or child battering, and postoperative causes secondary to surgical trauma. Pseudocysts of the pancreas constitute a common complication.

5. *Vascular.* Vascular disease does not seem to play a significant role in pediatric patients. There has been, however, a report of pancreatitis in a patient with periarteritis nodosa secondary to vasculitis and thrombosis of the pancreatic blood vessels.

6. *Allergic.* In some instances allergy may play a role in the development of pancreatitis.

7. *Idiopathic.* If no cause of pancreatitis is ascertained, it is assumed to be idiopathic.

Regardless of the cause, patients present with abdominal pain, vomiting, fever, leukocytosis and, occasionally, jaundice. Shortness of breath may be associated with pleural effusions or elevation of the diaphragm secondary to ascites. Delayed symptoms of polyarthritis and subcutaneous nodules associated with intramedullary fat necrosis also have been reported.

Recurring Chronic Pancreatitis

Recurrent chronic pancreatitis is assumed to be a disease of adults, rarely occurring in children. In recent years, however, recognition of hereditary pancreatitis as a major cause of recurrent chronic pancreatitis in the 1st decade of life has altered this concept. Differential diagnosis of recurrent pancreatitis in children includes hereditary pancreatitis, ascariasis, hereditary hyperparathyroidism, hyperlipoproteinemia, cystic fibrosis and idiopathic pancreatitis.

HEREDITARY PANCREATITIS. — Hereditary pancreatitis is the most common cause of recurrent pancreatitis in childhood. It is transmitted as an autosomal dominant condition and is characterized by recurring episodes of severe abdominal pain. The underlying defect in hereditary pancreatitis is unknown but is unlikely to be the result of an inborn error of metabolism. It may be the result of an anatomical defect, such as stenosis of the pancreatic duct or hypertrophy of the sphincter of Oddi. Pathologically, the pancreas shows extensive interstitial fibrosis with near-total loss of acinar tissue but relative preservation of islet cells and evidence of dilatation of major and minor ducts. The pathological picture is similar to that commonly seen in cystic fibrosis.

Although the onset of hereditary pancreatitis is in early childhood, the disease may not be recognized until adult life, when pancreatic calcification, pancreatic insufficiency and intestinal malabsorption occur. Episodes of abdominal pain may occur as often as twice a month, or with symptom-free intervals of several years. Each exacerbation lasts 1–3 days and is similar to those in chronic recurring pancreatitis in adults. However, in hereditary pancreatitis, in addition to a family history there are definite differences, such as age of onset (earlier), absence of other etiological factors (alcoholism or gallstones) and an equal sex incidence. All reported cases of hereditary pancreatitis have been in whites. When pancreatic calcification develops, patients are at greater risk for the development of pancreatic carcinoma. It appears that extensive chronic inflammation (manifested by pancreatic calcification) predisposes to the development of pancreatic malignancy in adult life. Other causes of pancreatic calcification include cystic fibrosis, alcoholism, hyperparathyroidism, kwashiorkor and idiopathic pancreatic calcification.

ASCARIASIS.—This condition may cause pancreatic duct obstruction with secondary pancreatitis but it is rare in the United States.

HEREDITARY HYPERPARATHYROIDISM.—This is an autosomal dominant disease that may cause recurrent pancreatitis. However, only a small number of patients with hereditary hyperparathyroidism have recurrent pancreatitis in childhood.

FAMILIAL HYPERLIPOPROTEINEMIA.—This is another rare cause of recurrent pancreatitis in childhood. The disease is probably inherited as an autosomal recessive and in the pediatric age group is the result of lipoprotein lipase deficiency.

CYSTIC FIBROSIS.—Cystic fibrosis is a hereditary disease that probably is due to an inborn error of metabolism; it is transmitted as a mendelian recessive trait and is associated with generalized dysfunction of the exocrine glands. The triad of chronic pulmonary disease, pancreatic insufficiency and elevation of sweat chloride levels is present in most of these patients. The disease is fairly common and is most often seen in whites; it is rare in blacks. About 80% of patients with cystic fibrosis have complete exocrine pancreatic deficiency; 10% have a partial pancreatic enzyme deficiency; and 10% have no clinical or laboratory evidence of pancreatic deficiency.

Hepatic cirrhosis, intestinal obstruction, nasal polyps, sinusitis, rectal prolapse, hypertrophic pulmonary osteoarthopathy and retarded growth and maturation are some of the other manifestations of cystic fibrosis. Most of the symptoms are probably due to obstruction of the organ passages (such as bronchioles, pancreatic ducts and biliary ducts) as a result of thick mucus production. In about 15% of patients, meconium ileus is present at birth. The meconium ileus equivalent may be seen in older children and is probably related to cessation of exogenous pancreatic enzyme therapy. The small bowel and colon appear abnormal in contrast studies, with the small bowel showing thickened mucosal folds and the colon showing multiple small filling defects.

Except for rare calcifications secondary to pancreatitis, cystic fibrosis produces no demonstrable roentgenographic findings localized to the pancreas. In contrast, ultrasonography and computerized tomography clearly demonstrate the gross pathological changes in the pancreas. Pathologically, the pancreas is small, thinner and firmer than normal. The pancreatic ducts are dilated and there is secondary degeneration of the parenchyma. After several years, the pancreas becomes atrophic, fibrotic and replaced with fat. The islets of Langerhans are usually normal. Most of the pathological changes are thought to be secondary to obstruction of the glands and ducts by accumulation and precipitation of abnormal secretions (e.g., pancreas and intrahepatic bile ducts). Ultrasonographically, the pancreas may be markedly echogenic, with dilatation of the main pancreatic duct.

GENETIC PANCREATIC DEFICIENCIES NOT DUE TO CYSTIC FIBROSIS. — Although most of the children with pancreatic achylia have cystic fibrosis, several other entities have been recognized in which pancreatic insufficiency is a part of the clinical picture.

Congenital hypoplasia of the exocrine pancreas associated with pancreatic achylia and malnutrition has been described in patients who have fatty replacement of the pancreas but no evidence of fibrosis or ductal dilatation. Another form has been reported in patients with pancreatic achylia, short stature and hematologic abnormalities such as anemia, thrombocytopenia and neutropenia (Schwachman-Diamond syndrome). All these patients have had normal sweat tests with no pulmonary disease. Metaphyseal dysostosis, Hirschsprung's disease and hepatic fibrosis have been present in some of these patients.

Trypsinogen deficiency (reported in 2 infants), enterokinase deficiency (reported in 3 infants) and pancreatic deficiency associated with Klinefelter's syndrome are other extremely rare forms of pancreatic deficiency.

CYSTS OF THE PANCREAS

Congenital Cysts

Congenital pancreatic cysts are extremely rare and of unknown etiology. They may be solitary or multiple. Multiple asymptomatic cysts are frequently associated with polycystic disease of the kidney and liver.

Pseudocysts

Pseudocysts lack an epithelial lining, are usually unilocular and are the result of blunt abdominal trauma (accident or battered child) in as many as 50–75%
of patients. They are the result of a collection of necrotic tissue, blood and pancreatic secretions that extrude from the pancreas following an injury and usually loculate in the lesser sac. Occasionally, these contents may dissect into the mediastinum or retroperitoneum. The inflammatory reaction that follows encapsulates the pseudocyst with a fibrous wall.

Other causes of pseudocysts include the various causes of pancreatitis mentioned above. The age range of children reported with pseudocysts varies from 6 months to 15 years. The majority of the patients are boys. The diagnosis of a pseudocyst should be suspected in any child that has abdominal pain, vomiting and an abdominal mass following trauma. Since there may be associated injuries to adjacent organs, such as the kidney, liver and spleen, these organs should be carefully screened initially by ultrasonography. Because the body and tail, rather than the head, of the pancreas are in close proximity to the vertebrae, they are more often affected by blunt abdominal trauma.

TUMORS OF THE PANCREAS

Carcinoma of the pancreas is rare in children but has been reported as early as 3 months of age. Initial symptoms are usually an abdominal mass, enlarged liver, weight loss, jaundice and distal metastases. The tumor may arise from the ducts or islets of Langerhans. Carcinomas of the islet cells are rarely functional but may cause hypoglycemia.

A cystadenoma of the pancreas is rare at any age, but particularly in children. They are usually multilocular cystic neoplasms that are manifested as a large abdominal mass with displacement of adjacent organs.

Adenomas of the islets of Langerhans may or may not have hormonal function. Since most of the tumors in children are small, they are difficult to detect. Angiographically, islet cell tumors of any type show as a round, well-circumscribed, dense staining during the capillary and venous phase.

Functioning islet cell tumors can give rise to a number of clinical syndromes, such as the following:

1. *Hyperinsulinism.* The majority of islet cell neoplasms associated with excessive secretion of insulin are benign adenomas. The predominant cellular constituent is the β cell. In some cases, adenomas of other endocrine glands are also present, which is termed multiple endocrine adenomatosis (Wermer's syndrome). Multiple endocrine adenomatosis is characterized by adenomas of the parathyroid glands, pancreas and pituitary gland and is probably inherited as an autosomal dominant trait. This syndrome usually manifests itself in the 3d or 4th decade of life.

2. *Zollinger-Ellison syndrome.* This syndrome is characterized by peptic ulcers secondary to excessive gastric secretion and islet cell tumors. In contrast to insulinomas, over half of these tumors are malignant. The tumor originates from the non-β-cell component of the islet cells and is usually located in the body or tail of the gland.

3. *Pancreatic cholera.* These patients have non-β-cell tumors of the pancreas but no evidence of excessive gastrin activity or peptic ulcers. They have overwhelming diarrhea and electrolyte imbalance.

4. *Glucagon-producing islet cell tumors.* These tumors appear to derive from α cells and produce glucagon, which causes hyperglycemia and diabetes.

REFERENCES

Arey, J. B.: Tumors of the Pancreas, in Nelson, W. E. (ed.): *Textbook of Pediatrics* (Philadelphia: W. B. Saunders Co., 1975).

Barkin, J., et al.: Computerized tomography, diagnostic ultrasound, and radionuclide scanning: Comparison of efficacy in diagnosis of pancreatic carcinoma, J.A.M.A. 238: 2040, 1977.

Belber, J. P., et al.: Fusion anomalies of the pancreatic ductal system: Differentiation from pathologic states, Radiology 123:637, 1977.

Berenson, J. E., et al.: The abdominal fat necrosis sign, Radiology 100:567, 1971.

Blumenthal, H. T., et al.: Acute pancreatitis in the newborn, in infancy and in childhood, Am. Surg. 27:533, 1961.

Bongiovi, J. J., et al.: Pancreatic pseudocyst occurring in the battered-child syndrome, J. Pediatr. Surg. 4:220, 1969.

Buchta, R. M., et al.: Zollinger-Ellison syndrome in a 9-year-old child: A case report and review of this entity in childhood, Pediatrics 47:594, 1971.

Carroll, B., et al.: Pancreatic cystadenocarcinoma: CT body scan and gray-scale ultrasound appearance, A.J.R. 131: 339, 1978.

Clouse, M. E., et al.: Subselective angiography in localizing insulinomas of the pancreas, A.J.R. 128:741, 1977.

Conrad, M. R., et al.: Pancreatic pseudocysts: Unusual ultrasound features, A.J.R. 130:265, 1978.

Crade, M., et al.: Water distension of the gut in the evaluation of the pancreas by ultrasound, A.J.R. 131:348, 1978.

DeGraaff, C. S., et al.: Gray-scale echography of the pancreas: Re-evaluation of normal size, Radiology 129:157, 1978.

DiMagno, E. P., et al.: A prospective comparison of current diagnostic tests for pancreatic cancer, N. Engl. J. Med. 297:737, 1977.

Di Sant' Agnese, P. A.: The Pancreas, in Nelson, W. E. (ed.): *Textbook of Pediatrics* (Philadelphia: W. B. Saunders Co., 1975).

Di Sant' Agnese, P. A., et al.: Pathogenesis and physiopathology of cystic fibrosis of the pancreas: Fibrocystic disease of the pancreas (mucoviscidosis), N. Engl. J. Med. 277:1287, 1967.

Di Sant' Agnese, P. A., et al.: Pathogenesis and physiopathology of cystic fibrosis of the pancreas (continued): Fibrocystic disease of the pancreas (mucoviscidosis), N. Engl. J. Med. 277:1344, 1967.

Di Sant' Agnese, P. A., et al.: Pathogenesis and physiopathology of cystic fibrosis of the pancreas (concluded): Fibrocystic disease of the pancreas (mucoviscidosis), N. Engl. J. Med. 277:1399, 1967.

Doust, B. D., et al.: Gray-scale ultrasonic properties of the normal and inflamed pancreas, Radiology 120:653, 1976.

Eaton, S. B., et al.: *Radiology of the Pancreas and Duodenum* (Philadelphia: W. B. Saunders Co., 1973).

Eklof, O., et al.: Ectopic pancreas, Pediatr. Radiol. 1:24, 1973.

Feinberg, S. B., et al.: Comparison of ultrasound pancreatic scanning and endoscopic retrograde cholangiopancreatograms: A retrospective study, J. Clin. Ultrasound 5: 96, 1977.

Fellman, K., et al.: Unusual bone changes in exocrine pancreas insufficiency with cyclic neutropenia, Acta Radiol. Diagn. 12:428, 1972.

Filly, R. A., et al.: Echographic diagnosis of pancreatic lesions: Ultrasound scanning techniques and diagnostic findings, Radiology 96:575, 1970.

Frey, C., et al.: Inflammatory lesions of the pancreas in infancy and childhood, Pediatrics 32:93, 1963.

Galligan, J. J., et al.: Pancreatic pseudocysts in childhood, Am. J. Dis. Child. 112:479, 1966.

Ghorashi, B., et al.: Gray-scale sonographic anatomy of the pancreas, J. Clin. Ultrasound 5:25, 1977.

Goldberg, B. B., et al.: Ultrasonic evaluation of masses in pediatric patients, A.J.R. 116:677, 1972.

Goldstein, H. M., et al.: Prone view ultrasonography for pancreatic tail neoplasms, A.J.R. 131:231, 1978.

Gosink, B. B., et al.: The dilated pancreatic duct: Ultrasonic evaluation, Radiology 126:475, 1978.

Grosfeld, J. L., et al.: Pancreatic and gastrointestinal trauma in children, Pediatr. Clin. North Am. 22:365, 1975.

Gross, J. B., et al.: Hereditary pancreatitis: Description of a 5th kindred and summary of clinical features, Am. J. Med. 33:358, 1962.

Haaga, J. R., et al.: Computed tomography of the pancreas, Radiology 120:589, 1976.

Harris, R. D., et al.: Aneurysms of the small pancreatic arteries: A cause of upper abdominal pain and intestinal bleeding, Radiology 115:17, 1975.

Kalwinsky, D., et al.: Pancreatitis presenting as unexplained ascites, Am. J. Dis. Child. 128:734, 1974.

Kattwinkel, J., et al.: Hereditary pancreatitis: Three new kindreds and a critical review of the literature, Pediatrics 51:55, 1973.

Keating, J. P., et al.: Pancreatitis and osteolytic lesions, J. Pediatr. 81:350, 1972.

Kilman, J. W., et al.: Pancreatic pseudocysts in infancy and childhood, Surgery 55:455, 1964.

Kirchner, S. G., et al.: Pancreatic pseudocyst of the mediastinum, Radiology 123:37, 1977.

Kreel, L.: Computerized tomography of the pancreas, J. Comput. Tomogr. 1:287, 1977.

Kreel, L., et al.: Computed tomography of the normal pancreas, J. Comput. Assist. Tomogr. 1:290, 1977.

Kressel, H. Y., et al.: CT scanning and ultrasound in the evaluation of pancreatic pseudocysts: A preliminary comparison, Radiology 126:153, 1978.

Lawson, T. L.: Sensitivity of pancreatic ultrasonography in the detection of pancreatic disease, Radiology 128:733, 1978.

Lee, J. K. T., et al.: Pancreatic imaging by ultrasound and computed tomography: A general review, Radiol. Clin. North Am. 17:105, 1979.

Leopold, G. R.: Pancreatic echography: A new dimension in the diagnosis of pseudocyst, Radiology 104:365, 1972.

Levin, D. C., et al.: Arteriography in the evaluation of pancreatic pseudocysts, A.J.R. 129:243, 1977.

Lucaya, J., et al.: Ectopic pancreas in the stomach, J. Pediatr. Surg. 11:101, 1976.

MacMahon, H., et al.: Erect scanning of pancreas using a gastric window, A.J.R. 132:587, 1979.

Mah, P-T., et al.: Pancreatic acinar cell carcinoma in childhood, Am. J. Dis. Child. 128:101, 1974.

Meyers, M. A., et al.: Effects of pancreatitis on the small bowel and colon: Spread along mesenteric planes, A.J.R. 119:151, 1973.

Moss, A. A., et al.: The effect of Gastrografin and glucagon on CT scanning of the pancreas: A blind clinical trial, Radiology 126:711, 1978.

Moynan, R. W., et al.: Pancreatic carcinoma in childhood, J. Pediatr. 65:711, 1964.

Nelman, H. L., et al.: Angiographic features of peripancreatic malignant lymphoma, Radiology 115:589, 1975.

Pena, S. D. J., et al.: Child abuse and traumatic pseudocyst of the pancreas, J. Pediatr. 83:1026, 1973.

Rickham, P. P.: Islet cell tumors in childhood, J. Pediatr. Surg. 10:83, 1975.

Sarti, D. A.: Rapid development and spontaneous regression of pancreatic pseudocysts documented by ultrasound, Radiology 125:789, 1977.

Seidelmann, F. E., et al.: CT demonstration of the splenic vein-pancreatic relationship: The pseudodilated pancreatic duct, A.J.R. 129:17, 1977.

Seymour, E. Q.: Unreliability of an increased gastrocolic measurement in the diagnosis of acute pancreatitis, Radiology 123:527, 1977.

Shwachman, H., et al.: Recurrent acute pancreatitis in patients with cystic fibrosis with normal pancreatic enzymes, Pediatrics 55:86, 1975.

Singleton, E. B., et al.: Radiologic evaluation of pancreatic disease in children, Semin. Roentgenol. 3:267, 1968.

Stephens, D. H., et al.: Diagnosis and evaluation of retroperitoneal tumors by computed tomography, A.J.R. 129:395, 1977.

Taybi, H., et al.: Metaphyseal dysostosis and the associated syndrome of pancreatic insufficiency and blood disorders, Radiology 93:563, 1969.

Viamonte, M.: Morphologic-radiographic correlations of the pancreas, Radiol. Clin. North Am. 17:119, 1979.

Weill, F., et al.: Ultrasonography of the normal pancreas, Radiology 123:417, 1977.

Weistein, D. P., et al.: Ultrasonic demonstration of the pancreatic duct: An analysis of 41 cases, Radiology 130:729, 1979.

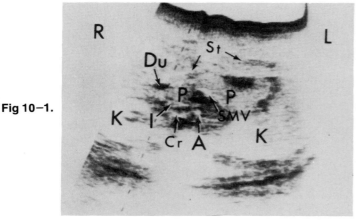

Fig 10–1.

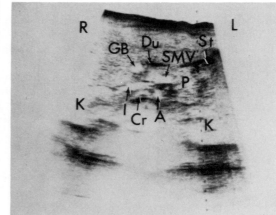

Fig 10–2.

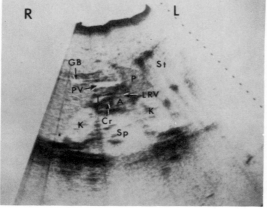

Fig 10–3.

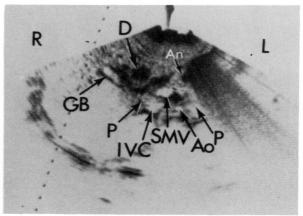

Fig 10–4.

Figs 10–1 to 10–4.—Normal neonatal pancreas. Normal pancreas can usually be seen in the neonate. In transverse scans by angling the transducer caudally, using the left lobe of liver as acoustic window, segments of body and tail of pancreas can usually be visualized. Close attention should be paid to various vascular landmarks, including superior mesenteric vein, portal vein and superior mesenteric artery (Figs 10–1 and 10–2). One may also see left renal vein coursing between superior mesenteric artery and aorta (Fig 10–3). It is always important to delineate as much of stomach and duodenal bulb as possible as these may mimic masses of pancreas (Fig 10–4).

Normal echogenicity of neonatal pancreas is very similar to liver. Occasionally pancreas is slightly more echogenic than liver in this age group. R = right; L = left; Du = duodenum; K = kidney; St = stomach; P = pancreas; I and IVC = inferior vena cava; Cr = crus of diaphragm; A and Ao = aorta; SMV = superior mesenteric vein; LRV = left renal vein; PV = portal vein; GB = gallbladder; D = duodenal bulb; Sp = spine; An = antrum.

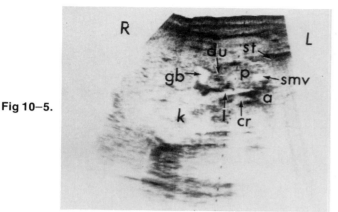

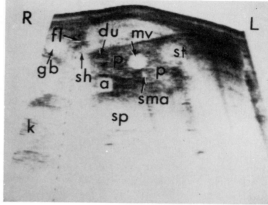

Fig 10–5.

Fig 10–6.

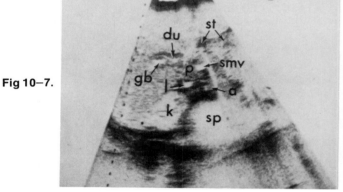

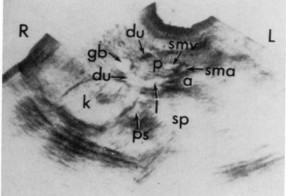

Fig 10–7.

Fig 10–8.

Figs 10–5 to 10–8. — Normal neonatal pancreas. Head of pancreas may also be visualized in the neonate but requires even closer anatomical analysis; specifically, gallbladder, superior mesenteric vein, superior mesenteric artery, inferior vena cava and aorta should be identified. Most difficult aspect of head of pancreas to define is right lateral margin. In neonate precise landmarks of common bile duct and gastroduodenal artery cannot usually be visualized. Therefore, duodenal sweep is used to define lateral margin of pancreas, in the form of echogenic mucosa or acoustical shadowing secondary to intraluminal gas in 1st or 2d portion of duodenum. R = right; L = left; gb = gallbladder; du = duodenum; st = stomach; p = pancreas; smv = superior mesenteric vein; a = aorta; k = kidney; l = inferior vena cava; cr = crus of diaphragm; sp = spine; sma = superior mesenteric artery; sh = shadowing; fl = falciform ligament; mv = mesenteric vein; ps = psoas muscle.

Fig 10–9.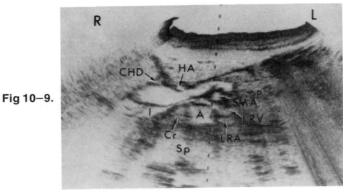

Fig 10–10.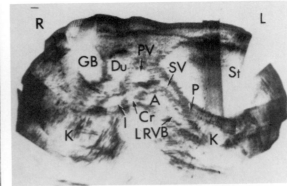

Fig 10–11.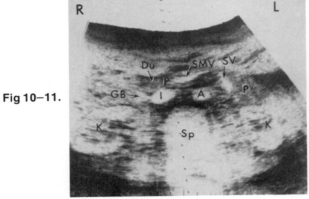

Fig 10–12.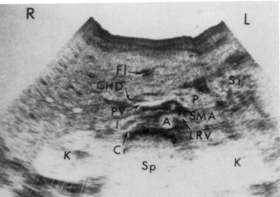

Figs 10–9 to 10–12.—Normal pancreas in older child. Similar type of anatomical analysis is used to identify pancreas in older child. In body-tail region, careful attention to vascular landmarks, including hepatic artery, portal vein, splenic vein, superior mesenteric artery, left renal vein and left renal artery, are necessary for proper identification. Gas in stomach remains a problem. More recently, utilizing oral fluid and rescanning with patient in upright position has enabled better visualization of body-tail region of pancreas. Similarly, if one is able to scan prone with water tank system now commercially available, many problems related to gas in stomach can be avoided. R = right; L = left; CHD = common hepatic duct; HA = hepatic artery; I = inferior vena cava; SMA = superior mesenteric artery; A = aorta; Cr = crus of diaphragm; Sp = spine; LRA = left renal artery; LRV = left renal vein; P = pancreas; St = stomach; GB = gallbladder; Du = duodenum; PV = portal vein; K = kidney; LRVB = left renal vascular bundle; SV = splenic vein; SMV = superior mesenteric vein; Fl = falciform ligament.

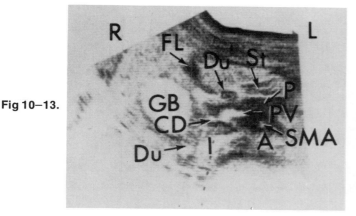

Fig 10–13.

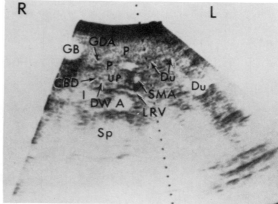

Fig 10–14.

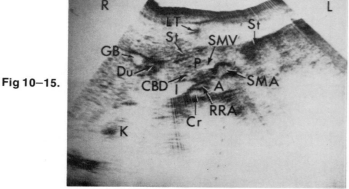

Fig 10–15.

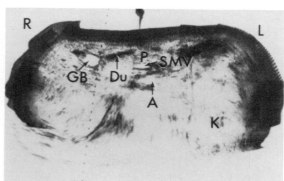

Fig 10–16.

Figs 10–13 to 10–16.—Normal pancreas in older child. Head of normal pancreas can usually be well demonstrated in older child. Medial aspect of head is identified by surrounding vascular landmarks, including superior mesenteric vein, superior mesenteric artery, portal vein, inferior vena cava, left renal vein and aorta. Most difficult portion of pancreas to define is lateral aspect of head. Sonographic patterns of duodenal sweep can be utilized but, in addition, gastroduodenal artery and common bile duct may be identified in older children. Gas within duodenal bulb may still be a problem in some children, but using oral fluids and various patient positions usually enables adequate visualization of the lateral margin of pancreas. R = right; L = left; FL = falciform ligament; Du = duodenum; St = stomach; P = pancreas; GB = gallbladder; CD = common duct; PV = portal vein; SMA = superior mesenteric artery; A = aorta; I = inferior vena cava; GDA = gastroduodenal artery; CBD = common bile duct; UP = uncinate process of pancreas; LRV = left renal vein; DW = duct of Wirsung; SMV = superior mesenteric vein; LT = ligamentum teres; Cr = crus of diaphragm; RRA = right renal artery; K = kidney; Sp = spine.

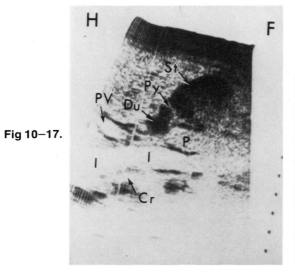

Fig 10–17.

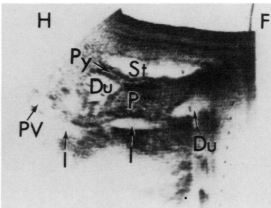

Fig 10–18.

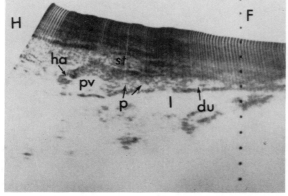

Fig 10–19.

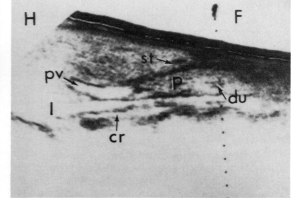

Fig 10–20.

Figs 10–17 to 10–20.—Normal pancreas. Longitudinal scans are equally important in defining various aspects of pancreas. Cephalic margin of pancreatic head is best defined by the point where portal vein almost touches inferior vena cava. Posterior aspect of pancreatic head is usually related to inferior vena cava. Anterior and inferior margins of pancreatic head are best identified by localizing stomach and duodenal sweep. These may have a variety of patterns, including totally mucus echogenic pattern, fluid-type pattern if fluid techniques are utilized and bull's-eye-type pattern. H = head; F = feet; PV = portal vein; I = inferior vena cava; Cr = crus of diaphragm; Du = duodenum; Py = pylorus; St = stomach; P = pancreas; ha = hepatic artery.

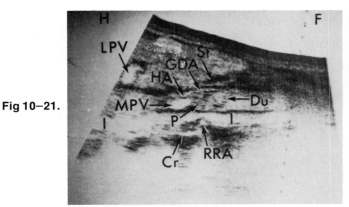

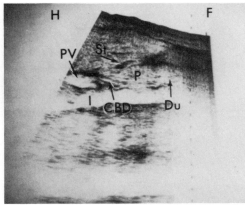

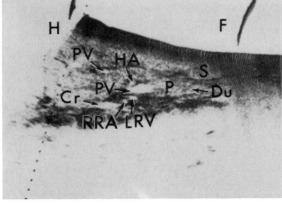

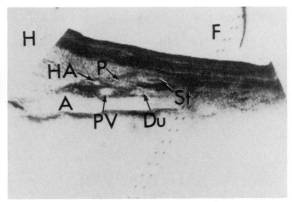

Figs 10–21. **Fig 10–22.**

Fig 10–23. **Fig 10–24.**

Figs 10–21 to 10–24.—Normal pancreas. In older child, head of pancreas can be further defined on longitudinal scans by identification of hepatic and gastroduodenal artery as well as common bile duct. Arteries course on anterior aspect of head of pancreas, whereas common bile duct passes posteriorly (Figs 10–21 and 10–22). In some patients head of pancreas is situated between inferior vena cava and aorta (Figs 10–23 and 10–24). In this location portal vein will be more posteriorly located and hepatic artery cephalically located. Additional posterior landmarks are left renal vein and right renal artery. One should also search for stomach anteriorly and duodenum posteriorly as caudal landmarks. H = head; F = feet; LPV = left portal vein; MPV = main portal vein; I = inferior vena cava; HA = hepatic artery; P = pancreas; GDA = gastroduodenal artery; St and S = stomach; Du = duodenum; Cr = crus of diaphragm; RRA = right renal artery; PV = portal vein; CBD = common bile duct; LRV = left renal vein; A = aorta.

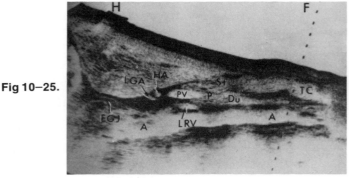

Fig 10—25.

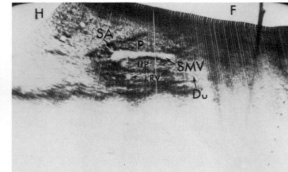

Fig 10—26.

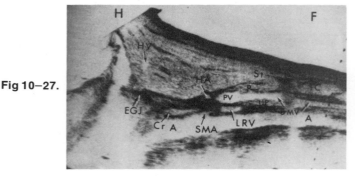

Fig 10—27.

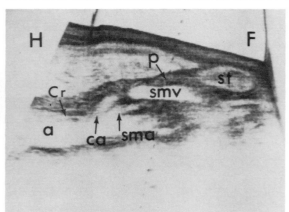

Fig 10—28.

Figs 10—25 to 10—28. — Normal pancreas. In the region of pancreatic neck and uncinate process, more on midline longitudinal scans, variety of anatomical landmarks can be identified. Frequently, origins of celiac and superior mesenteric arteries are helpful cephalic and dorsal landmarks, as is origin of superior mesenteric vein. It should be emphasized that uncinate process of pancreas may in fact be posterior to superior mesenteric vein. Left renal vein will be seen coursing posterior to pancreas. Attempt should be made to identify 3d portion of duodenum; however, this is frequently difficult because it is collapsed by its tight course between superior mesenteric artery and aorta. One may occasionally see an additional vessel superior to pancreas, adjacent to hepatic or splenic artery, representing left gastric artery. Portion of crus of diaphragm may also be seen as prominent structure anterior to aorta between esophagogastric junction and origin of celiac artery. H = head; F = feet; LGA = left gastric artery; HA = hepatic artery; EGJ = esophagogastric junction; A = aorta; PV = portal vein; LRV = left renal vein; P = pancreas; St = stomach; Du = duodenum; TC = transverse colon; SA = splenic artery; UP = uncinate process; SMV = superior mesenteric vein; Cr = crus of diaphragm; SMA = superior mesenteric artery; ca = celiac artery.

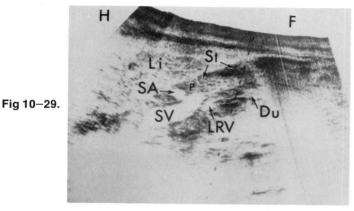

Fig 10–29.

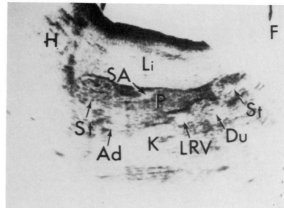

Fig 10–30.

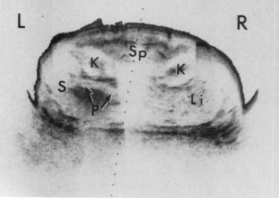

Fig 10–31.

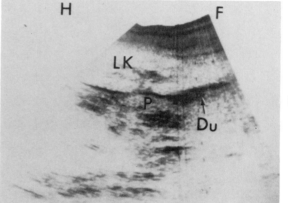

Fig 10–32.

Figs 10–29 to 10–32.—Normal pancreas. Parasagittal scans to left of midline may frequently delineate portions of body and tail of pancreas (Figs 10–29 and 10–30). Pancreas will be bracketed by splenic artery superiorly, splenic vein and left renal vein posteriorly, stomach anteriorly and 4th portion of duodenum inferiorly. Occasionally left adrenal gland is seen slightly cephalic to deep aspect of pancreas, and gastric cardia identified directly superior to pancreas.

When parasagittal scans are unsuccessful, one may identify pancreas by scanning in prone position (Figs 10–31 and 10–32). Pancreas lies anterior to the left kidney, but anatomical landmarks are less reliable in this position. H = head; F = feet; L = left; R = right; Li = liver; St = stomach; P = pancreas; SA = splenic artery; SV = splenic vein; LRV = left renal vein; Du = duodenum; K = kidney; Ad = adrenal gland; S = spleen; LK = left kidney.

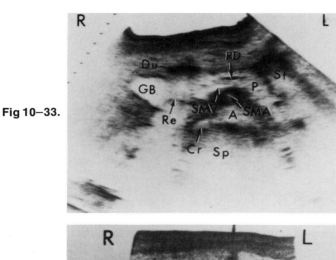

Fig 10–33.

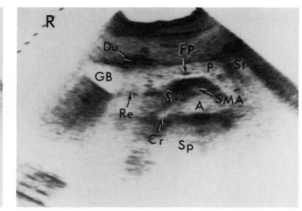

Fig 10–34.

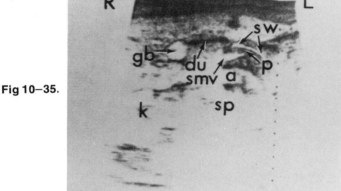

Fig 10–35.

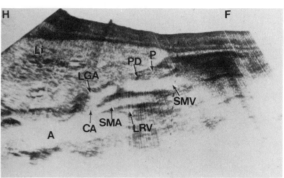

Fig 10–36.

Figs 10–33 to 10–36.—Normal pancreatic duct. Normal pancreatic duct can be identified in a number of patients, particularly in neck region (Fig 10–33). However, for proper identification of pancreatic duct one must exclude echogenic line immediately anterior to splenic vein representing a thin fat pad (Fig 10–34). In addition, posterior wall of stomach may create tubular sonolucent region that mimics dilated pancreatic duct (Fig 10–35). Pancreatic duct may also be visualized on longitudinal scans as echogenic dot surrounded by pancreatic tissue anterior to superior mesenteric vein (Fig 10–36). R = right; L = left; H = head; F = feet; GB = gallbladder; Du = duodenum; Re = reverberation artifact; FP = fat pad; SV = splenic vein; Cr = crus of diaphragm; Sp = spine; A = aorta; P = pancreas; SMA = superior mesenteric artery; St = stomach; SMV = superior mesenteric vein; PD = pancreatic duct; SW = stomach wall; K = kidney; Li = liver; LGA = left gastric artery; CA = celiac artery; LRV = left renal vein. Figures 10–33 and 10–34 are courtesy of Drs. David and Barbara Weinstein, Philadelphia.

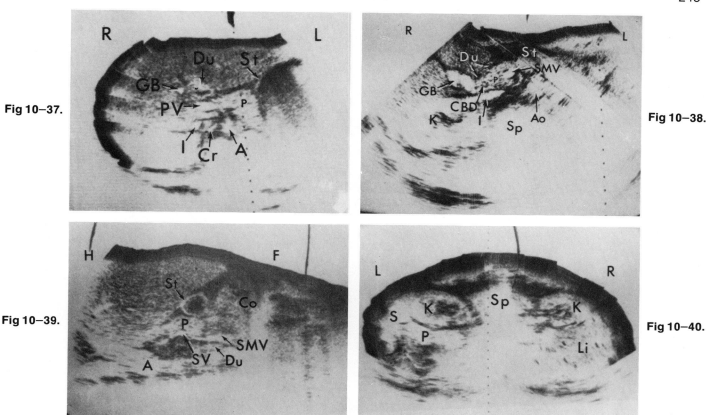

Figs 10–37.

Fig 10–38.

Fig 10–39.

Fig 10–40.

Figs 10–37 to 10–40.—Acute pancreatitis. Acute pancreatitis can be demonstrated in neonate and young child by either texture change or enlargement of pancreas. Usually entire pancreas is involved, although enlargement occasionally is localized to pancreatic head. Major texture alteration is loss of echogenicity compared to liver. If pancreatitis is severe, superior mesenteric and splenic venous systems may be difficult to identify. R = right; L = left; H = head; F = feet; GB = gallbladder; Du = duodenum; PV = portal vein; St = stomach; I = inferior vena cava; Cr = crus of diaphragm; A and Ao = aorta; P = pancreas; CBD = common bile duct; K = kidney; Sp = spine; SMV = superior mesenteric vein; Co = colon; SV = splenic vein; Li = liver; S = spleen.

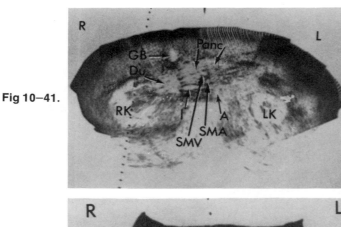

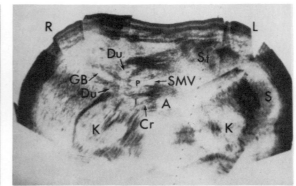

Fig 10–41.

Fig 10–42.

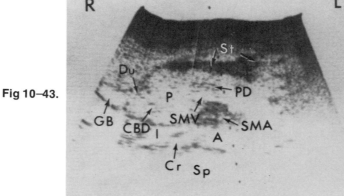

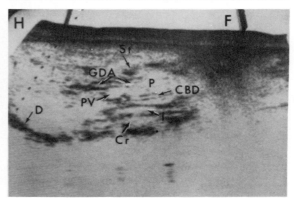

Fig 10–43.

Fig 10–44.

Figs 10–41 to 10–44. —Acute pancreatitis. In older child acute pancreatitis is manifested by loss of normal pancreatic texture as well as enlargement. In addition, one may visualize some enlargement of biliary system or pancreatic duct. These are frequently transient phenomena that will return to normal after resolution of pancreatitis. When comparing texture of pancreas to liver, it is important to compare at same depths from transducer. In addition, one must be certain that liver is not inherently involved with disease process that might change its texture. R = right; L = left; H = head; F = feet; GB = gallbladder; Du = duodenum; RK = right kidney; LK = left kidney; I = inferior vena cava; A = aorta; SMA = superior mesenteric artery; SMV = superior mesenteric vein; P and Panc = pancreas; Cr = crus of diaphragm; K = kidney; St = stomach; S = spleen; CBD = common bile duct; PD = pancreatic duct; GDA = gastroduodenal artery; D = diaphragm; PV = portal vein; Sp = spine.

Fig 10–45.

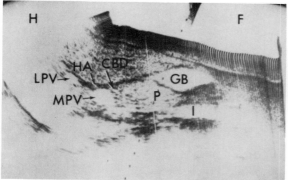

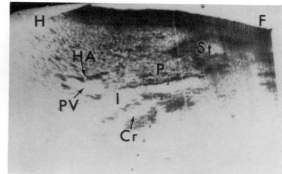

Fig 10–46.

Fig 10–47.

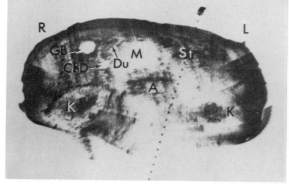

Figs 10–45 to 10–47.—Follow-up of acute pancreatitis. Ultrasound is an excellent modality to follow up patients with acute pancreatitis. Serial examinations in uncomplicated cases will show gradual reversal to a normal size and echogenicity, as well as disappearance of any minor dilatation of biliary or pancreatic ductal systems (Figs 10–45 and 10–46). However, pancreatitis may be complicated by development of pseudocyst, which is easily demonstrated with ultrasonography (Fig 10–47). H = head; F = feet; R = right; L = left; MPV = main portal vein; LPV = left portal vein; HA = hepatic artery; CBD = common bile duct; P = pancreas; I = inferior vena cava; GB = gallbladder; Cr = crus of diaphragm; St = stomach; A = aorta; K = kidney; Du = duodenum; M = pancreatic pseudocyst; PV = portal vein.

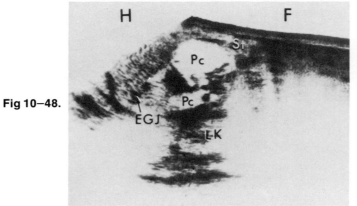

Fig 10–48.

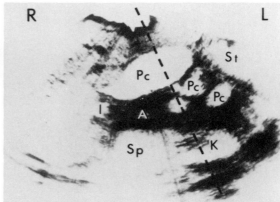

Fig 10–49.

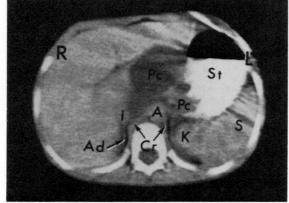

Fig 10–50.

Figs 10–48 to 10–50. – Pseudocysts of pancreas. More than half of the cases of pseudocysts of pancreas in children are the result of trauma. Ultrasonography is an excellent method for evaluation of pancreatic laceration and development of pseudocysts. They appear as thin- or thick-walled fluid collection usually confined to pancreatic region. However, they may extend beyond confines of pancreas into superior retroperitoneum, anterior pararenal space, lower abdomen or even into the mediastinum. In addition to ultrasonography (Figs 10–48 and 10–49), computed tomog-raphy (Fig 10–50) can be used to diagnose pseudocysts; however, this modality may best be utilized in clinical setting of a suspected pancreatic abscess. It has advantage of demonstrating extraluminal air, confirming diagnosis of abscess. H = head; F = foot; R = right; L = left; LK = left kidney; EGJ = esophagogastric junction; Pc = pseudocyst of pancreas; St = stomach; S = spleen; Sp = spine; K = kidney; A = aorta; I = inferior vena cava; Ad = adrenal gland; Cr = crus of diaphragm.

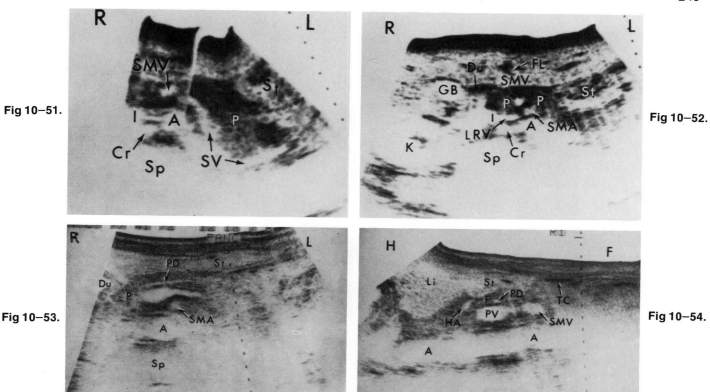

Figs 10–51 to 10–54.—Chronic pancreatitis. One of the most difficult diagnoses to make on ultrasonograms is chronic pancreatitis. This may be seen as complication of hereditary pancreatitis or association with cystic fibrosis. Although fibrofatty infiltration of pancreas increases the echogenicity (Figs 10–51 and 10–52), this unfortunately overlaps biological echogenic variation of normal pancreas. As a result, a more significant finding is presence of dilated pancreatic duct (Figs 10–53 and 10–54). More data and experience are needed to know exactly how dilated a pancreatic duct must become before it is reliably visualized and definitely abnormal. R = right; L = left; H = head; F = feet; SMV = superior mesenteric vein; SV = splenic vein; P = pancreas; St = stomach; A = aorta; I = inferior vena cava; Cr = crus of diaphragm; Sp = spine; Du = duodenum; GB = gallbladder; FL = falciform ligament; LRV = left renal vein; K = kidney; SMA = superior mesenteric artery; PD = pancreatic duct; PV = portal vein; Li = liver; HA = hepatic artery; TC = transverse colon.

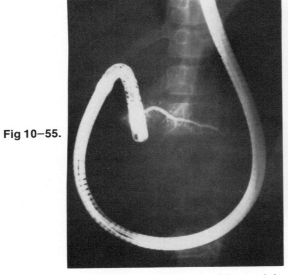

Fig 10–55.

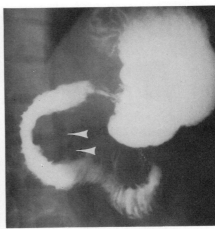

Fig 10–56.

Figs 10–55 to 10–60.—Other roentgenographic modalities in evaluation of pancreas. Pancreatic duct may be evaluated by ERCP (Fig 10–55). This procedure is more difficult in children than in adults. Contrast study of gastrointestinal tract might demonstrate changes of duodenum as result of acute pancreatitis (Fig 10–56) with spiculation of folds, or may show areas of calcification *(arrowheads),* which in children is usually result of cystic fibrosis or hereditary pancreatitis. Pseudocysts of pancreas may also be demonstrated roentgenographically on abdominal film (Fig 10–57), excretory urogram (Fig 10–58, *arrowheads*), upper gastrointestinal series (Fig 10–59) or direct injection of cyst (Fig 10–60).

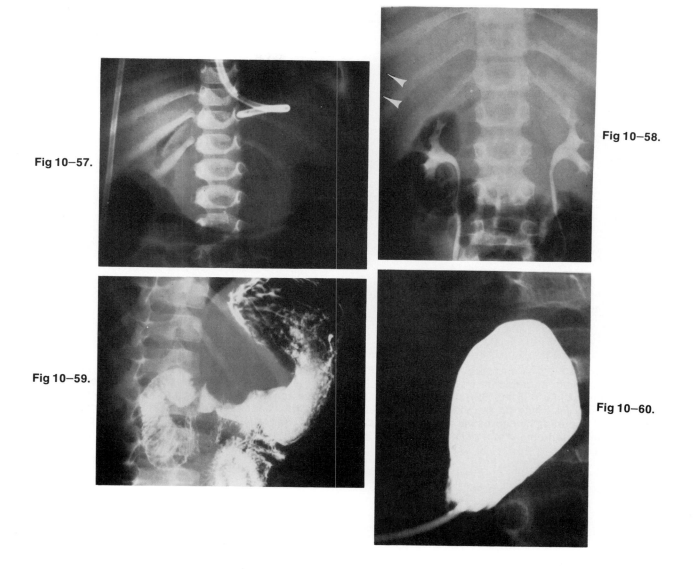

Fig 10—57.

Fig 10—58.

Fig 10—59.

Fig 10—60.

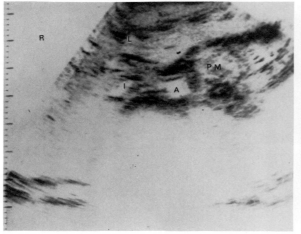

Fig 10–61.

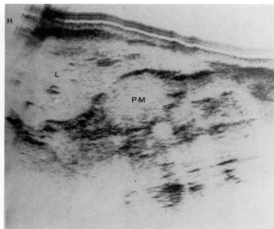

Fig 10–62.

Figs 10–61 and 10–62.—Pancreatic masses in children. Pancreatic masses can be demonstrated in transverse (Fig 10–61) and longitudinal (Fig 10–62) ultrasonograms. Enlargement of pancreas could be secondary to pancreatitis or infiltration of pancreas by neoplastic process. This case shows pancreatic enlargement in a patient with Wegener's granulomatosis.

Since neoplastic diseases of pancreas are rare in children, angiography of pancreas plays a minor diagnostic role in this age group. However, if angiography is performed it may provide more accurate means of making specific diagnosis (see text). H = head; L = liver; PM = pancreatic mass; R = right; I = inferior vena cava; A = aorta.

11

Peritoneum, Mesentery and Bowel

PERITONEUM

THE PERITONEAL CAVITY includes the greater sac, the lesser sac, rectouterine pouch of Douglas, paracolic gutters and the subphrenic spaces.

Ascites

The appearance of ascites within the peritoneal cavity depends on several factors: amount of ascitic fluid, presence of adhesions, fat in the mesentery and air vs. fluid-filled bowel loops.

The smallest amount of detectable ascitic fluid by sonography is 100 ml. With the lesser amounts, fluid collects in the colonic gutters and pelvis; with larger amounts, accumulation occurs laterally and around the liver, spleen, hepatorenal angle and in the lesser sac.

Rapid fluid movement to the dependent side represents free intraperitoneal fluid. Loculated ascites is usually due to adhesions. Malignant ascites is indistinguishable from the benign variety unless there are nodules along the peritoneum or an uneven distribution of fluid due to loculations.

Fluid in the colon can mimic ascites in the flank at ultrasound, but it does not move with position, and an x-ray film taken with the patient erect or in the decubitus position will show the air fluid levels in the colon.

Acute hemoperitoneum and ascites are indistinguishable.

Abscess

Plain abdominal films taken with the patient in the supine and upright positions are the initial means of investigation for abscess evaluation. Air bubbles in an unusual location that do not move with a change in position, an area of increased density or loss of the normal fascial planes can all suggest an abscess, but in most cases these findings are not present.

Gallium citrate-67 scanning, diagnostic ultrasound and computerized tomography all have the ability to detect abscesses, although one modality is usually favored, depending on clinical circumstances, and, if necessary, confirmed in equivocal cases by another, complementary modality.

Diagnostic ultrasound has the potential advantage of providing immediate results without ionizing radiation, determining volume and specifying the spatial location. Although this modality is extremely sensitive to detection of fluid collections, the type of fluid depicted is not specific, and abscess, hematoma, lymphocele and urinoma can appear similar. Fluid-filled bowel loops usually can be differentiated from abscess with real-time ultrasound studies.

Gallium citrate-67 isotope is not specific in that it localizes in abscesses and inflammatory processes as well as in some tumors, wounds, bowel involved with regional enteritis, incisions and colostomies. False negative results can occur if the target-to-background ratio is low or if the abnormal activity is adjacent to the liver or spleen, two organs that normally accumulate the isotope in the pediatric patient. Other normal areas of increased activity in the pediatric population are the epiphyseal plates, thymus, nasopharynx, lacrimal glands and bowel.

Deferoxamine mesylate is being investigated as an

abscess-detecting agent. Deferoxamine labeled with Indium[111] appears, in rats and rabbits, to have abscess-detection abilities similar to ^{67}Ga-citrate.

Computerized tomography combines some of the advantages and disadvantages of ultrasound and gallium imaging. With a narrow collimated x-ray beam, transverse cross-sectional images are obtained equally well in all portions of the body, with almost immediate image reconstruction. Although anatomical detail is excellent, as with ultrasound, the nature of the fluid collection is not specific, and subacute and chronic hematomas, lymphoceles, urinomas and complex cysts may appear similar. Abscesses are usually low-density lesions (0–30 Hounsfield units), although the periphery may have a higher density and occasionally become slightly enhanced after contrast infusion. Air fluid levels or air bubbles are highly suggestive of abscess formation; however, opacification of the bowel by oral contrast material is necessary in most cases to confirm the extraluminal location of the suspected abscess. Abscesses can also thicken or obliterate the fascial planes and displace normal adjacent structures. In general, computerized tomography is reserved for confirmation of equivocal results, confirmation of a preceding imaging modality in a patient in whom abscess is strongly suspected, or for planning of a surgical route of drainage when more anatomical detail is necessary.

Subdiaphragmatic abscesses, most commonly a problem in the postoperative patient, can be visualized by ultrasound under the right hemidiaphragm if they are at least 1–2 cm, except for the most laterally located abscesses. The left subphrenic space is characteristically obscured by bowel gas in the left upper quadrant. Performing the examination with the patient in a right lateral decubitus position, using the spleen as an ultrasonic window, allows a limited examination of this left subphrenic space. Diaphragmatic movement is quickly assessed by ultrasound, albeit more easily in evaluation of the right hemidiaphragm. Although fluoroscopy of the diaphragms will document lack of movement, ultrasound has the additional ability to search for a possible etiology.

[67]Ga-citrate has some limited success in subdiaphragmatic abscess localization. Small to moderate abscess detection by gallium suffers from relative obscuration by normal ^{67}Ga-citrate liver and spleen activity, although on occasion an increased yield results from combined gallium and ^{99m}Tc-sulfur colloid scans.

Retroperitoneal abscesses are discussed in chapter 12; pelvic abscesses in chapter 14.

Hematomas

Hematomas may be posttraumatic, occur spontaneously in patients with altered coagulation states or be iatrogenic. When detected by ultrasound they may be indistinguishable from abscesses or tumors. The shape is ovoid to spherical when intra-abdominal in location, and lentiform when in the abdominal wall or subcapsular. Walls vary from smooth to irregular and, initially, the internal contents are anechoic because of unclotted blood; however, usually within the first month they develop strong internal echoes due to clot formation. Beyond this time, the internal echoes usually diminish, correlating with clot lysis. Occasionally, septae and fluid-fluid levels are noted. Hematomas are discussed further in chapter 13.

CYSTIC ABDOMINAL MASSES

Abdominal distention, especially when painless and chronic, should first be evaluated by plain roentgenograms of the abdomen. An ultrasound study should be performed as one of the initial diagnostic procedures to determine the nature of the distention: whether there is a mass, whether it is cystic or solid, and its organ of origin. If the determination of origin is not possible, the relationship to and the visualization of normal structures can quickly narrow the diagnostic possibilities.

Omental and Mesenteric Cysts

Twenty-five percent of mesenteric and omental cysts occur in patients less than 10 years of age, 50% are within the small-bowel mesentery and, of these, 50% lie in the mesentery of the ileum (Mittelstaedt,

1975). Usually there is painless abdominal enlargement, unless there are complications of hemorrhage, torsion, pressure and rupture.

These cysts are palpable and the unilocular or multilocular cysts contain serous more often than chylous fluid. The omental cyst lies anterior to the bowel beneath the skin, conforming to instead of distending the abdominal wall. Mesenteric cysts are more spherical and deeper, but both meet the ultrasonic criteria of cysts except when complications such as hemorrhage or infection intervene, creating internal echoes.

Duplication Cysts

The majority of the duplication cysts are diagnosed in patients up to 2 years of age, and most frequently in the right lower quadrant near the terminal portion of the ileum. Most duplication cysts do not communicate with the bowel and may be similar to mesenteric cysts.

The mucosal-lined cavity can create an echogenic internal rim and there may be a finite wall thickness due to muscle fibers. Like other cystic structures, complications can occur that will create complex internal echoes. In colonic duplications there is an increased incidence of genitourinary anomalies.

Cystic Lymphangiomas

Cystic lymphangiomas, also known as cystic hygromas, occur primarily under 2 years of age. They appear as a palpable mass and are frequently multicystic. They are uncommon and almost always benign.

Cystic lymphangioma is composed of multiple dilated endothelial-lined cystic spaces of uncertain etiology, which probably are congenitally malformed lymphatic vessels that dilate as the result of increased intraluminal pressure. As the cystic spaces enlarge, there is rupture and bleeding into cysts, which ultimately results in necrosis and fibrosis. Ridge-like projections of connective tissue and deep trabeculations of the cyst walls indicate previous rupture of cysts with fusion or communication, resulting in a multicystic mass. Lymphangiography, although only occasionally warranted, is diagnostic, demonstrating contrast droplets entering the tumor.

Cystic lymphangiomatosis. — Lymphangiomatosis is a rare, tumor-like condition characterized by smooth muscle proliferation involving major lymphatic trunks in the mediastinum and retroperitoneum. Characteristically occurring in females of reproductive age, the older pediatric population is at risk for this multifocal or diffuse process. Ultrasound examination demonstrates thick-walled cystic periaortic and pericaval structures of variable size that are contiguous and septated. Occasionally, dependent internal echoes signifying debris are present.

Cystic Meconium Peritonitis

This large meconium cyst is lined by a thick membrane containing multiple calcium deposits and plaques. It is found in the newborn and distinguished on plain film by a well-defined, round, soft tissue abdominal mass with or without air. Calcium deposits may be speckled, blotchy or globular within or outside the cyst wall. Medical attention is usually immediate because of massive abdominal distention.

Pelvic cystic lesions are discussed in chapter 14.

BOWEL DILATATION

A frequent cause of abdominal distention is dilated bowel loops. Bowel distention can be divided into congenital and acquired causes.

Congenital Dilatations

Neonatal abdominal distention is frequently associated with bowel dilatation. Intestinal obstruction is observed in approximately 1 of 1,500 newborn infants and is characterized by a triad of vomiting, abdominal distention and the failure to pass meconium. The lower the level of obstruction, the greater the number of distended bowel loops and the degree of abdominal distention. Normally air should reach the colon 4–6 hours after birth.

Atresia and stenosis. — These account for one-third of intestinal obstructions. Atresia is twice as common as stenosis in the ileum and jejunum and may be multiple in 15% of cases. The ileum is the most frequent portion of the bowel involved in atresia and stenosis and then, in decreasing order, are the duodenum, jejunum and colon.

INTERNAL WEBS OR DIAPHRAGMS.—These constitute another cause of obstruction that occurs primarily in the duodenum and esophagus, and, rarely, in the pyloris. The degree of obstruction and luminal narrowing are directly related. Associated malformations are common.

MALROTATION AND MIDGUT VOLVULUS.—These constitute another cause of intestinal obstruction. Malrotation should be correctly termed arrested or incomplete rotation. In patients with malrotation, the mesentery is free so that the entire pedicle can twist on itself, leading to duodenal obstruction and infarction of the midgut since the superior mesenteric vessels are included in the pedicle. This is a more serious consequence of incomplete rotation since vomiting decompresses the small bowel and distention of the abdomen occurs only as a late manifestation, following circulatory compromise.

Other causes of intestinal obstruction include Meckel's diverticulum as the leading point of an intussusception, intra-abdominal and extra-abdominal hernias and imperforate anus.

MECONIUM PLUGS.—These are among functional causes of obstruction and usually cause a very distal obstruction in the colon, although rarely the plugs may lodge elsewhere in the intestinal tract. The plugs are usually dislodged following a meglumine diatrizoate enema.

MECONIUM ILEUS.—Unlike meconium plugs, meconium ileus is always associated with cystic fibrosis. Because of the lack of normal pancreatic enzymes, an abnormal meconium forms, becomes inspissated and obstructs the terminal portion of the ileum. The loops of dilated proximal small bowel vary in width, unlike the evenly dilated appearance of those loops in atresia. A granular appearance may be present on plain roentgenograms at the place of heaviest meconium concentration. There is an absence of colonic air and a paucity of air fluid levels on the films taken with the patient in the upright or decubitus position. The diagnosis is suggested by demonstration of a microcolon at barium enema examination. Some patients, however, have a complicated meconium ileus with segmental volvulus, atresia, stenosis or a chemical peritonitis following perforation. When perforation occurs, multiple calcifications can be noted on plain films of the abdomen.

HIRSCHSPRUNG'S DISEASE.—This implies agenesis of the parasympathetic ganglion cells between the mucosa and submucosa and between the muscular layers of the involved segment of bowel. In this predominantly male disease, the sigmoid colon and rectum are most frequently involved. Less than 5% of patients have the entire colon involved. A barium enema is required for diagnosis, although rectal biopsy is mandatory for confirmation.

Acquired Causes of Bowel Dilatations

The acquired causes of bowel dilatations are due both to mechanical and to nonmechanical obstruction. The most frequent pediatric cause of "paralytic" ileus or nonmechanical obstruction is pneumonia in infants and peritonitis in the older child. Other causes include recent operation, trauma, drugs and hypokalemia.

Incarcerated inguinal hernias and intussusception are the most frequent causes of mechanical obstruction. Intussusception most commonly occurs in males in the 3- to 11-month age group. The majority are ileocolic, but some may be ileoileocolic or ileoileal. Specific causes can be found in less than 10% of these patients. A Meckel's diverticulum, bowel tumor, duplication or ectopic pancreas nodule can serve as a leading mass.

Foreign bodies, traumatic hematomas and adhesions may all obstruct the bowel.

REFERENCES

Altemeier, W. A., et al.: Retroperitoneal abscess, Arch. Surg. 83:512, 1961.

Aronberg, D. J., et al.: Evaluation of abdominal abscess with computed tomography, J. Comput. Assist. Tomogr. 2:384, 1978.

Bernardino, M. E., et al.: Computed tomography diagnosis of mesenteric masses, A.J.R. 132:33, 1979.

Brasch, R. C., et al.: Computed body tomography in children: Evaluation of 45 patients, A.J.R. 131:21, 1978.

Caffey, J.: *Pediatric X-Ray Diagnosis* (7th ed.; Chicago: Year Book Medical Publishers, Inc., 1978).

Chandra, R., et al.: In-desferal: A new radiopharmaceutical for abscess detection, Radiology 128:697, 1978.

Churchill, R. J., et al.: CT imaging of the abdomen: Methodology and normal anatomy, Radiol. Clin. North Am. 17:13, 1979.

Doust, B. D., et al.: Ultrasonic distinction of abscesses from other intra-abdominal fluid collections, Radiology 125:213, 1977.

Doust, B. D., et al.: Ultrasonography of abdominal fluid collections, Gastrointest. Radiology 3:273, 1978.

Haller, J. O., et al.: Sonographic evaluation of mesenteric and omental masses in children, A.J.R. 130:269, 1978.

Handmaker, H., et al.: Gallium imaging in pediatrics, J. Nucl. Med. 18:1057, 1977.

Harvey, W. C., et al.: [67]Gallium in 68 consecutive infection searches, J. Nucl. Med. 16:2, 1975.

Hill, M., et al.: Gray-scale B-scan characteristics of intra-abdominal cystic masses, J. Clin. Ultrasound 6:217, 1978.

Hopkins, G. B., et al.: Gallium-67 and subphrenic abscesses: Is delayed scintigraphy necessary? J. Nucl. Med. 16:609, 1975.

Kangarloo, H., et al.: Ultrasonic evaluation of abdominal gastrointestinal tract duplication in children, Radiology 131:191, 1979.

Kolawole, T. M., et al.: Meconium peritonitis presenting as giant cysts in neonates, Br. J. Radiol. 46:964, 1973.

Korobkin, M., et al.: Comparison of computed tomography, ultrasonography, and gallium-67 scanning in the evaluation of suspected abdominal abscess, Radiology 129:89, 1978.

Kressel, H. Y., et al.: Ultrasonographic appearance of gas-containing abscesses in the abdomen, A.J.R. 130:71, 1978.

Leonidas, J. C., et al.: Cystic retroperitoneal lymphangioma in infants and children, Radiology 127:203, 1978.

Levitt, R. G., et al.: Computed tomography and ^{67}Ga citrate radionuclide imaging for evaluating suspected abdominal abscess, A.J.R. 132:529, 1979.

McQuown, D. S., et al.: Abdominal cystic lymphangiomatosis: Report of a case involving the liver and spleen and illustration of 2 cases with origin in the greater omentum and root of the mesentery, J. Clin. Ultrasound 3:291, 1975.

Mittelstaedt, C.: Ultrasonic diagnosis of omental cysts, Radiology 117:673, 1975.

Moncada, R., et al.: Normal vascular anatomy of the abdomen on computed tomography, Radiol. Clin. North Am. 17:25, 1979.

Nelson, W. E., et al.: *Textbook of Pediatrics* (9th ed.; Philadelphia: W. B. Saunders Co., 1969).

Oliff, M., et al.: Retroperitoneal iliac fossa pyogenic abscess, Radiology 126:647, 1978.

Roy, C. C., et al.: *Pediatric Clinical Gastroenterology* (St. Louis: C. V. Mosby Co., 1975).

Rudolph, A. M.: *Pediatrics* (16th ed.; New York: Appleton-Century-Crofts, 1977).

Sample, W. F.: Normal abdominal anatomy defined by gray-scale ultrasound, Radiol. Clin. North Am. 17:3, 1979.

Sample, W. F., et al.: Computed body tomography and gray-scale ultrasonography: Anatomic correlations and pitfalls in the upper abdomen, Gastrointest. Radiol. 3:243, 1978.

Walsh, J., et al.: Gray-scale ultrasonography in retroperitoneal lymphangiomyomatosis, A.J.R. 129:1101, 1977.

Wicks, J. D., et al.: Giant cystic abdominal masses in children and adolescents: Ultrasonic differential diagnosis, A.J.R. 130:853, 1978.

Yeh, H. C., et al.: Ultrasonography in ascites, Radiology 124:783, 1977.

Fig 11–1.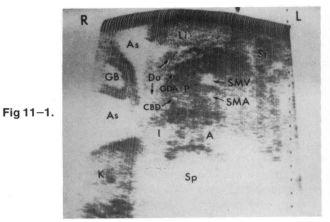

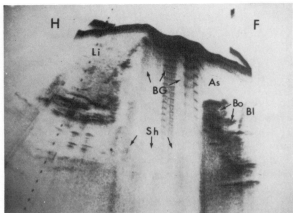 **Fig 11–2.**

Fig 11–3.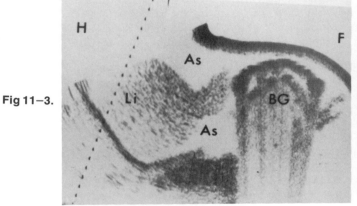

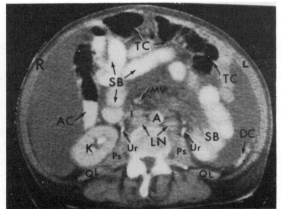 **Fig 11–4.**

Figs 11–1 to 11–4.—Ascites. Ascites can be demonstrated equally well by ultrasound or computed tomography. In both modalities gallbladder wall may appear thickened since fluid is present on either side. Although in some patients retroperitoneal detail can be satisfactorily displayed on ultrasonograms, in the presence of ascites (Fig 11–1), in many patients pooling of bowel in midline with subsequent shadowing artifacts from gas obscure mid and lower retroperitoneum (Figs 11–2 and 11–3). As a result, in patients with marked ascites, it is frequently advantageous to study them with computed body tomography (Fig 11–4). Various portions of gastrointestinal tract can be highlighted with oral iodinated contrast material and portions of renal collecting system can similarly be seen with judicious use of intravenous contrast material. H = head; F = feet; R = right; L = left; Li = liver; BG = bowel gas; Sh = shadowing; As = ascites; Bo = bowel; Bl = bladder; GB = gallbladder; K = kidney; Du = duodenum; GDA = gastroduodenal artery; CBD = common bile duct; I = inferior vena cava; A = aorta; Sp = spine; SMV = superior mesenteric vein; SMA = superior mesenteric artery; St = stomach; TC = transverse colon; AC = ascending colon; DC = descending colon; SB = small bowel; MV = mesenteric vessel; Ur = ureter; LN = lymph node; Ps = psoas muscle; QL = quadratus lumborum; P = pancreas.

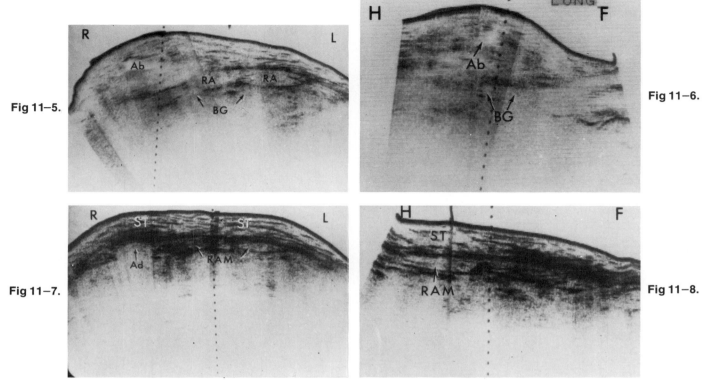

Figs 11–5 to 11–8. — Abdominal abscess. Both abdominal wall and intraperitoneal abscesses can frequently be identified by ultrasonography. With newer instrumentation a variety of patterns are demonstrated. Usually an irregular sonolucent fluid collection can be delineated. Serial examination will often show resolution with adequate drainage or antibiotic therapy. Figs 11–5 and 11–6 are initial scans of a patient with subcutaneous abscess, and Figs 11–7 and 11–8 are the scans of same patient one week following therapy. R = right; L = left; H = head; F = feet; Ab = abscess, RA and RAM = rectus abdominus muscle; BG = bowel gas; ST = subcutaneous tissue; Ad = adhesion.

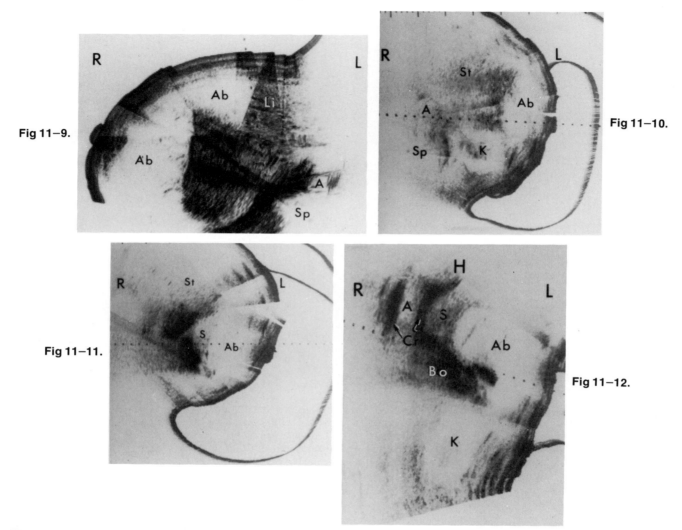

Figs 11–9 to 11–12. — Intra-abdominal abscesses. Ultrasound may be very effective in identifying intra-abdominal abscesses, particularly those around liver and spleen. Nongas-containing abscesses may have a variety of acoustical patterns from sonolucent regions to areas with low to medium echoes. A gas-containing abscess with microbubbles may be extremely echogenic. Abscesses containing large pockets of gas may be completely missed on ultrasound and misinterpreted as loops of bowel. As a result, normal ultrasonogram does not rule out presence of abscess and may warrant further evaluation with either computed body tomography or gallium scan. Choice between these 3 modalities depends on clinical condition of patient and whether there are any specific physical findings to point to given area. R = right; L = left; Ab = abscess; Sp = spine; A = aorta; St = stomach; K = kidney; S = spleen; H = head; Cr = crus of diaphragm; Bo = bowel; Li = liver.

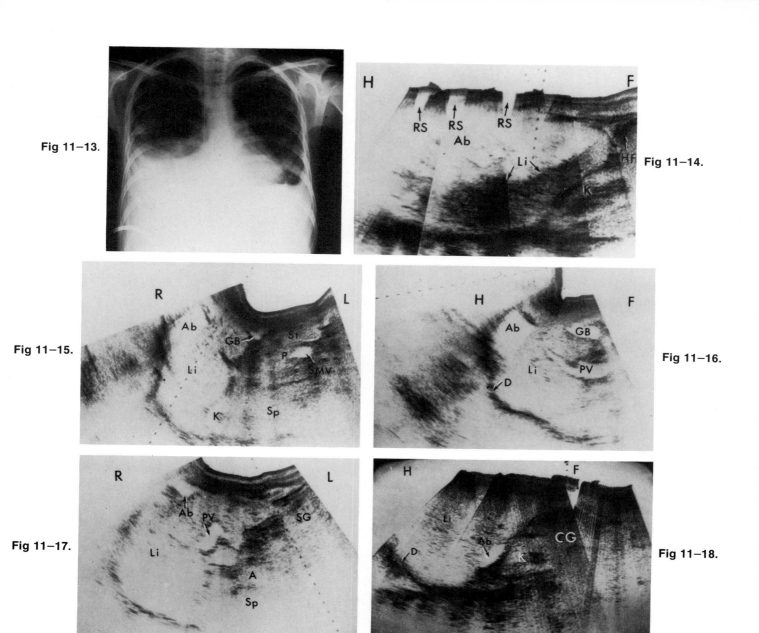

Figs 11–13 to 11–18. — Intra-abdominal abscesses. Plain films of abdomen or chest may suggest diagnosis of subdiaphragmatic abscess by presence of pleural fluid (Fig 11–13). Nevertheless, since diaphragm cannot be visualized, another modality is usually necessary to better localize an infradiaphragmatic process. A very flexible approach to the right upper quadrant is necessary to study all potential subdiaphragmatic and subhepatic spaces with ultrasound.

Fluid collections may be seen along right lateral aspect of liver (Fig 11–14), along superior aspect of liver (Figs 11–15 to 11–17) and in subhepatic space (Fig 11–18). H = head; F = feet; R = right; L = left; RS = rib shadow; Ab = abscess; Li = liver; HF = hepatic flexure; K = kidney; GB = gallbladder; Sp = spine; SMV = superior mesenteric vein; P = pancreas; St = stomach; PV = portal vein; D = diaphragm; A = aorta; SG = stomach gas; CG = colon gas.

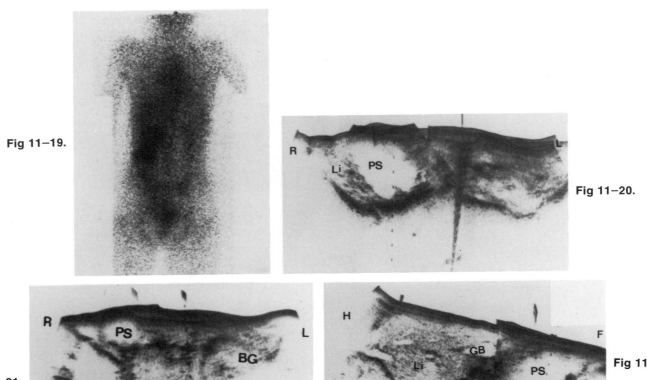

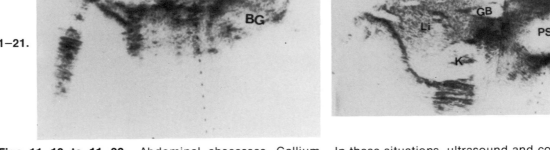

Figs 11–19 to 11–22.—Abdominal abscesses. Gallium scans are excellent way to search for abscesses, particularly when patient has no specific signs or symptoms pointing to an area and clinical condition warrants 1- to 3-day wait, which is necessary for complete gallium scan. However, an area of increased uptake may be confused with normal bowel and precise anatomical location may not be possible. In these situations, ultrasound and computed body tomography can be utilized to locate more precisely the organs involved. Psoas abscesses have rather classical appearance on gallium scan (Fig 11–19) as well as on ultrasonograms (Figs 11–20 to 11–22). R = right; L = left; H = head; F = feet; Li = liver; BG = bowel gas; PS = psoas abscess; K = kidney; GB = gallbladder.

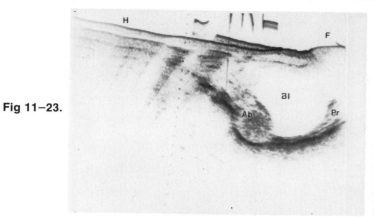

Fig 11–23.

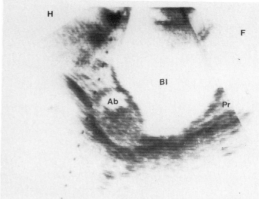

Fig 11–24.

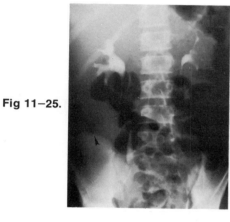

Fig 11–25.

Figs 11–23 to 11–25.—Appendiceal abscess. Although abscesses involving bowel are not frequently diagnosed specifically by ultrasound, occasionally an appendiceal abscess will extend into the pelvic region and, particularly in a male, substantiate the diagnosis. Appendiceal abscesses can similarly present as pelvic masses in females, mimicking the more usual pelvic inflammatory disease. When these abscesses contain significant air they may appear as very echogenic masses (Figs 11–23 and 11–24), requiring correlation with either abdominal films (Fig 11–25, *arrow*) or computed body tomograms. H = head; F = feet; Bl = bladder; Ab = abscess; Pr = prostate.

Fig 11–26.

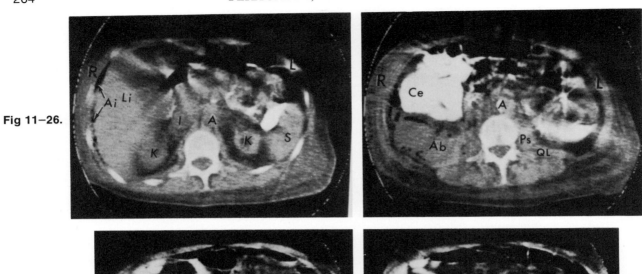

Fig 11–27.

Fig 11–28.

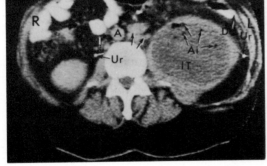

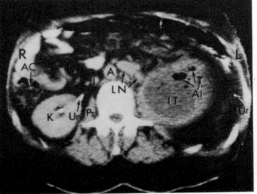

Fig 11–29.

Figs 11–26 to 11–29.—Abscesses. A major strength of computed body tomography is its ability to detect extraluminal gas. The presence of such a finding virtually cinches the diagnosis of abscess. When air exists around liver (Fig 11–26) or in retroperitoneal tissues (Figs 11–27 to 11–29), little confusion exists with normal bowel. However, in search for abscesses, both small and large bowel should be specifically identified by using oral iodinated contrast material. R = right; L = left; Ai = air; Li = liver; K = kidney; A = aorta; I = inferior vena cava; S = spleen; Ab = abscess; Ce = cecum; Ps = psoas muscle; QL = quadratus lumborum muscle; Ur = ureter; LN = lymph nodes (arrows); IT = infected tumor; DC = descending colon; AC = ascending colon.

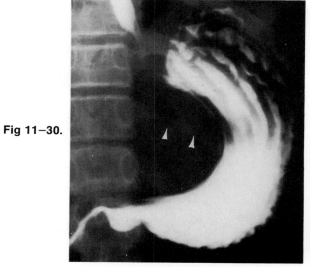

Fig 11–30.

Fig 11–31.

Figs 11–30 to 11–31. — Lesser sac abscess. Lesser sac abscess will be seen as mass lesion that may contain air and may displace stomach. Although lesser sac abscess can be demonstrated roentgenographically, this method should be reserved for situations in which computed tomography and ultrasound are not available. In computed tomography and ultrasound, not only may the abscess be identified but the exact origin of lesion can also be assessed. Arrowheads in Figures 11–30 and 11–31 indicate air in the lesser sac abscess.

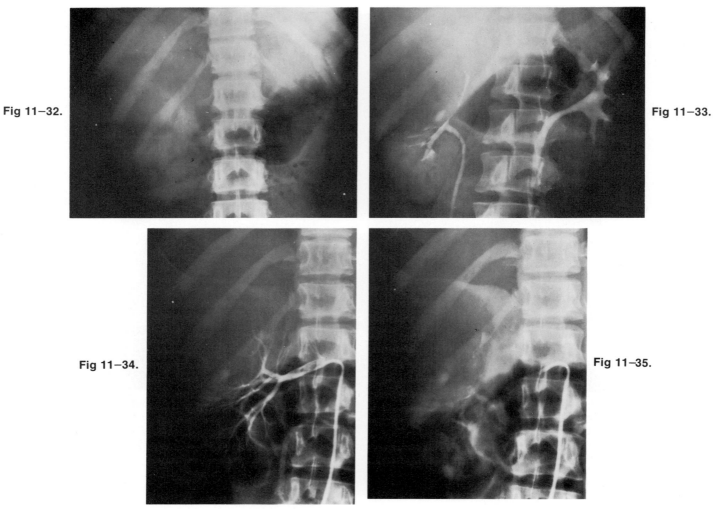

Fig 11–32.

Fig 11–33.

Fig 11–34.

Fig 11–35.

Figs 11–32 to 11–35. — Renal abscess. Conventional radiography, particularly excretory urogram, plays a significant role in detection of renal abnormalities, including renal abscess (Figs 11–32 and 11–33). Diagnosis can be made accurately in conjunction with clinical history and ultrasonography. Occasionally, arteriography may be used to establish diagnosis (Figs 11–34 and 11–35).

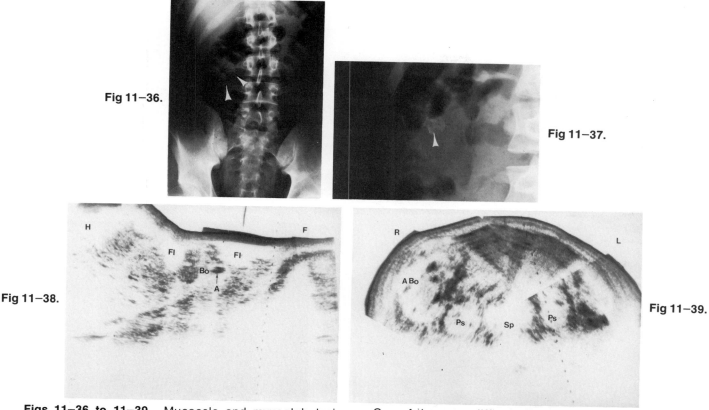

Fig 11–36.

Fig 11–37.

Fig 11–38.

Fig 11–39.

Figs 11–36 to 11–39.—Mucocele and myxoglobulosis. Myxoglobulosis is a rare type of mucocele of the appendix, characterized by a cluster of calcifications. Both mucocele and myxoglobulosis are usually asymptomatic but can appear as acute appendicitis. Wall calcifications are linear (Figs 11–36 and 11–37, *arrowheads*), but if contents of myxoglobulosis calcify, diagnosis can be established on plain film of abdomen.

One of the more difficult diagnoses using ultrasound is identifying abscesses related to bowel. Gas patterns within bowel may obscure the area entirely or mimic extraluminal gas collections. Nevertheless, abnormal fluid areas or an abnormal bowel pattern frequently can be identified in the suspected areas (Figs 11–38 and 11–39). H = head; F = feet; Fl = fluid; Bo = bowel; A = air; ABo = abnormal bowel; Ps = psoas muscle; Sp = spine; R = right; L = left.

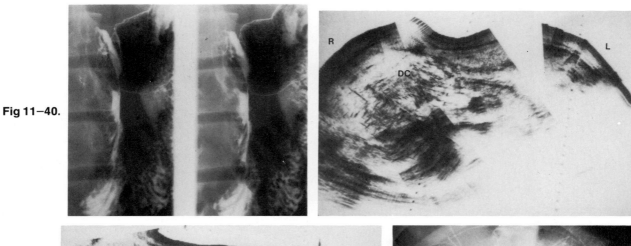

Fig 11–40.

Fig 11–41.

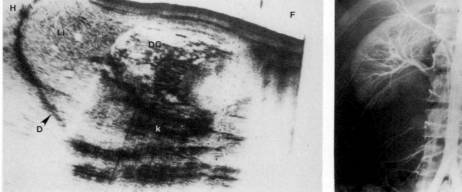

Fig 11–42.

Fig 11–43.

Figs 11–40 to 11–43.—Duodenal duplication cysts. Contrast studies of upper gastrointestinal tract may show extrinsic compression by duodenal duplication cyst (Fig 11–40). Also, sonographically, this mass may appear markedly echogenic, which is due to bleeding, inspissated material or infection of the cyst (Figs 11–41 and 11–42).

Angiographically (Fig 11–43), duplication cysts appear as an avascular mass with stretching of vessels and displacement of adjacent organs. R = right; L = left; DC = duplication cyst; D = diaphragm; Li = liver; k = kidney; H = head; F = foot.

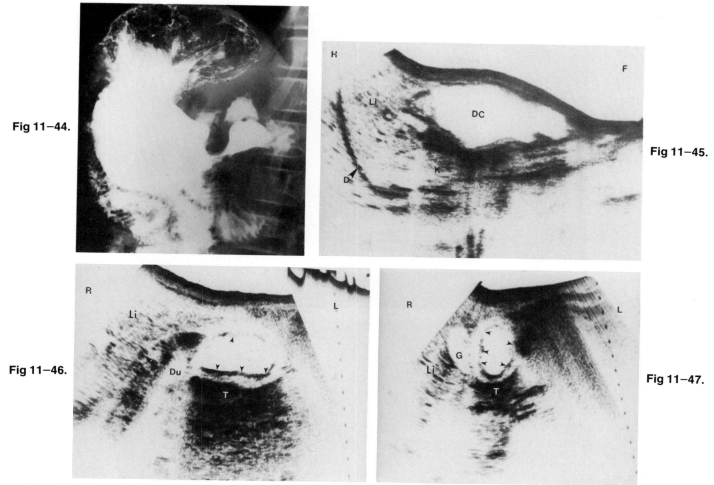

Figs 11–44 to 11–47.—Antral duplication cysts. Again, contrast studies on the upper gastrointestinal tract may show extrinsic compression on the antrum and duodenum (Fig 11–44) by the cyst. Uncomplicated duplication cysts would appear as a sonolucent mass (Figs 11–45 to 11–47). Visualization of mucosal lining *(arrowheads)* is highly suggestive of this diagnosis. R = right; L = left; H = head; F = foot; Li = liver; DC = duplication cyst; D = diaphragm; K = kidney; T = through transmission; Du = duodenum; G = gallbladder.

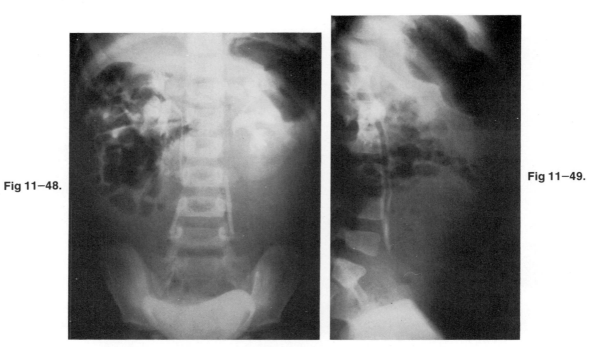

Fig 11-48.

Fig 11-49.

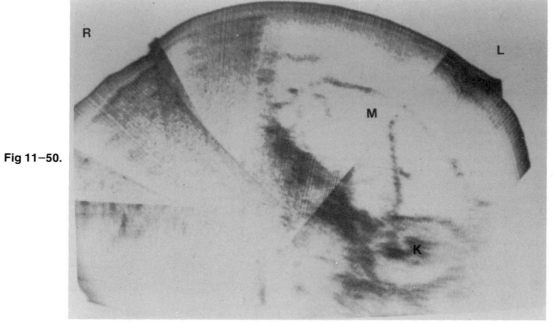

Fig 11-50.

270

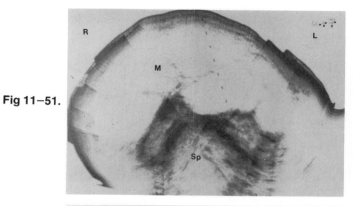

Fig 11—51.

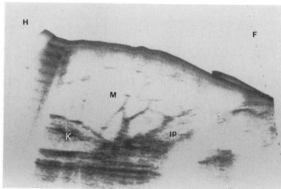

Fig 11—52.

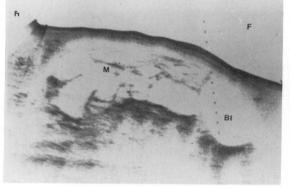

Fig 11—53.

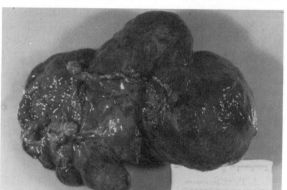

Fig 11—54.

Figs 11–48 to 11–54. — Cystic lymphangioma. Many times clinical examination or other imaging procedures, such as excretory urogram (Figs 11–48 and 11–49), will indicate intra-abdominal mass and further characterization is warranted. Ultrasonography of the region can determine cystic, complex or solid nature of the process and relate it to other intra-abdominal structures (Figs 11–50 to 11–53). The pathological specimen in this case of cystic lymphangioma is illustrated for morphologic comparison (Fig 11–54). R = right; L = left; H = head; F = feet; M = mass; K = kidney; Sp = spine; IP = iliopsoas muscle; Bl = bladder.

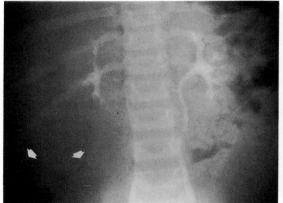

Fig 11—55.

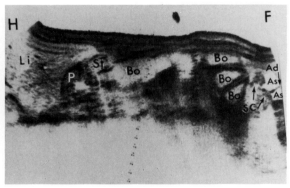

Fig 11—56.

Figs 11—55 and 11—56.— Mesenteric cyst. Relatively large mesenteric cyst, displacing right kidney, can be seen in excretory urogram (Fig 11–55, *arrowhead*) but cannot be sep-

arated from liver. Ultrasonography (Fig 11–56) shows the large fluid collection separate from liver. H = head; F = feet; FM = fluid mass.

Fig 11—57.

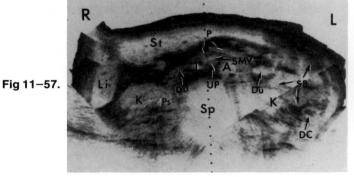

Fig 11—58.

Figs 11—57 to 11—62.— Distended bowel. A difficult diagnosis to make on ultrasonograms is bowel distended with either fluid or feces (Fig 11–57). Careful scanning technique may delineate mucosal lining of such fluid-filled masses, allowing for proper identification (Figs 11–58 and 11–59). In addition, real-time examination may allow the sonographer to detect peristaltic waves (Fig 11–60) or to watch movement of air bubbles. Alternatively, one may watch changes in position of movable portions of bowel with real-time as the patient's position is altered. When bowel is distended with stool and food contents, it may have a bizarre type of mixed echogenic pattern. In children, this

may be encountered in Hirschsprung's disease (Fig 11–61). Calcified fecaloma in the cecum strongly suggests diagnosis of Hirschsprung's disease in this patient (Fig 11–62). R = right; L = left; H = head; F = feet; St = stomach; Li = liver; K = kidney; P = pancreas; SMV = superior mesenteric vein; I = inferior vena cava; A = aorta; UP = uncinate process; Du = duodenum; SB = small bowel; Sp = spine; Ps = psoas muscle; DC = descending colon; GB = gallbladder; PC = peristaltic contraction; MV = mesenteric vein; Bo = bowel; As = ascites; Ad = adnexa; SC = sigmoid colon; Ca = cardia of stomach; TP = tail of pancreas; SV = splenic vein; Bl = bladder; BG = bowel gas.

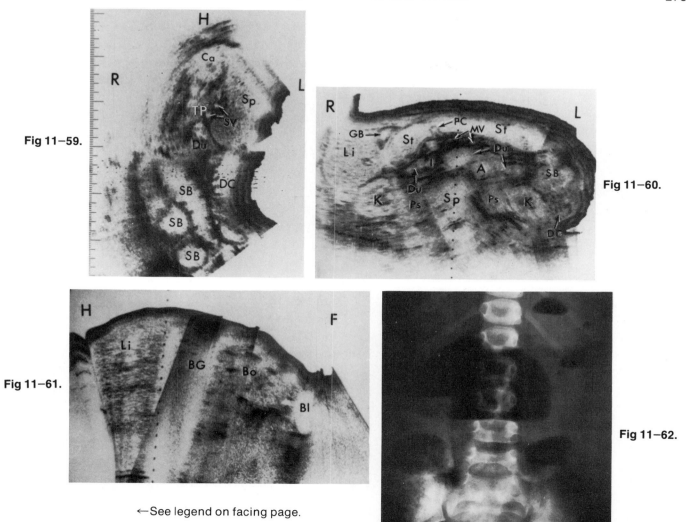

Fig 11–59.

Fig 11–60.

Fig 11–61.

Fig 11–62.

←See legend on facing page.

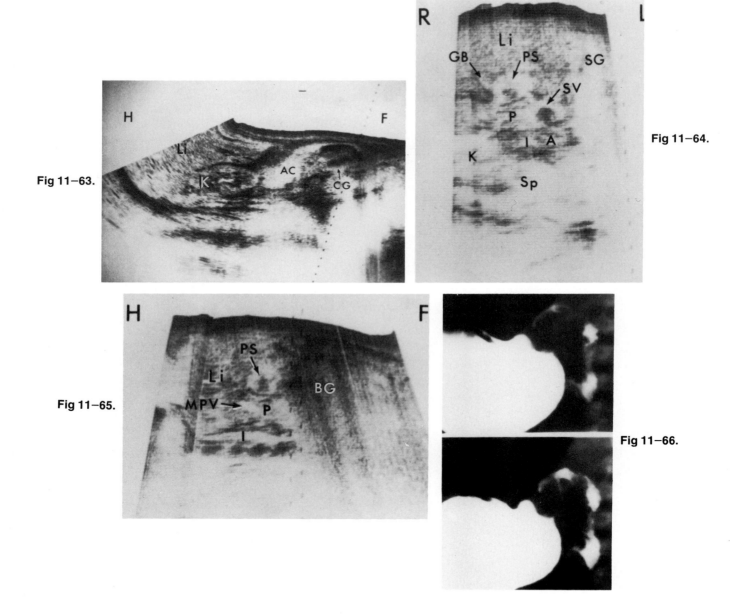

Fig 11–63.

Fig 11–64.

Fig 11–65.

Fig 11–66.

Figs 11–63 to 11–66.—Abnormal bowel. In some cases, presence of abnormal bowel can be suggested on ultrasonograms. By means of careful attention to gas or mucosa patterns, an abnormality such as Crohn's disease of the colon can be suspected (Fig 11–63). Similarly, duodenal bulb and pylorus can frequently be identified on ultrasonograms. When muscular layer becomes thickened, this region attains a size greater than 1 cm and the muscular-mucosal disproportion can be appreciated, suggesting diagnosis of pyloric stenosis (Figs 11–64 and 11–65). When these abnormalities are suggested on ultrasonograms, the proper gastrointestinal tract study can be recommended, such as an upper gastrointestinal series in the case of pyloric stenosis (Fig 11–66). H = head; F = feet; R = right; L = left; K = kidney; Li = liver; AC = ascending colon; CG = colon gas; Ps = psoas muscle; GB = gallbladder; PS = pyloric stenosis; P = pancreas; SV = splenic vein; SG = stomach gas; I = inferior vena cava; A = aorta; K = kidney; Sp = spine; MPV = main portal vein; BG = bowel gas.

12

Retroperitoneum

WILMS' TUMOR and neuroblastoma are the major retroperitoneal tumors in the pediatric patient and these are discussed in chapters 6 and 7. Teratoma, lymphangioma, enterogenous cyst, xanthogranuloma, giant lymph node hyperplasia (Castleman's disease), lymphoma, metastasis and inflammatory masses are found in the retroperitoneum. Embryonal rhabdomyosarcoma and fibromatosis involving only the retroperitoneum are uncommon.

TUMORS

Lymphomas

Malignant lymphomas are relatively rare, constituting about 10% of all childhood neoplasms. They are usually divided into Hodgkin's lymphoma and non-Hodgkin's lymphoma (NHL). Hodgkin's disease is rare before the age of 5, with a gradual rise of cases until adolescence when a striking increase is noted through age 30. Male pediatric patients predominate. Non-Hodgkin's lymphomas are heterogeneous by histopathology, site of origin and clinical manifestations. In children, NHL is 3 to 4 times more common than Hodgkin's lymphoma and differs in many respects from the adult form. In childhood NHL, the malignant cells are poorly differentiated, infiltration is diffuse, therapy is less effective and there is earlier dissemination.

Accurate staging of lymphoma is a prerequisite for subsequent therapy. Prior to the advent of computerized tomography and ultrasound, lymphangiography and laparotomy were the cornerstones of diagnosis and staging.

The para-aortic nodes are commonly involved in Hodgkin's lymphoma and somewhat less frequently so in NHL. Fifty percent of patients with NHL have mesenteric lymph node involvement at initial diagnosis. The splenic hilar nodes are involved in only a small percentage of Hodgkin's disease patients but in more than 50% of patients with NHL.

Gallium citrate-67 scanning, lymphangiography, computerized body scanning, ultrasound, chest roentgenology and conventional tomography are the usual tools of investigation. Depending on the site of lymphomatous disease, one modality is often superior to the others, and usually at least two complementary studies are performed prior to surgery. Laparotomy with lymph node biopsy and splenectomy are still undertaken for diagnosis and staging. Splenic involvement indicates a high probability of microscopic disease in the liver and/or bone marrow. This information is critical in the determination of therapy.

Retroperitoneal Metastasis

Metastatically involved nodes usually are seen as a single or discrete mass or as multiple, conglomerate masses in the para-aortic region or other nodal locations. Lymphangiography will be diagnostic, but in a patient with a known primary tumor in whom retroperitoneal metastases are suspected, demonstration of these nodes by ultrasound or, if necessary, computerized tomography is sufficient.

Retroperitoneal Hemangioma

Multiple small calcific densities in the retroperitoneum are suggestive of the diagnosis on plain films of the abdomen, but ultrasound or computerized tomography may be required to document the size and extent of the lesion.

Retroperitoneal Liposarcoma

Gallium scans do not always detect retroperitoneal liposarcoma since frequent hemorrhage and necrosis impair gallium uptake. Ultrasound will image a mass, but the echogenicity depends on the amount of fat and degree of necrosis and hemorrhage. Computerized tomography in some cases may be able to suggest the specific diagnosis because of the fat content, since fat has a characteristic attenuation number (0–90 Hounsfield units).

Retroperitoneal Teratoma

This entity is usually identified on a plain film of the abdomen, demonstrating fat and bone elements. It may be located above, medial to or below the kidney, with concomitant displacement of the kidney. It is called fetus in fetu if there is a recognizable trunk and limbs.

NONTUMOROUS RETROPERITONEAL MASSES

Inflammatory Masses

The incidence of retroperitoneal abscesses has decreased in recent years, but they constitute a serious problem, for the mortality is 40–50%. Pyelonephritis, bowel perforation, trauma, surgery and tuberculosis are predisposing factors. The excretory urogram may be normal, the gallium scan should be abnormal, but ultrasound and, if necessary, computerized tomography are the modalities of choice for direct visualization, rapid diagnosis and estimation of location and size. The images of abscesses are similar to those found elsewhere in the body, and blood, pus and urine can all have a similar appearance.

Hemorrhage

In the pediatric population, trauma is the most common cause of hemorrhage and may be present in spite of normal plain film findings, including normal iliopsoas borders or no renal displacement. Fresh hemorrhage is sonolucent at the time of initial ultrasound examination, but as it ages into a hematoma, echoes begin to appear, reflecting clot formation. With time and lysis of the clot, the echoes will again disappear. A fresh hematoma on computerized tomographic evaluation has an attenuation value of approximately 20–40 Hounsfield units, decreasing as the hematoma ages to as low as 12 Hounsfield units in one month's time (−1,000 to +1,000 scale). The hematoma may obscure, displace or compress normal retroperitoneal structures.

Fibrosis

Retroperitoneal fibrosis can produce ureteral obstruction and has rarely been noted in children. The distribution of fibrosis varies in extent and location, but the majority of cases are located over the anterior sacrum and inferior part of the lumbar spine at the sacral promontory. The cause may be idiopathic or related to previous surgery or drugs, and the diagnosis of retroperitoneal fibrosis is suspected on the clinical signs and symptoms of backache, abdominal pain, leg edema and hydrocele. At the time of excretory urography, typically there is hydronephrosis and ureterectasis limited to the upper ureter, with medial deviation of the ureters.

The ultrasound appearance is one of a relatively echo-free, smooth, bordered mass with subtle low-level gray tones within the mass. Lymphomatous retroperitoneal nodes elevate the aorta and vena cava from the spine.

REFERENCES

Arger, P. H., et al.: Retroperitoneal fibrosis: An analysis of the clinical spectrum and roentgenographic signs, A.J.R. 119:812, 1973.

Bekerman, C., et al.: Scintigraphic evaluation of childhood malignancies by ^{67}Ga-citrate, Radiology 127:719, 1978.

Brasch, R. C., et al.: Computed body tomography in children: Evaluation of 45 patients, A.J.R. 131:21, 1978.

Brascho, D. J., et al.: The accuracy of retroperitoneal ultrasonography in Hodgkin's disease and non-Hodgkin's lymphoma, Radiology 125:485, 1977.

Breiman, R. S., et al.: CT-pathologic correlations in Hodgkin's disease and non-Hodgkin's lymphoma, Radiology 126:159, 1978.

Cabanillas, F., et al.: Comparison of lymphangiograms and gallium scans in the non-Hodgkin's lymphomas, Cancer 39:85, 1977.

Caffey, J.: *Pediatric X-Ray Diagnosis* (7th ed; Chicago: Year Book Medical Publishers Inc., 1978).

Castellino, R. A., et al.: Lymphographic accuracy in Hodgkin's disease and malignant lymphoma with a note on the "reactive" lymph node as a cause of most false-positive lymphograms, Invest. Radiol. 9:155, 1974.

Dehner, L. P., et al.: Soft Tissue, Peritoneum, and Retroperitoneum, in *Pediatric Surgical Pathology* (St. Louis: C. V. Mosby Co., 1975).

Edeling, C. J.: Tumor visualization using [67]gallium scintigraphy in children, Radiology 127:727, 1978.

Farrer, J.: Idiopathic retroperitoneal fibrosis: Report of first case observed in a child, Pediatrics 30:225, 1962.

Glatstein, E., et al.: The value of laparotomy and splenectomy in the staging of Hodgkin's disease, Cancer 24:709, 1969.

Goffinet, D. R., et al.: Staging laparotomies in unselected previously untreated patients with non-Hodgkin's lymphomas, Cancer 32:672, 1973.

Handmaker, H., et al.: Gallium imaging in pediatrics, J. Nucl. Med. 18:1057, 1977.

Hoffer, P. B., et al.: The utility of gallium-67 in tumor imaging: A comment on the final reports of the cooperative study group, J. Nucl. Med. 19:1082, 1978.

Johnston, G. S., et al.: Gallium-67 citrate imaging in Hodgkin's disease: Final report of cooperative group, J. Nucl. Med. 18:692, 1977.

Kaplan, H. S., et al.: Hodgkin's disease: Multidisciplinary contributions to the conquest of a neoplasm, Radiology 123:551, 1977.

Laing, F. C., et al.: Value of ultrasonography in the detection of retroperitoneal inflammatory masses, Radiology 123:169, 1977.

Lee, R. K. T., et al.: Accuracy of computed tomography in detecting intra-abdominal and pelvic adenopathy in lymphoma, A.J.R. 131:311, 1978.

Martin, D. W., et al.: Hodgkin's disease, West. J. Med. 127:487, 1977.

Nelson, W. E., et al.: *Textbook of Pediatrics* (9th ed; Philadelphia: W. B. Saunders Co., 1969).

Peterson, A. S., et al.: Retroperitoneal fibrosis and gluteal pain in a child, J. Pediatr. 85:228, 1974.

Pilepich, M. V., et al.: Contribution of computed tomography to the treatment of lymphomas, A.J.R. 131:69, 1978.

Redman, H. C., et al.: Computed tomography as an adjunct in the staging of Hodgkin's disease and non-Hodgkin's lymphomas, Radiology 124:381, 1977.

Rochester, D., et al.: Ultrasound in the staging of lymphoma, Radiology 124:483, 1977.

Sagel, S. S., et al.: Detection of retroperitoneal hemorrhage by computed tomography, A.J.R. 129:403, 1977.

Sample, W. F.: Normal abdominal anatomy defined by gray-scale ultrasound, Radiol. Clin. North Am. 17:3, 1979.

Sample, W. F., et al.: Computed body tomography and gray-scale ultrasonography: Anatomic correlations and pitfalls in the upper abdomen, Gastrointest. Radiol. 3:243, 1978.

Sanders, R. C., et al.: Sonography in the diagnosis of retroperitoneal fibrosis, J. Urol. 118:944, 1977.

Stephens, D. H., et al.: Diagnosis and evaluation of retroperitoneal tumors by computed tomography, A.J.R. 129:395, 1977.

Stevenson, E. O., et al.: Retroperitoneal space abscesses, Surg. Gynecol. Obstet. 128:1202, 1969.

Zelch, M. G., et al.: Clinical comparison of computed tomography and lymphangiography for detection of retroperitoneal lymphadenopathy, Radiol. Clin. North Am. 17:157, 1979.

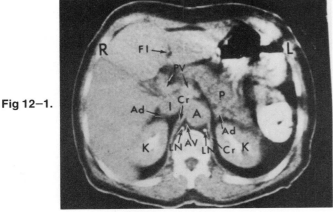

Fig 12–1.

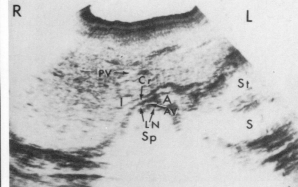

Fig 12–2.

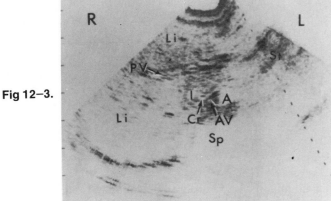

Fig 12–3.

Figs 12–1 to 12–3.—Normal retroperitoneum. Both computed body tomography (Fig 12–1) and ultrasonography (Figs 12–2 and 12–3) are important imaging modalities for retroperitoneum. With faster computerized tomographic scanners and improved gray-scale ultrasound instrumentation, an incredible amount of detail can be imaged. In high retroperitoneum, crura of diaphragm can be imaged with both modalities. Where crus decussates in front of aorta, portions of lymphatic system as well as azygos venous system can be seen with both modalities. Although size criteria have not been established for children, in adults these structures should normally reach a diameter no greater than 5 mm. If a mass is encountered in retrocrural area greater than 5 mm in diameter, it can arise from either lymphatic or vascular system. Alternatively, primary retroperitoneal tumors can appear in this region. R = right; L = left; Fl = falciform ligament; PV = portal vein; Ad = adrenal gland; K = kidney; I = inferior vena cava; A = aorta; Cr = crus of diaphragm; P = pancreas; LN = lymph nodes; Sp = spine; S = spleen; St = stomach; Li = liver; AV = azygos vein.

Fig 12–4.

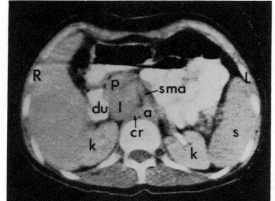

Fig 12–5.

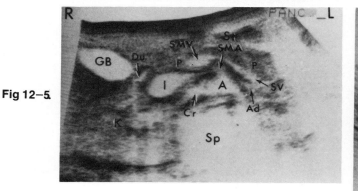

Fig 12–6.

Figs 12–4 to 12–6.—Normal retroperitoneum. As one progresses caudally in upper retroperitoneum, right crus of diaphragm may become quite prominent, wedged between inferior vena cava and aorta. This portion of crus may reach a size of 1–1.5 cm and must be specifically identified in patients on both computed body tomograms (Fig 12–4) and ultrasonograms (Figs 12–5 and 12–6). In addition, various branches of aorta and inferior vena cava should be individually identified as one progresses caudally. If all the anatomy in this region is identified, then small abnormal masses can be identified. R = right; L = left; P = pancreas; Du = duodenum; I = inferior vena cava; A = aorta; Cr = crus of diaphragm; k = kidney; SMA = superior mesenteric artery; s = spleen; GB = gallbladder; Sp = spine; Ad = adrenal gland; SV = splenic vein; St = stomach; PV = portal vein; HA = hepatic artery; SMV = superior mesenteric vein.

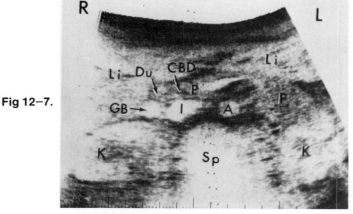

Fig 12–7.

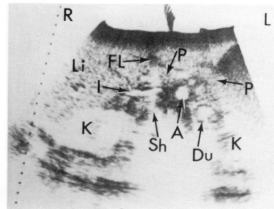

Fig 12–8. →

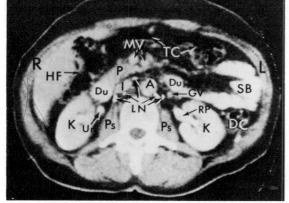

Fig 12–9.

Figs 12–7 to 12–9. — Normal retroperitoneum. In the region of head of pancreas, a variety of patterns in gallbladder and duodenum may be encountered. The most confusing variation is the presence of the gallbladder in Morison's pouch (Fig 12–7). The 2d and particularly the 4th portion of duodenum may be difficult to identify on all ultrasonograms. Occasionally, echogenic mucus and sometimes fluid pattern can be identified (Fig 12–8). The 2d and 4th portions of duodenum are usually far better identified on computed body tomograms when they are scanned after oral ingestion of iodinated contrast agents (Fig 12–9). These portions of duodenum may reside at same level as lymph nodes, indicated in this patient by their high density, which is a consequence of previously administered lym-phangiographic contrast material. Also noted in the computed body tomogram is round structure in left mid retroperitoneum representing prominent gonadal vein. This structure can also reach a size of 1 cm in some patients and must not be mistaken for a pathological process. R = right; L = left; Li = liver; Du = duodenum; GB = gallbladder; CBD = common bile duct; P = pancreas; K = kidney; I = inferior vena cava; A = aorta; Sp = spine; FL = falciform ligament; Sh = shadowing; HF = hepatic flexure of colon; MV = mesenteric vessels; Ur = ureter; Ps = psoas muscle; LN = lymph node; GV = gonadal vein; SB = small bowel; DC = descending colon; TC = transverse colon; RP = renal pelvis.

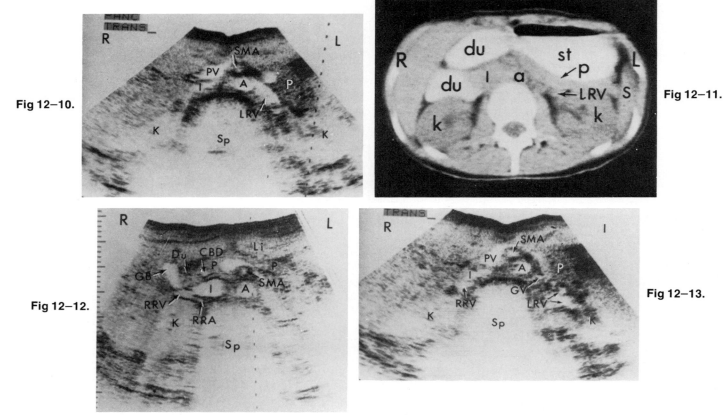

Figs 12–10 to 12–13. — Normal retroperitoneum. As one scans caudally in the retroperitoneum, additional normal structures that may appear as prominent masses are renal vessels. The left renal vein, particularly in supine positions with patient holding his breath in Valsalva's maneuver, may be partially enlarged as it passes between superior mesenteric artery and aorta. Proximal segment in left side of retroperitoneum may be quite sizable and may be mistaken for a retroperitoneal mass (Figs 12–10 to 12–13). Similarly, on the right, the renal vein or the renal artery, particularly in patients with ptotic kidneys, may appear as a rounded structure (see Fig 12–12) that can attain a size close to 1 cm. Carefully tracing these back to origin from prevertebral vessels will eliminate confusion. Similarly, gonadal vein on left side may represent prominent structure that must not be confused with retroperitoneal mass (see Fig 12–13). R = right; L = left; PV = portal vein; I = inferior vena cava; A = aorta; P = pancreas; LRV = left renal vein; K or k = kidney; Sp = spine; Du or du = duodenum; st = stomach; S = spleen; GB = gallbladder; CBD = common bile duct; Li = liver; RRV = right renal vein; RRA = right renal artery; SMA = superior mesenteric artery; GV = gonadal vein.

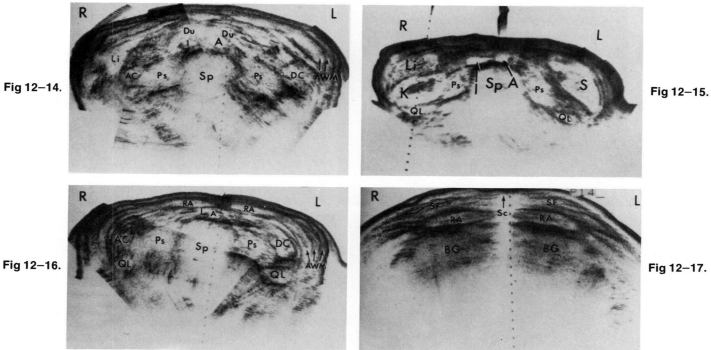

Fig 12–14.

Fig 12–15.

Fig 12–16.

Fig 12–17.

Figs 12–14 to 12–17.—Normal retroperitoneum. Mid to lower retroperitoneum is a difficult area to examine by ultrasound. Only in very thin patients with collapsed bowel can high-detail scans be obtained (Figs 12–14 and 12–15). In these situations many layers of the abdominal wall can be specifically identified (Fig 12–16). In addition, prevertebral vessels can be clearly seen, as well as retrofascial muscles (psoas and quadratus lumborum). Nevertheless, in many patients loops of bowel adjacent to prevertebral vessels may mimic retroperitoneal masses (Fig 12–17). With advent of high-resolution real-time systems, these may be identified specifically by peristalsis or air bubbles. R = right; L = left; Li = liver; Du = duodenum; I = inferior vena cava; A = aorta; AC = ascending colon; Ps = psoas muscle; Sp = spine; DC = descending colon; AWM = abdominal wall muscle; S = spleen; K = kidney; QL = quadratus lumborum muscle; RA = rectus abdominus muscle; SF = subcutaneous fat; BG = bowel gas; Sc = scar.

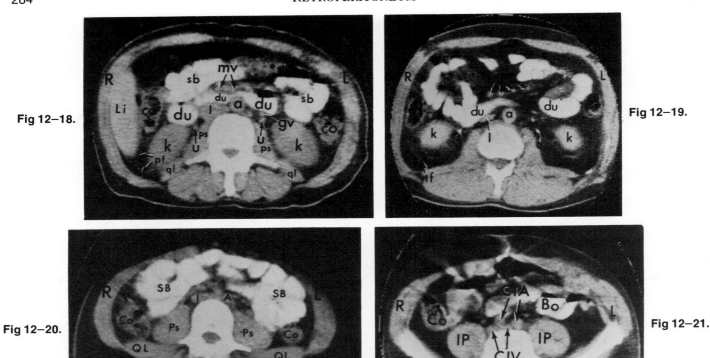

Fig 12–18.

Fig 12–19.

Fig 12–20.

Fig 12–21.

Figs 12–18 to 12–21.—Normal retroperitoneum. Mid to lower retroperitoneum is frequently far better visualized on computed body tomograms (Figs 12–18 to 12–21). Bowel can be specifically identified by gas pattern in colon and by oral iodinated contrast material in small bowel or colon. The 2d, 3d and 4th portions of duodenal sweep course surprisingly close to lymph-node-bearing regions and are more easily identified on computed body tomograms (Figs 12–18 and 12–19). In addition, ureters can be specifically identified by means of intravenous contrast material. In fat patients, anterior and posterior pararenal fascia representing divisions of transversalis fascia can be specifically identified. As a result, perinephric and anterior and posterior paranephric spaces can be specifically delineated. One potentially confusing area, however, is at the bifurcation of aorta and inferior vena cava (Fig 12–21). The aorta branches into common iliac arteries anteriorly and somewhat cephalically to the branching of the inferior vena cava into common iliac veins. This, in conjunction with ureters and gonadal vein, can lead to a number of round structures normally present in this area. R = right; L = left; Li = liver; Co or co = colon; k = kidney; pf = pararenal fascia; QL or ql = quadratus lumborum; u = ureter; Ps = psoas muscle; du = duodenum; SB or sb = small bowel; I = inferior vena cava; a = aorta; mv = mesenteric vein; gv = gonadal vein; tf = transversalis fascia; CIA = common iliac arteries; IP = iliopsoas muscles; Bo = bowel; CIV = common iliac veins.

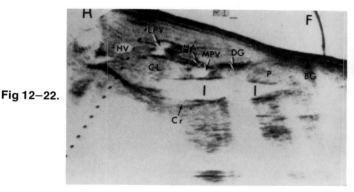

Fig 12–22.

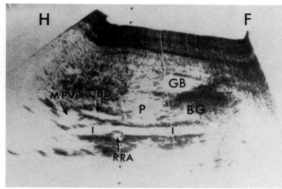

Fig 12–23.

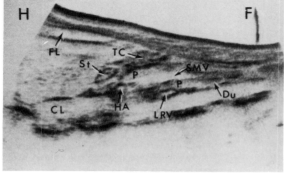

Fig 12–24.

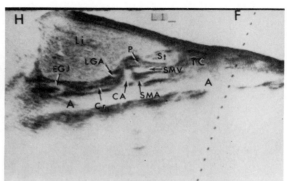

Fig 12–25.

Figs 12–22 to 12–25. — Normal retroperitoneum. Longitudinal parasagittal ultrasonograms performed with patient in supine position are critical to adequate evaluation of the retroperitoneum. In region of inferior vena cava, crus of the diaphragm lies posteriorly (Fig 12–22). In addition, right renal artery may notch undersurface of inferior vena cava (Fig 12–23). Portions of main portal vein, common bile duct and 3d portion of duodenum should be specifically identified since they can appear as apparent retroperitoneal masses. Similarly, anterior to the pancreas, both stomach and transverse colon should be identified to avoid mistaking them for mesenteric masses (Fig 12–24). Main branches of aorta, as well as their subsequent first-order branches, should be specifically identified (Fig 12–25). Uncinate process of pancreas passing underneath superior mesenteric vessel should not be mistaken for retroperitoneal mass. Similarly, decussating portion of crus between esophagogastric junction and celiac artery may be quite prominent and mimic a retroperitoneal mass. H = head; F = feet; HV = hepatic vein; LPV = left portal vein; CL = caudate lobe; Cr = crus of diaphragm; I = inferior vena cava; HA = hepatic artery; MPV = main portal vein; DG = duodenal gas; P = pancreas; BG = bowel gas; CBD = common bile duct; RRA = right renal artery; GB = gallbladder; FL = falciform ligament with properitoneal fat pad; TC = transverse colon; St = stomach; SMV = superior mesenteric vein; LRV = left renal vein; Du = duodenum; EGJ = esophagogastric junction; Li = liver; LGA = left gastric artery; CA = celiac artery; A = aorta; SMA = superior mesenteric artery.

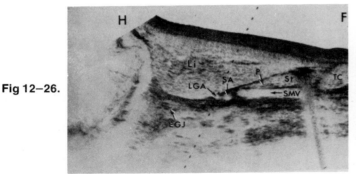

Fig 12–26.

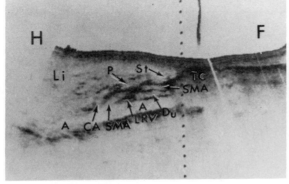

Fig 12–28.

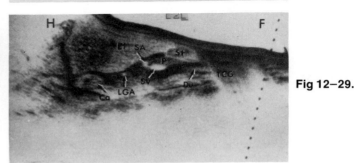

Fig 12–27.

Fig 12–29.

Figs 12–26 to 12–29. — Normal retroperitoneum. A variety of patterns of vasculature can be seen in any one section on longitudinal parasagittal ultrasonogram. Furthermore, if one is having difficulty identifying a specific structure, scanning more medially or laterally on longitudinal scans will usually determine origin of structure and whether it represents a normal or abnormal structure in retroperitoneum. Specific attention should be paid to patterns of bowel in esophagogastric junction, stomach and transverse colon areas (Fig 12–26). Attempts should be made to specifically identify left gastric artery, splenic artery, celiac artery, superior mesenteric artery, left renal vein, superior mesenteric vein and other prevertebral vessels (Figs 12–27 to 12–29). Prominent portions of crus of diaphragm should be identified. Finally, one of the more difficult areas to delineate is 3d portion of duodenum, which may mimic a midretroperitoneal mass (Figs 12–28 and 12–29). H = head; F = feet; Li = liver; EGJ = esophagogastric junction; LGA = left gastric artery; SA = splenic artery; P = pancreas; St = stomach; TC = transverse colon; SMV = superior mesenteric vein; Cr = crus of diaphragm; A = aorta; CA = celiac artery; SMA = superior mesenteric artery; IMA = inferior mesenteric artery; Du = duodenum; LRV = left renal vein; Ca = cardia of stomach; TCG = transverse colon gas; SV = splenic vein.

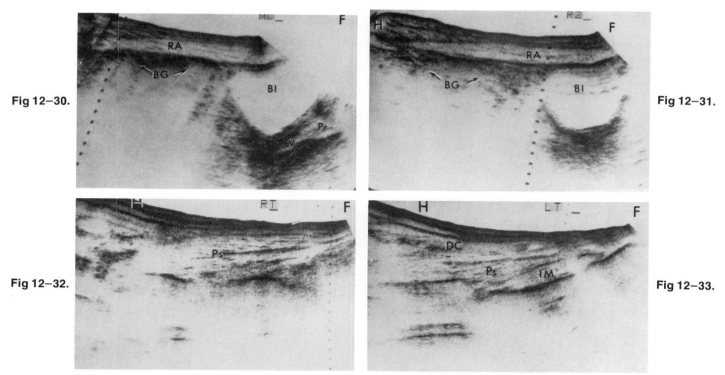

Figs 12–30.   **Fig 12–31.**

Fig 12–32.   **Fig 12–33.**

Figs 12–30 to 12–33.—Normal retroperitoneum. Even on longitudinal parasagittal scans, the mid to lower abdomen may be obscured by gas. Nevertheless, portions of rectus abdominus muscle as well as psoas muscle may be easily identified, particularly if pressure is applied with the transducer. The two components to iliopsoas muscle may be specifically identified, particularly in thin, muscular patients (Figs 12–30 to 12–33). One should utilize a full bladder to at least visualize portions of retroperitoneum as the muscles extend down into pelvis. In male patients, one can usually identify prostate and seminal vesicles (Fig 12–30); in females, both ovaries and uterus. H = head; F = feet; RA = rectus abdominus muscle; BG = bowel gas; Bl = bladder; SV = seminal vesicles; Pr = prostate; Ps = psoas muscle; IM = iliac muscle; DC = descending colon.

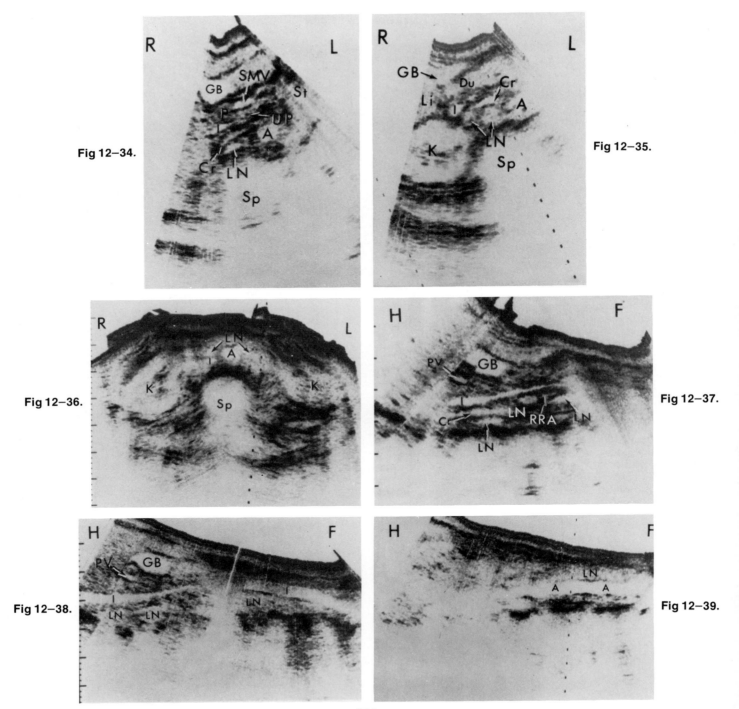

Fig 12–34.

Fig 12–35.

Fig 12–36.

Fig 12–37.

Fig 12–38.

Fig 12–39.

288

Figs 12–34 to 12–39. — Lymphadenopathy. Subtle degrees of adenopathy, whether from primary lymphoma or metastatic disease, can be detected if close attention is paid to anatomical detail. In and about the regions of the crus, nodes 1 to 2 cm in diameter can be detected as long as crus of the diaphragm can be specifically identified (Figs 12–34 and 12–35). In middle to lower retroperitoneum, adenopathy has to be more extensive to distinguish it as separable and distinct from bowel (Fig 12–36). Sometimes longitudinal scans can show the subtlest forms of adenopathy (Figs 12–37 to 12–39). Careful attention to the course of inferior vena cava and its distance from spine may indicate adenopathy. Diagnosis is more assured if one can identify specifically crus of diaphragm and right renal artery. Aorta may also be lifted from spine by a distance greater than 1 cm and is frequently associated with extension of the mass anteriorly (see Fig 12–39). Since aneurysms rarely occur in children, this is not often a diagnostic consideration. However, in adults one must pay close attention to configuration of mass surrounding aorta and its extension and obliteration of psoas muscles in order to make the correct diagnosis. R = right; L = left; H = head; F = feet; GB = gallbladder; SMV = superior mesenteric vein; P = pancreas; St = stomach; I = inferior vena cava; A = aorta; UP = uncinate process; Cr = crus of diaphragm; LN = lymph node; Sp = spine; Du = duodenum; K = kidney; Li = liver; RRA = right renal artery; PV = portal vein.

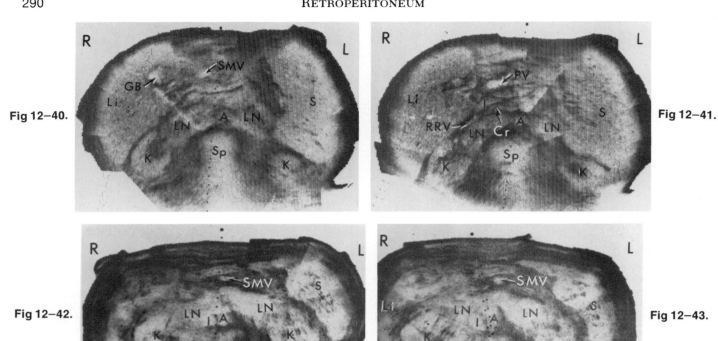

Figs 12–40. **Fig 12–41.** **Fig 12–42.** **Fig 12–43.**

Figs 12–40 to 12–43.—Lymphadenopathy. As lymphadenopathy in the retroperitoneum becomes more extensive, it is easier to diagnose on ultrasonograms. A number of patterns for lymph node enlargement have been observed and depend somewhat on cause of the process. In lymphoma (Figs 12–40 to 12–43) common pattern is mantle-shaped mass obliterating prevertebral vessels and tissue planes along psoas margins and kidneys. Alternatively, a number of small masses may be distinguishable (see Fig 12–41). As lymph node masses increase in size, more and more retroperitoneal vasculature will be visibly deviated. In lymphoma, one may note additional findings, such as splenomegaly. R = right; L = left; Li = liver; GB = gallbladder; SMV = superior mesenteric vein; LN = lymph node; A = aorta; S = spleen; K = kidney; Sp = spine; RRV = right renal vein; PV = portal vein; Cr = crus of diaphragm; I = inferior vena cava.

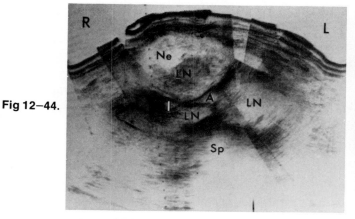

Fig 12–44.

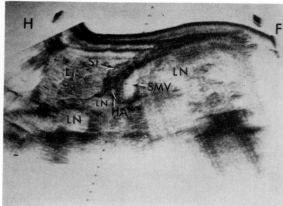

Fig 12–45.

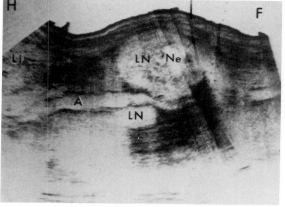

Fig 12–46.

Figs 12–44 to 12–46. —Lymphadenopathy. When massive lymphadenopathy occurs, it is readily detectable clinically as well as on ultrasonograms (Figs 12–44 to 12–46). Texture patterns, however, frequently change with areas of central necrosis (Figs 12–44 and 12–46). This is particularly true of metastatic disease, whereas it is uncommon with lymphoma. When large masses with central necrosis are identified, primary or metastatic retroperitoneal sarcoma must also be considered. R = right; L = left; H = head; F = feet; Ne = necrosis; LN = lymph node; A = aorta; I = inferior vena cava; Sp = spine; Li = liver; St = stomach; HA = hepatic artery; SMV = superior mesenteric vein.

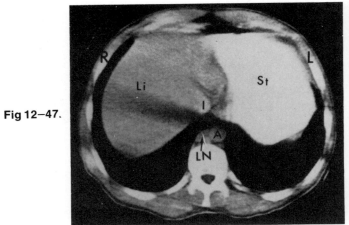

Fig 12–47.

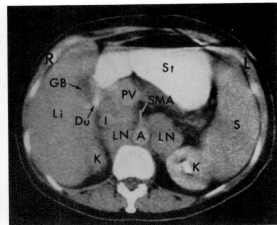

Fig 12–48.

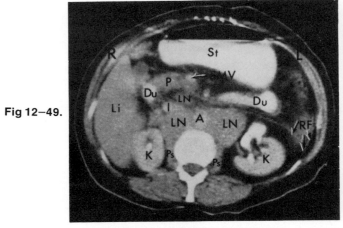

Fig 12–49.

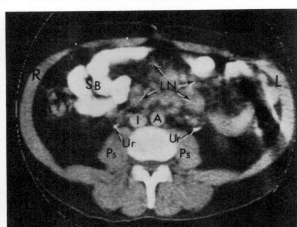

Fig 12–50.

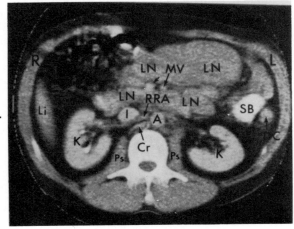

Fig 12–51.

Figs 12–47 to 12–51.—Lymphadenopathy. In older children, sufficient retroperitoneal fat is usually present so that computed tomography may be the procedure of choice in evaluating the retroperitoneum for lymphadenopathy. Extent of adenopathy into lower thorax can frequently be better appreciated by additional masses in the posterior mediastinum and retrocrural area (Fig 12–47). Findings of lymphadenopathy on computed tomograms in high and midretroperitoneum are similar to those of ultrasound (Figs 12–48 to 12–51). Computed body tomography has advantage of better delineating bowel by means of oral iodinated contrast material. Vessels that are frequently isodense with lymph nodes may be visualized by use of intravenous iodinated contrast material. Computed tomography also has possible advantage of better separating adenopathy that is in the mesentery vs. that in the retroperitoneal space. R = right; L = left; Li = liver; St = stomach; I = inferior vena cava; A = aorta; LN = lymph node; GB = gallbladder; PV = portal vein; Du = duodenum; SMA = superior mesenteric artery; K = kidney; S = spleen; P = pancreas; RF = renal fascia; SB = small bowel; Ur = ureters; Ps = psoas muscle; Cr = crus of diaphragm; RRA = right renal artery; MV = mesenteric vein; DC = descending colon; SMV = superior mesenteric vein.

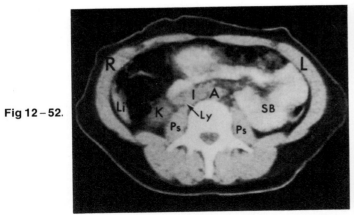

Fig 12–52.

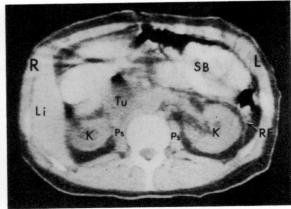

Fig 12–53.

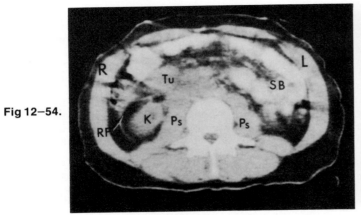

Fig 12–54.

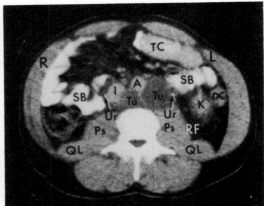

Fig 12–55.

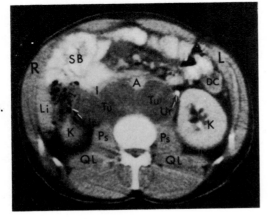

Fig 12–56.

Figs 12–52 to 12–56. – Lymphadenopathy. In the older child, computed tomography has a number of advantages over ultrasonography in evaluation of retroperitoneal disease. First, small bowel may normally reside very close to retroperitoneal structures and mimic masses on ultrasound. Bowel can be specifically highlighted on computed tomograms by means of oral iodinated contrast material administration. Subtle losses of fat planes can then be better appreciated. (Fig 12–52). In addition, anterior and posterior pararenal fascia can be visualized normally in a number of patients. Thickening of this fascia may indicate extension of a malignant process and can be detected with computed tomograms (Figs 12–53 and 12–54). This observation is not specific for malignancy; it can be observed in various inflammatory processes as well as the phlegmon associated with pseudocysts.

Computed tomography also has the advantage of better delineating ureters and determining whether their deviation is a normal variant or related to presence of tumor masses (Figs 12–55 and 12–56). Differential enhancement by intravenous iodinated contrast material has been noted in some metastases, specifically those arising from testicular primaries. R = right; L = left; Li = liver; K = kidney; I = inferior vena cava; A = aorta; Ps = psoas muscle; Ly = lymphoma; SB = small bowel; Tu = tumor; RF = renal fascia; Ur = ureter; QL = quadratus lumborum muscle; TC = transverse colon; DC = descending colon.

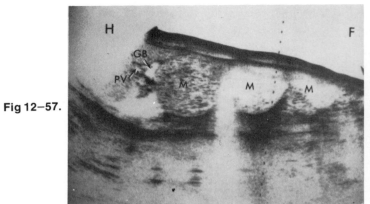

Fig 12—57.

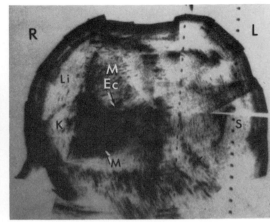

Fig 12—58.

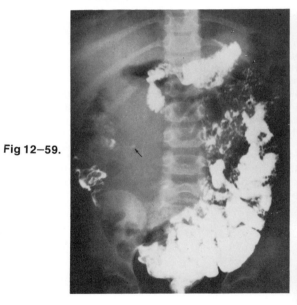

Fig 12—59.

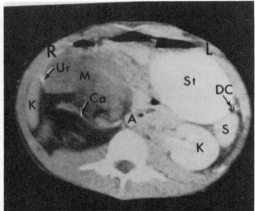

Fig 12—60.

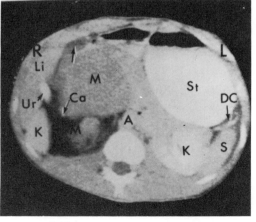

Fig 12—61.

296

Figs 12–57 to 12–61.—Retroperitoneal benign teratoma. Ultrasound may be utilized to characterize other retroperitoneal masses. In benign cystic teratomas, a variety of tissue components may be present. Cystic elements can readily be detected. When these tumors contain fat, hair or skeletal tissues, they usually appear as highly echogenic regions. This type of mixed pattern is very suggestive of teratomatous process (Figs 12–57 and 12–58). However, when these masses become quite large it may be difficult to identify all of the specific elements. Correlation with plain films or other routine radiological procedures (Fig 12–59, *arrow* points to calcification) may aid in differential diagnosis. Alternatively, one can use computed tomography for the advantages of defining specifically calcium and fat-containing areas (Figs 12–60 and 12–61). H = head; F = feet; R = right; L = left; GB = gallbladder; PV = portal vein; M = mass; Li = liver; K = kidney; S = spleen; Ec = echogenic region; Ur = ureter; Ca = calcification; A = aorta; St = stomach; DC = descending colon; F = fat; Sp = spine.

Fig 12–62.

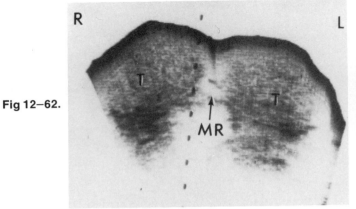

Fig 12–63.

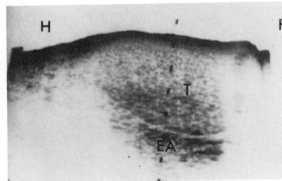

Fig 12–64.

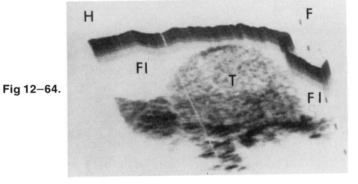

Fig 12–65.

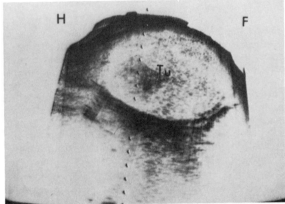

Figs 12–62 to 12–65. — Testicular ultrasound. Testicular ultrasound has become a very reliable adjunct to diagnosis of scrotal masses. In addition, in cases of retroperitoneal adenopathy where the primary lesion is unknown, ultrasound may be used to screen the scrotum for primary tumor. Testes are examined in both transverse and longitudinal scans (Figs 12–62 and 12–63). The normal testis has very homogeneous texture of medium echogenicity. The epididymis is not normally visualized. Distinction between extratesticular or testicular mass can reliably be made in approximately 85% of cases. In addition, fluid (Fig 12–64) vs. complex vs. solid aspects to a mass may give differential diagnostic information. Tumors in general have been less echogenic than normal testis (Fig 12–65) except in cases where there is central necrosis. Some of these acoustical texture patterns do overlap with benign disease of the testis, such as torsion and abscess. R = right; L = left; H = head; F = feet; T = testis; MR = median raphe; EA = epididymal area; Fl = fluid; Tu = tumor.

13

Trauma

BLUNT ABDOMINAL TRAUMA, the most common form of abdominal trauma, comprises 2–5% of all childhood accidents and occurs in two peak periods, 5 to 7 years and adolescence. If isolated to the abdomen, 80% of traumas are due to falls; if multiple injuries are involved, 60% are related to traffic accidents, with a male predominance. Children are generally more vulnerable than adults to the effects of comparable injury because of the relatively larger size of the viscera, lack of intra-abdominal and extra-abdominal fat and relatively pliable bones.

The spleen has the highest incidence of abdominal visceral injury, followed by the liver, kidneys, mesentery and bowel. The methods of investigation depend primarily on the site or sites of suspected injury and the clinical status of the patient. Although attention is focused more commonly on one organ, ultrasound and computerized tomography offer the significant advantage of rapid multiorgan evaluation and should be the initial means of investigation in many cases.

SPLEEN

In a child with severe blunt abdominal trauma, certain plain roentgenographic findings demand specific evaluation of the spleen. These include elevation of the left hemidiaphragm, medial displacement of the stomach, enlarged splenic shadow and fractured ribs.

Detailed examination of the spleen may be achieved by using ultrasound, radioisotope scanning, computerized tomography or angiography. Ultrasound and radioisotope scans are preferred in the pediatric age group; other investigative modalities are reserved for cases where diagnosis of splenic injury cannot be made accurately by ultrasonography or isotope scanning.

Recently, conservative management has been proposed by many pediatric surgeons when a relatively small splenic hematoma is present, since there is a markedly increased risk of postsplenectomy sepsis associated with a high mortality in the pediatric patient. Moreover, there is evidence that the traumatized spleen is capable of healing itself, and attempts are being made in those patients requiring splenic surgery to preserve functional tissue by primary repair and hemostatic agents. The conservative nonoperative approach requires close clinical monitoring and a watch for delayed rupture, the most serious consequence of nonintervention. Approximately 75% of delayed ruptures occur within the first 2 weeks after trauma, with the incidence falling rapidly after the first 4–5 days. The incidence of delayed rupture is 2–16%. If a hematoma is documented at the baseline study, follow-up examinations are required.

LIVER

The liver is the most commonly injured organ in penetrating abdominal trauma and is injured about half as frequently as the spleen in blunt abdominal trauma. The majority of patients with significant hepatic injury are admitted to the emergency room in profound shock. Penetrating hepatic injury even without significant clinical findings justifies surgical intervention to prevent subsequent massive hemorrhage. Blunt, closed abdominal trauma to the right upper quadrant on occasion may cause significant injury and yet be relatively silent to the examining physician. It is in these cases that ultrasound, radionuclide scanning, computerized tomography and arteriography can aid in patient management.

HEMATOBILIA

Immediate hematobilia occurs when the traumatized liver communicates directly with the biliary system. Delayed hematobilia follows development of an ischemic hepatic region that became necrotic and developed communication between the biliary system and the hepatic vein, hepatic artery or portal vein. The gastrointestinal bleeding that is the end result may therefore occur 3 days to 4 weeks following the initial trauma. Colicky pain and jaundice are the usual accompaniments.

BILE DUCT INJURY

Rupture of the extrahepatic ducts, although rare, has a high associated mortality when it occurs. Direct impact may squeeze bile from a full gallbladder into the ducts, causing rupture. Alternatively, a severe blow to the liver may cause the hepatoduodenal ligament to be wrenched superiorly and the duct to be torn away from its fixed duodenal attachments. Most ruptures occur in the retroduodenal area at the pancreatic margin. An operative cholangiogram is required when free bile is noted to be within the peritoneal cavity. A partial tear of the extrahepatic biliary system can result in extravasation and delayed ductal stenosis.

PANCREAS

Blunt abdominal trauma is the most frequent cause of pancreatic injury. Such injuries can be significant and include contusion, laceration, duct disruption and transection, as well as subsequent pseudocyst formation. The mechanism of injury is directly related to a compressing force that crushes the body of the gland against the vertebral column. Persistent amylase level elevations and a developing palpable mass are hallmarks of pseudocyst formation.

RENAL TRAUMA

When a history of blunt trauma, especially applied posteriorly, is associated with hematuria, investigation of the kidneys is mandatory. Suggestive plain film findings of injury include transverse process or lower rib fracture, loss of the renal contour and a contiguous soft tissue mass. At times a reflex ileus may obscure the kidneys.

The high-dose excretory urogram with nephrotomography is the initial means of investigation, and one of its most important results is the demonstration of a contralateral normal kidney.

Types of Renal Injury*

Renal contusion is the most common injury and the excretory urogram demonstrates little or no evidence of decreased function.

Cortical laceration may be suggested by a palpable mass or loss of psoas outline but the excretory urogram shows an intact collecting system.

Calyceal laceration: the excretory urogram demonstrates pericalyceal distortion with an intact renal outline and may have an intrarenal extravasation of contrast material or intraluminal calyceal filling defect representing a clot.

_____

*Adapted from Reid, 1973.

Complete fracture implies separation of the renal parenchyma from the pelvis or calyces or separation from the capsule with extravasation of contrast material into the perirenal tissues on the excretory urogram.

Pedicle injuries denote serious injury to the renal vascular supply and the excretory urogram demonstrates nonfunction of some parts or all of the kidney.

Although renal contusion is the most common injury, unless it is severe the excretory urogram may be normal. In those unusual circumstances in which the examination is nondiagnostic because of obscuring bowel gas or when a kidney is not visualized after injection, renal ultrasonography, isotope scanning, arteriography or computerized tomography should be judiciously utilized. The differential diagnosis of a nonvisualizing kidney includes contralateral solitary kidney, vascular pedicle disruption, thrombosis of the renal artery and severe renal contusion. To differentiate the possibilities, the renal isotope scan is a safe, rapid examination that often can be done portably in the emergency room using a technetium-labeled compound such as ^{99m}Tc-pentetic acid, ^{99m}Tc-dimercaptosuccinic acid (^{99m}Tc-DSMA) or ^{99m}Tc-glucoheptonate, and a high-resolution gamma camera. A flow study should be obtained at the time of injection to assess the status of the renal artery, and then static images should be obtained to assess the regional tubular function.

The place of arteriography in renal trauma is controversial. In the pediatric patient it requires technical skill, an available angiography team and sedation in the young child when it may be otherwise contraindicated. Arteriography is, however, an extremely accurate test usually reserved for those cases in which surgery is contemplated.

Demonstrating the positions of maximal functioning renal tissue is paramount in salvage of a portion of the kidney. Indications for arteriography include complete fracture and pedicle injuries. Delayed indications include persistent hematuria, renal artery bruit suggesting a possible pseudoaneurysm, and hypertension.

GASTROINTESTINAL TRACT AND MESENTERY

Gastric injuries are rare; if blunt abdominal trauma occurs with a distended, food-filled stomach, perforation may occur on the anterior wall.

Small-bowel injuries occur in 5–15% of children hospitalized for blunt abdominal trauma, with the most frequent sites of injury occurring at those points of relative fixation to the abdominal wall in the duodenum, adjacent to the ligament of Treitz and the terminal ileum.

The cecum and sigmoid colon are more susceptible to blunt trauma than the other portions of the colon. Partially covered by peritoneum, rupture may be intraperitoneal or extraperitoneal. Intramural hematomas, intraperitoneal perforations and retroperitoneal rupture are complications of blunt abdominal trauma.

Mesenteric lacerations and traumatic vascular injury can be identified at arteriography, but more commonly other coexisting serious injuries have forced immediate surgery.

PELVIC TRAUMA

Evaluation of the kidneys, ureters, bladder and urethra are imperative in cases of pelvic trauma. In the male, a modified retrograde examination can be performed through a Foley balloon catheter placed against the penis, and extravasation searched for at the time of injection.

Massive extraperitoneal arterial hemorrhage is a leading cause of death in patients with pelvic fracture. Active hemorrhage can be identified by the arteriographer and, in some instances, treated by embolization.

POSTTRAUMATIC OR POSTSURGICAL FLUID COLLECTIONS

Urinomas

Most cases of urinomas are a result of renal and ureteral trauma, although there are cases reported following surgical operations or diagnostic cystoscopic procedures involving inadvertent perforation. Rarely idiopathic, congenital obstruction or spontaneous perforation by a calculus can also result in urinoma formation.

A rent in calyces, renal pelvis or ureter allows urine to escape into the perirenal or periureteral tissues, causing irritation and a fibroblastic reaction and ultimately a pseudocyst that may not be recognized for several weeks or even months until pain and/or a palpable mass brings it to medical attention. Undetected intact urinomas may progress to abscess formation. Plain roentgenograms may reveal a unilateral mass usually displacing the kidney cephalad and laterally. The urinoma may lie next to a part of the kidney or may completely encompass the kidney similar to a hydrocele. Ultrasound examination will depict the relationship of the mass to the kidney, its size and its internal structure, and the clinical history should serve to differentiate it from a hematoma, abscess or lymphocele. If urinoma is suspected, the excretory urogram or renal scan is also necessary to evaluate renal function. Only rarely does contrast material fill the mass; more commonly, hydronephrosis is present with diminished renal function.

Lymphoceles

Lymphoceles are difficult to distinguish at ultrasound from abscesses and some hematomas, but should be among the diagnostic possibilities in the postsurgical, especially the renal transplant, patients. The ultrasound examination of lymphoceles usually shows irregular walls and internal echoes. Unlike abscesses, lymphoceles can have thin septae, but usually show no associated soft tissue changes or fluid-fluid levels, unless superimposed infection or hemorrhage has occurred.

Peritoneal Pseudocysts of Cerebrospinal Fluid

These are complications of ventricular peritoneal shunts and are associated with dysfunction of the shunt and increased intracranial pressure. A cyst is readily diagnosed by ultrasound, but localization of the shunt by plain films is necessary for conclusive diagnosis.

REFERENCES

Ahmed, S.: Bile duct injuries from non-penetrating abdominal trauma in childhood, Aust. N.Z. J. Surg. 46:109, 1976.

Asher, W. M., et al.: Echographic evaluation of splenic injury after blunt trauma, Radiology 118:411, 1976.

Babbitt, D. P., et al.: Intramural duodenal hematoma in children, Am. J. Dis. Child. 115:37, 1968.

Barbaric, Z. L., et al.: Control of renal arterial bleeding after percutaneous biopsy, Urology 8:108, 1976.

Burrington, J. D.: Surgical repair of a ruptured spleen in children, Arch. Surg. 112:417, 1977.

Caffey, J.: Pediatric X-Ray Diagnosis (7th ed; Chicago: Year Book Medical Publishers, Inc., 1978).

Chafen, L. T., et al.: Spontaneous perforation of the extrahepatic bile-duct, Br. J. Radiol. 49:798, 1976.

Charters, A. C., et al.: Intrahepatic bile duct rupture following blunt abdominal trauma, Arch. Surg. 113:873, 1978.

Cleveland, H. C., et al.: Retroperitoneal rupture of the duodenum due to non-penetrating trauma, Surg. Clin. North Am. 43:413, 1963.

Cockett, A. T. K., et al.: Recent advances in the diagnosis and management of blunt renal trauma, J. Urol. 113:750, 1975.

Cornell, W. P., et al.: X-ray diagnosis of penetrating wounds of the abdomen, J. Surg. Res. 5:142, 1965.

Douglas, G. J., et al.: The conservative management of splenic trauma, J. Pediatr. Surg. 6:565, 1971.

Ein, S. H., et al.: Nonoperative management of traumatized spleen in children, how and why, J. Pediatr. Surg. 13:117, 1978.

Emanuel, B., et al.: Renal trauma in children, J. Trauma 17:275, 1977.

Felson, B., et al.: Intramural hematoma of the duodenum, Radiology 63:823, 1954.

Flickinger, F. W., et al.: Radionuclide scan findings in delayed splenic rupture, Radiology 129:763, 1978.

Foley, L. C., et al.: Ultrasound of epigastric injuries after blunt trauma, A.J.R. 132:593, 1979.

Gilday, D. L., et al.: Scintigraphic evaluation of liver and spleen injury, Semin. Nucl. Med. 4:357, 1974.

Gold, R. E., et al.: Radiologic evaluation of splenic trauma, CRC Crit. Rev. Radiol. Sci. 3:453, 1972.

Gould, R. J., et al.: Retroperitoneal rupture of the duodenum due to blunt non-penetrating abdominal trauma, Radiology 80:743, 1963.

Griffin, L. H., et al.: The influence of radioisotope imaging on current treatment of blunt spleen trauma, Ann. Surg. 44:318, 1978.

Grosfeld, J. L., et al.: Pancreatic and gastrointestinal trauma in children, Pediatr. Clin. North Am. 22:365, 1975.

Harris, J. H., et al.: The roentgen diagnosis of pelvic extra-peritoneal effusion, Radiology 125:343, 1977.

Howman-Giles, R., et al.: Splenic trauma: Nonoperative management and long-term follow-up by scintiscan, J. Pediatr. Surg. 13:121, 1976.

Izant, R. J., et al.: Duodenal obstruction due to intramural hematoma in children, J. Trauma 4:797, 1964.

Javadpour, N., et al.: Renal trauma in children, Surg. Gynecol. Obstet. 136:237, 1973.

Kakos, G. S., et al.: Small bowel injuries in children after blunt abdominal trauma, Ann. Surg. 174:238, 1971.

Korobkin, M., et al.: Computed tomography of subcapsular splenic hematoma, Radiology 129:441, 1978.

Lang, E. K.: The role of arteriography in trauma, Radiol. Clin. North Am. 14:353, 1976.

McCort, J. J.: Abdominal Trauma, in Margulis, A. R. (ed.): *Alimentary Tract Roentgenology* (2d ed.; St. Louis: C. V. Mosby Co., 1973).

Nelson, W. E., et al:. *Textbook of Pediatrics* (9th ed; Philadelphia: W. B. Saunders, Co., 1969).

Parrish, R. A., et al.: Duodenal and biliary obstruction secondary to intramural hematoma, Am. J. Surg. 108:428, 1964.

Peters, P. C., et al.: Blunt renal injuries, Urol. Clin. North Am. 4:17, 1977.

Ratner, M. H., et al.: Surgical repair of the injured spleen, J. Pediatr. Surg. 12:1019, 1977.

Reid, I. S.: Renal trauma in children: A ten-year review, Aust. N.Z. J. Surg. 42:260, 1973.

Resnicoff, S. A., et al.: Retroperitoneal rupture of the duodenum due to blunt trauma, Surg. Gynecol. Obstet. 125:77, 1967.

Saad, S. A., et al.: Traumatic hematocele of the gallbladder with hemobilia, J. Trauma 19:67, 1979.

Sandblom, P.: Hemobilia, Surg. Clin. North Am. 53:1191, 1973.

Schiller, M., et al.: Diagnosis of experimental renal trauma, J. Pediatr. Surg. 7:187, 1972.

Scully, R. E., et al.: Weekly clinicopathological exercises: Case 9-1978, N. Engl. J. Med. 298:558, 1978.

Singer, D. B.: Postsplenectomy sepsis, Perspect. Pediatr. Pathol. 1:285, 1973.

Talbert, J. L., et al.: Acute abdominal injuries in children, Pediatr. Ann. 5:35, 1976.

Thomas, J. L., et al.: Echographic detection and characterization of abdominal hemorrhages: In patients with altered coagulation states, Arch. Intern. Med. 138:1392, 1978.

Tonnesen, P.: Rupture of extra-hepatic biliary ducts from blunt external trauma, Dan. Med. Bull. 17:238, 1970.

Trimble, C., et al.: Sinography of abdominal stab wounds, Am. J. Surg. 117:426, 1969.

Wicks, J. D., et al.: Gray-scale features of hematomas: An ultrasonic spectrum, A.J.R. 131:977, 1978.

Williams, J. E.: Radiology now. Renal trauma: The place of arteriography, Br. J. Radiol. 49:743, 1976.

Wynn, W. W., et al.: Comparison of arteriography, venography, and pyelography in experimental renal trauma, Invest. Urol. 16:62, 1978.

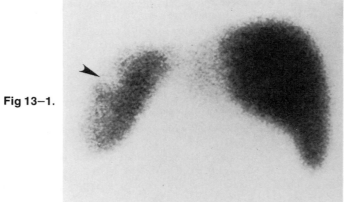

Fig 13–1.

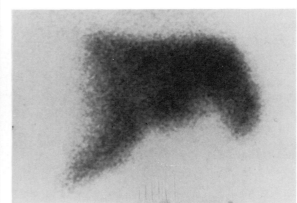

Fig 13–2.

Fig 13–3.

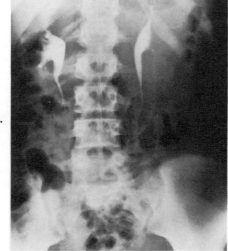

Figs 13–1 to 13–3.—Hematomas. A variety of modalities may be used to detect injured organs. These should be chosen according to clinical findings in a given patient. Splenic (Fig 13–1, *arrowhead*) and hepatic (Fig 13–2) hematomas can easily be identified with ^{99m}Tc-sulfur colloid scans. Renal and perirenal hematomas (Fig 13–3) may be detected roentgenographically. The best screening procedure in an injured child is probably ultrasonography, and further diagnostic modalities can follow initial ultrasonographic findings.

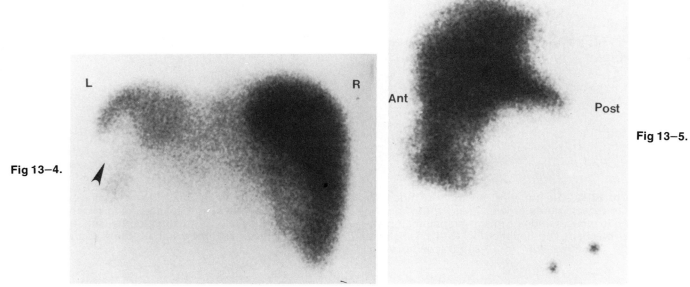

Fig 13-4.

Fig 13-5.

Figs 13—4 to 13—8.—Hematomas. Although ^{99m}Tc-sulfur colloid liver/spleen scan has acceptable accuracy for detecting splenic (Fig 13–4, *arrowhead*) and liver (Fig 13–5) hematomas, imaging modalities that can look at organs in addition to liver and spleen in trauma cases are preferable as screening procedures. Both ultrasound and computed tomography can serve this function, but in the pediatric age group ultrasound is preferred in order to minimize radiation. Furthermore, trauma to other areas may prevent moving the patient into the computed tomography gantry. On ultrasonograms, hematomas have variable acoustical texture that overlaps with other pathologic processes such as abscesses and tumors. As a result, clinical correlation is usually necessary to specifically suggest the diagnosis. Acoustical texture depends on the duration of the hematoma. L = left; R = right; Ant = anterior; Post = posterior.

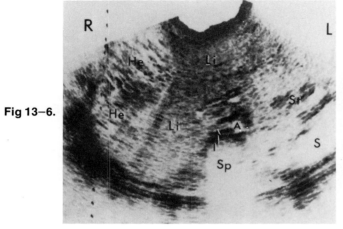

Fig 13–6.

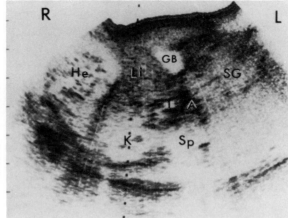

Fig 13–7.

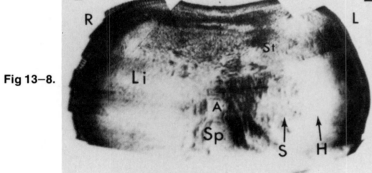

Fig 13–8.

Early on, hematomas may have variable echogenic pattern ranging from low-level to moderate-level echoes (Figs 13–6 and 13–7). After the liquefaction process begins, hematoma will take on more classical appearance of fluid collection (Fig 13–8). R = right; L = left; He = hematoma; Li = liver; Sp = spine; I = inferior vena cava; A = aorta; St = stomach; S = spleen; GB = gallbladder; SG = stomach gas; K = kidney; H = hematoma; Ant = anterior.

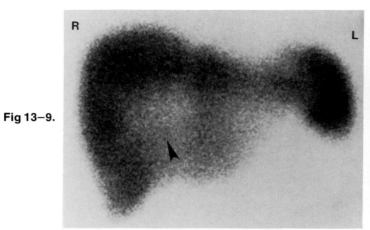

Fig 13–9.

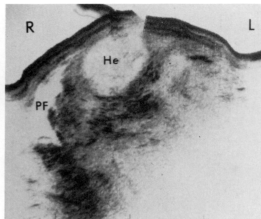

Fig 13–10.

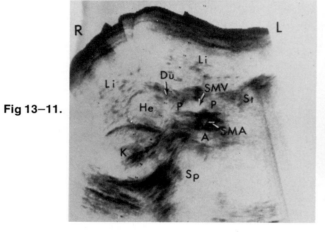

Fig 13–11.

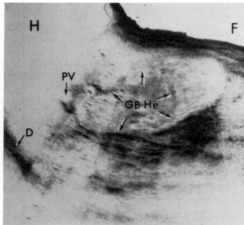

Fig 13–12.

Figs 13–9 to 13–12.—Hematomas. Technetium-99m-sulfur colloid liver/spleen scan may suggest hepatic or gallbladder hematoma by appropriate decrease in uptake of isotope in these regions (Fig 13–9, *arrowhead*). However, ultrasound may show additional information. Hematomas within gallbladder will usually demonstrate irregular echogenicity that may be partially mixed with bile or may completely fill gallbladder (Figs 13–10 to 13–12). Precise anatomical localization can be obtained by utilizing both transverse and longitudinal scans. In addition, ancillary findings such as free peritoneal fluid, as well as trauma to additional organs, may be found. R = right; L = left; He = hematoma; PF = peritoneal fluid; Li = liver; Du = duodenum; K = kidney; P = pancreas; SMV = superior mesenteric vein; SMA = superior mesenteric artery; A = aorta; Sp = spine; St = stomach; PV = portal vein; D = diaphragm; GBHe = gallbladder hematoma; H = head; F = feet.

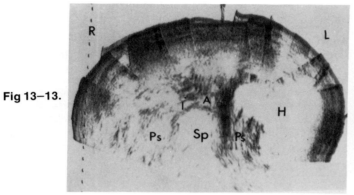

Fig 13–13.

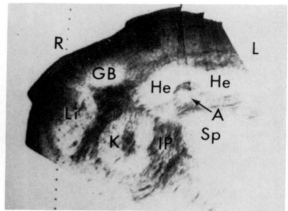

Fig 13–14.

Figs 13–13 to 13–17.—Hematomas. One of the advantages of ultrasound is ability to look at retroperitoneum as well as specific abdominal organs (Figs 13–13 to 13–15). By utilizing multiple patient positions, irregular fluid areas, with variable degrees of echogenicity may be observed in retroperitoneal and retrofascial spaces. Specific diagnosis that frequently can be made on ultrasound is a rectus hematoma (Fig 13–16). In some situations, an angiogram may be desirable in addition to the ultrasound. This additional modality is most frequently utilized in trauma to kidneys (Fig 13–17). R = right; L = left; I = inferior vena cava; A = aorta; Sp = spine (Figs 13–13 and 13–14, and spleen, Fig 13–15); Ps = psoas muscle; H and He = hematoma; Li = liver; GB = gallbladder; K = kidney; IP = iliopsoas muscle; LK = left kidney; RA = rectus abdominus muscle; RH = rectus hematoma; BG = bowel gas.

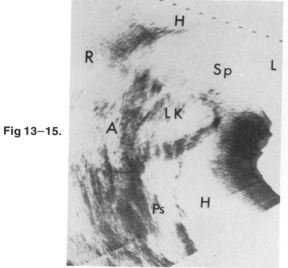

Fig 13–15.

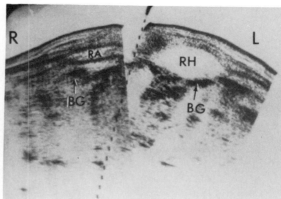

Fig 13–16.

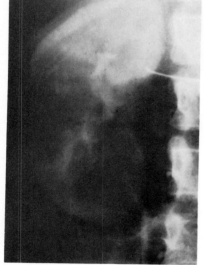

Fig 13–17.

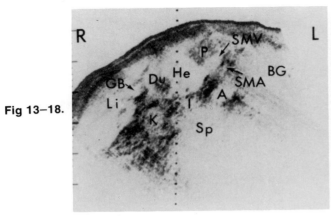

Fig 13–18.

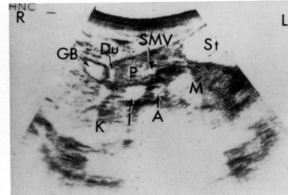

Fig 13–19.

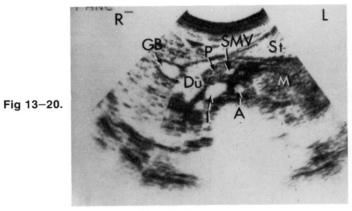

Fig 13–20.

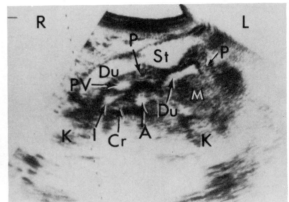

Fig 13–21.

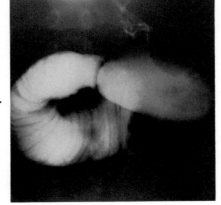

Fig 13–22.

Figs 13–18 to 13–22.—Hematomas. In some cases of blunt abdominal trauma, hematomas of the duodenal sweep can be specifically identified. Proximal to a duodenal hematoma, frequently fluid is present within the bowel secondary to the accompanying partial bowel obstruction. Figures 13–18 to 13–21 represent ultrasonograms demonstrating hematomas of 2d and 4th portions of duodenum, respectively. Multiple patient positions to move fluid around the duodenal sweep are frequently necessary to demonstrate the lesion. If suspicions are high, then upper gastrointestinal series can be performed to document the diagnosis and follow resolution of process (Fig 13–22). R = right; L = left; GB = gallbladder; Li = liver; K = kidney; Du = duodenum; He = hematoma; I = inferior vena cava; Sp = spine; A = aorta; P = pancreas; SMV = superior mesenteric vein; SMA = superior mesenteric artery; BG = bowel gas; M = hematoma; St = stomach; Cr = crus of diaphragm; PV = portal vein.

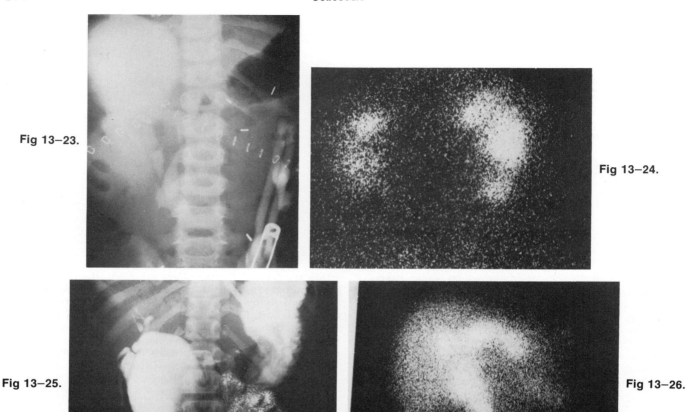

Fig 13–23.

Fig 13–24.

Fig 13–25.

Fig 13–26.

Figs 13–23 to 13–28. – Abnormal fluid collections follow-ing surgery. Various modalities may be utilized to make the diagnosis of abnormal fluid collection following operations. Figure 13–23 demonstrates large urinoma on the right side following operation for bilateral Wilms' tumor. Figure 13–24 is 26- to 28-second renal scan in another patient that demonstrates an area of increased activity in midportion of right kidney that subsequently was proved to be a urinoma.

Figure 13–25 is an upper gastrointestinal series in a child following surgical correction of a choledochal cyst. This study shows a large amount of contrast material in dilated duodenum and biliary tracts. Figure 13–26 is 131I-sodium rose bengal scan in another patient who had surgical correction of a choledochal cyst. This study also demon-strated a dilated bile duct and duodenum, with partial ob-struction of duodenum following surgery.

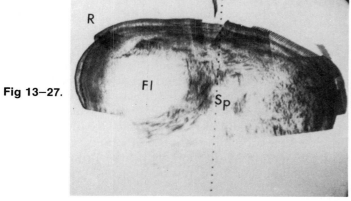

Fig 13–27.

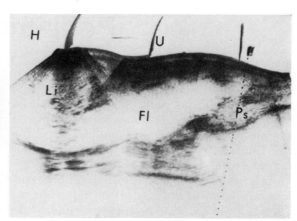

Fig 13–28.

Figures 13–27 and 13–28 are transverse and longitudinal scans of a patient in whom a lymphocele developed following retroperitoneal lymph node resection. R = right; H = head; U = umbilicus; Li = liver; Fl = fluid; Ps = psoas; Sp = spine.

14

Pediatric Pelvis

EVALUATION OF PELVIC MASSES in the pediatric population includes utilization of plain film, excretory urogram, barium enema, pelvic pneumography, conventional tomography, ultrasound and computerized tomography. A judicious combination of examinations results in rapid evaluation and diagnosis.

Bones, organ size, bowel gas pattern and abnormal calcifications are demonstrated by plain film, whereas renal function, kidney location and ureteral and bladder derangement are assessed by excretory urogram. During the initial phases of the excretory urogram, using high-dose contrast technique, differentiation between avascular and vascular pelvic lesions is often possible. Although this "total-body opacification" is more commonly performed in the evaluation of neonatal abdominal masses, this technique also has pelvic applications.

The ability to image the pediatric pelvis by ultrasound has condensed evaluation of pelvic masses and indirectly diminished overall gonadal irradiation. A full bladder is critical in the ultrasound examination.

Computerized tomography displays bone and soft tissue densities equally well. Computerized tomography presents the most information regarding the size and configuration of the tumor, which is useful for radiation therapy planning. Clips in the postoperative pelvis produce artifacts that may preclude adequate definition of tissue boundaries. On most conventional computerized tomographic body scanners, only a single transverse plane of examination is routinely available. Reconstructed longitudinal and coronal scans require additional software computer programs. The longitudinal and oblique scans for the most part are obtained routinely only by ultrasound. Reserved for the more complex situations, computerized tomography is discouraged as the primary diagnostic modality for the pelvis because of the associated radiation.

TECHNICAL CONSIDERATIONS

A 5.0-MHz or 3.5-MHz medium internal focus transducer is needed in the younger pediatric patients, and a 3.5-MHz long internal focus transducer in the adolescent patient. The distinction between cyst and solid is readily made in the larger masses, but as the masses reach a lower limit of 2 cm in diameter, the differentiation is more difficult. Beam width, transducer frequency and depth of the lesion are all determining factors in the ease of visualization of small lesions. When the cyst is superficial, 0.5–1.0 cm in diameter is the lower limit for this differentiation, and 1.0–2.0 cm when it is a deep cyst. The dynamic capabilities of real-time ultrasound should be taken advantage of when the question arises of pelvic abscess vs. multiple bowel loops.

Using a filled bladder, scans should first be performed in a transverse direction, the axis of the uterus determined, marked on the skin and longitudinal scans performed along this axis, angling the transducer to the right or left as necessary. Ovaries should be imaged in both the longitudinal and transverse scans, with the branch of the internal iliac vein posterior to the ovary as a confirmation of ovarian position.

The distinctness of the muscle borders is noteworthy, especially with regard to pelvic inflammatory disease, as discussed later in this chapter.

DEVELOPMENTAL ABNORMALITIES OF THE GENITAL TRACT

Early in fetal development, two pairs of parallel genital ducts are formed from the mesoderm, and are called the mesonephric or wolffian duct and the paramesonephric or müllerian duct. In the female fetus, the müllerian ducts fuse in the midportion to give rise to the uterus and the caudad portion forms the upper and midportion of the vagina. The most caudad portion of the vagina is formed from the urogenital sinus. The wolffian duct regresses and only remnants remain in the broad ligament, uterine wall and vagina. On occasion, there is failure of müllerian duct fusion and/or persistence of the septum between the ducts, or a combination of both, resulting in genital tract anomalies.

Congenital Absence of the Vagina

Absence of the middle and upper portions of the vagina that arises from the müllerian ducts is usually associated with the absence of the uterus and sometimes the fallopian tubes. The lower portion of the vagina, originating from the urogenital sinus, is usually present, although it may be hypoplastic.

The teenage patient, when first seen by the physician, usually has clinical evidence of amenorrhea, and hypoplasia or absence of the vagina is documented. Most cases are associated with the Mayer-Rokitansky-Kuster-Hauser syndrome. This syndrome is a relatively common cause of primary amenorrhea. The uterus varies from normal to the more common

finding of rudimentary or bicornuate cords with or without a lumen. Ovarian and serosal endometrial implants are common in those patients who lack only a vagina. Renal and skeletal abnormalities are also common. In one combined series, approximately one third of the patients had abnormal kidneys at excretory urogram; 74% had single agenesis or ectopia of one or both kidneys (Griffin et al., 1976). When hypoplasia or agenesis of the vagina is confirmed, an excretory urogram is mandatory. Of the various types of skeletal involvement, the axial skeleton and, to a lesser degree, the limbs and ribs demonstrate abnormalities.

Ultrasound delineates the presence of the uterus and is therefore instrumental in the planning of subsequent surgical repair.

Congenital Absence of the Cervix and Uterus

Although rare, uterine absence can be documented by ultrasound.

Congenital Anomalies of the Uterus

A unicornuate uterus results from a unilateral müllerian duct maldevelopment, whereas a unicornuate uterus with a rudimentary horn has partial development of the contralateral müllerian duct with or without communication of the horn to the uterus. Most rudimentary horns do not communicate but are connected by fibrous bands. If the endometrium in the rudimentary portion is functional, pain and an abdominal mass from blood rentention can occur at menarche.

Uterus didelphys refers to a complete duplication of the fallopian tubes, uterus, cervix and vagina. Variation does occur, resulting in a milder form of duplication, depending on the amount of müllerian duct fusion, persistence of the sagittal septum between the ducts, or a combination of both. Using acoustical texture information and careful scanning, 2 separate uterine cavities can be delineated. Caution is necessary not to interpret 1 of the uterine cavities as an adnexal mass, and the observation of the midline endometrial canal on longitudinal and transverse scans becomes important. Uterus duplex bicornis has 2 uterine cavities, 2 cervixes and 2 vaginas. This entity differs from uterus didelphys in that in uterus duplex bicornis there is fusion of the ducts but persistence of the septum.

Uterus bicornis unicollis indicates 2 separate uteri, 1 cervix, with 1 vagina. Milder bicornuate variations include uterus septus and subseptus, which result from a successful fusion of the ducts, creating a more normal uterine external contour but persistence of a part or all of the sagittal septum. Other variations include a single septated uterus with a double cervix and double vagina, as well as a single septated uterus with a single cervix and single vagina. The bicornuate uterus is relatively common among the anomalies, and careful transverse scanning from the vagina to the fundus of the broadened uterus will demonstrate a central canal in each horn. A hysterosalpingogram depicts the range of variations of the internal anatomy but cannot demonstrate the more rudimentary components, whereas ultrasound details the external uterine contour as well as the internal arrangement of the endometrial canal(s).

Bicornuate and unicornuate uteri are the common septation malformations of the female genital tract associated with unilateral renal agenesis. Any septation anomaly requires that a search be made by ultrasound and, if necessary, excretory urogram for both kidneys.

Skeletal anomalies of the vertebral column, scapulae and bony pelvis are also infrequently associated with septation anomalies.

AMBIGUOUS GENITALIA, HERMAPHRODITES

In infants with ambiguous genitalia, an immediate sex gender assignment is imperative. Ultrasound in a newborn female can consistently confirm the presence of a uterus, but this contrasts with the difficulty in demonstrating the newborn ovaries. In a normal infant, the ovaries may not have completely descended to below the pelvic rim, and an overdistended bladder is required. If ultrasound is not available, alternatively the internal genitalia can be demonstrated by pelvic pneumonography and a vaginogram.

Hermaphroditismus Verus

True hermaphroditism, although rare, can be present in the same individual, and the condition has 3 varieties: (1) Lateral. The testes is on one side, the ovary on the other. Usually the ovary is found on the left side. This variety accounts for approximately one third of the total cases. (2) Bilateral. Testicular and ovarian tissue is found bilaterally as an ovotestes. Approximately one fifth of the total cases are in this form. (3) Unilateral. Testicular and ovarian tissue is found on one side and testis or ovary is found on the other. This represents approximately one half of the cases.

Hermaphroditism in the true sense is rare, but the term is often used loosely to indicate a lack of consistency between gonadal morphology, external genitalia and secondary sexual characteristics. The complexity of the conditions and their causes has been well described (Pritchard, Novak).

Congenital Adrenal Hyperplasia

There is a varying degree of phallus development, with clitoral hypertrophy in a female. Virilization occurs in a genetically normal female as a result of an increased production of adrenocorticotropic hormone, which in turn stimulates and hypertrophies the reticular zone of the adrenal gland, resulting in an excess production of virilizing hormones. Early recognition of ambiguous genitalia and correct sex assignment using the diagnostic capabilities of ultrasound afford early treatment and subsequent normal female development at puberty.

Virilization from Maternal Hormonal Imbalance

Similarly, simple hypospadias and fusion of the scrotolabial folds are seen in newborn females whose mothers received progestins, androgenic steroids or had a virilizing ovarian tumor, including arrhenoblastoma, luteoma of pregnancy, Krukenberg's tumor and mucinous cystadenomas. Unlike congenital adrenal hyperplasia, these patients are not under continuous postnatal hormonal stimulation and will develop female secondary sexual characteristics at puberty. By delineation of the normal female neonatal internal anatomy, assignment to the male gender can be prevented.

Testicular Feminization

Testicular feminization, also known as the androgen insensitivity syndrome, escapes detection until later in life and at times is discovered in the evaluation of amenorrhea. This condition, a sex-linked recessive or male-limited autosomally dominated gene, results in a very normal-appearing female. The vagina ends in a blind pouch and the testes may be in the inguinal canal or in the labial folds, but are usually in the expected position of normal ovaries. Since testes in this circumstance are predisposed to malignant degeneration, ultrasound is useful in screening for tumors.

Partial Testicular Feminization

Partial testicular feminization is similar to complete testicular feminization, except that ambiguous genitalia are present at birth and some virilization occurs at puberty.

PRECOCIOUS PUBERTY, PSEUDOPUBERTY

True precocious puberty is always isosexual and indicates development of secondary sexual characteristics as well as an increased gonadal size and premature production of mature sperm or ova. Some pineal tumors, hypothalamic hamartomas, astrocytomas that occur with a male predominance, and Albright's syndrome, which has a female predominance, all are known causes of this condition. Idiopathic precocious puberty is the largest classification and has a marked female predominance.

In precocious pseudopuberty, the secondary sexual characteristics may be isosexual or heterosexual. The gonads may enlarge, but there is no gametogenesis. Ovarian tumors constitute a major etiological group in female patients with precocious pseudopuberty. The granulosa cell tumor is the most common ovarian neoplasm producing precocious pseudopuberty. Other ovarian causes are thecoma, arrhenoblastoma, lipoid cell tumor, embryonal teratoma, choriocarcinoma, chorioepithelioma and, rarely, benign ovarian cyst. Follicular cysts, common in childhood, are mostly nonfunctional. They are also commonly encountered in the ovaries of children with sexual precocity but usually are, with few exceptions, the result rather than the cause of the disorder. On rare occasions, removal of a benign-appearing cyst can result in cessation of precocious pubertal development. All of the abovementioned ovarian lesions are solid, except for the granulosa tumors, which can be purely cystic, mixed or entirely solid, and simple ovarian cysts. In young males, ectopic hormones can be produced by hepatoblastomas and in females by ovarian choriocarcinomas. Adrenal tumors, including adenomas and carcinoma, producing estrogens and androgens in children before puberty are rare. Adrenal glands, even in the neonate, are able to be visualized by ultrasound.

In the very young patient, the adrenal gland may have convex instead of the normal concave borders. Computerized tomography more consistently and reliably reveals the adrenal glands, and has even resolved tumors of 1 cm. Nuclear medicine with the use of ^{131}I-19 iodocholesterol isotope has correctly localized the side of the tumor, but has the disadvantage of the radiation dose and several days' imaging delay.

STEIN-LEVENTHAL SYNDROME

The exact pathogenesis of Stein-Leventhal syndrome, also known as polycystic ovaries, is not fully worked out. It is a disease of the neuroendocrine homeostatic control mechanism with distortion of the signal between the ovary and the hypothalamic-pituitary axis. The syndrome is characterized by bilateral polycystic ovaries in association with infertility and anovulatory menstrual irregularities, including amenorrhea, oligomenorrhea or dysfunctional uterine bleeding. An increase in the luteinizing hormone is present and usually there is mild to moderate hirsutism.

This condition lends itself to reliable diagnosis by ultrasound. Enlarged ovaries, usually 2–3 times the normal size, are present, with small horizontal echogenic lines representing small cysts that are beneath the limit of transducer resolution. Normal ovarian volume in a patient suspected of having Stein-Leventhal syndrome requires evaluation of the pituitary gland and adrenal glands to search for an extragonadal source of androgen production.

OVARIAN TUMORS

Simple cyst

A cyst can be of a simple follicular variety or it can be a corpus lutein cyst, which is formed from a follicle after the ovum is released and persists if fertilization and implantation occur. Theca lutein cysts, similar appearing, are most commonly associated with molar pregnancies and are frequently bilateral.

The obliterated vestigial remnants of the wolffian or mesonephric duct, referred to as Gartner's duct, extend from the broad ligament to the vagina and may be an incidental finding on a hysterosalpingogram. Cysts may arise from any portion of the duct and are called paraovarian cysts in the broad ligament and Gartner's duct cysts in the cervix or vagina. The latter are located in the anterolateral aspect of the cervix and vagina. Gartner's duct cysts, when examined by ultrasound, are thin-walled and sonolucent, with increased through transmission unless complicated by torsion or hemorrhage, with development of internal echoes signifying debris.

Benign Cystic Teratomas

Benign cystic teratomas or dermoid cysts make up a large proportion of ovarian tumors in young females. The average age of diagnosis in childhood varies from 13 to 15 years, although they have been present in children under 2 years of age. Initial confusion between the terms arose when dermoids were erroneously thought to form exclusively from ectodermal derivatives; however, mesoderm and, in some cases, endodermal derivatives are also present in these tumors. Benign cystic teratomas are presently considered to develop spontaneously from a totipotential ovum.

Bilateral in at least 10% of patients, most benign cystic teratomas are not discovered in the pediatric population until they produce a palpable mass, or pain from torsion on a pedicle, as this particular tumor is prone to do. Pelvic calcification or ossification on abdominal roentgenography occurs between 50% and 80% with observable teeth in 22–29% of these cases.

These tumors can have a relatively characteristic ultrasonic appearance, although they also can demonstrate the entire gamut of internal consistency from cystic to completely solid. Frequently they have discrete echogenic components. Malignant transformation of the mature cystic teratoma is almost unheard of in children.

Solid teratomas are more heterogeneous collections of tissues from the 3 germ layers, occur in a younger age group, that is, in the prepubertal female, and have a high incidence of malignant transformation.

Cystadenomas

Following puberty, cystadenomas are relatively common mucinous tumors, with respect to the serous variety. Approximately 5–10% of the mucinous cystadenomas are bilateral and on occasion grow to large proportions and undergo torsion with concomitant hemorrhage and necrosis. When a mucinous cystadenoma ruptures, the results are characterized by the presence of a sticky mucus substance throughout the peritoneal cavity produced by implanted mucus-producing cells.

Ultrasound can detect the presence of septae, which are found in both the mucinous and the serous cystadenomas, although more abundantly in the former. Papillary projections can on occasion be seen intermittently in the walls of the serous tumor.

Cystadenocarcinoma

Serous cystadenocarcinomas are more frequent than mucinous cystadenocarcinomas and both are relatively uncommon before the age of 14 years. The tumor can enlarge and reach into the upper part of the abdomen, but the patient is usually asymptomatic until the tumor reaches a size such that bladder irritation or a pressure sensation occurs. The intestines are rarely invaded by the tumor, but in later stages the lymph nodes are invaded. The relatively characteristic ultrasound image details septated cystic and solid components. Papillary projections, although occasionally seen in the benign variety, are more characteristic of the malignant serous ovarian tumor. Septations are present in both varieties but, especially in mucinous cystadenocarcinomas, the overall pattern is bizarre and distorted.

Granulosa Cell Tumors

A functioning ovarian tumor that may rarely be seen in the pediatric patient, granulosa cell tumor may be associated with isosexual precocious pseudopuberty. Although occasionally very small, the tumors tend to be large and associated with an increased abdominal growth, pressure sensation on the bladder and, in the young female, sexual precocity. Granulosa tumors are known to be rarely associated with malignancy. The majority of the tumors are solid, although some are partially or entirely cystic when examined by ultrasound. Ascites may be present.

Theca cell tumors, also functioning ovarian tumors, are less common in the pediatric patient and can also range in appearance from solid to cystic.

Arrhenoblastomas

Arrhenoblastomas are virilizing solid tumors and less than 5% are bilateral. These tumors are associated with defeminization and subsequent masculinization.

Dysgerminomas

Twenty-five percent of all dysgerminomas are seen in the adolescent and are associated with painless abdominal swelling. The average size of the tumor is 17 cm; it is bilateral in 10% of patients and may be associated with menstrual abnormalities. Dysgerminoma is a solid tumor with occasional associated ascites. Since the tumor metastasizes to the lymphatics, examination of the lymph nodes is necessary.

Endodermal Sinus Tumor

Endodermal sinus tumors are rare solid tumors, occurring primarily in young females and characterized by a rapid intra-abdominal growth and invasion of the retroperitoneal and intraperitoneal organs. At ultrasound the tumor may be mixed cystic and solid or purely solid.

Embryonal Carcinomas

Embryonal carcinomas are malignant and almost always fatal. They constitute approximately 6% of pediatric ovarian neoplasms, usually are detected in early adolescence and are characterized by progressive abdominal pain and an enlarging mass. The tumor is solid and nonspecific by ultrasound. Metastases are to the lungs, nodes, bone and liver.

Desmoid Tumors

Desmoid tumors are uncommon tumors that arise from the soft tissue and muscle and are classified as fibromatosis. Infrequently occurring in the pelvis, they can masquerade as ovarian tumors.

Gonadoblastomas

Gonadoblastomas are rare tumors found almost exclusively in the dysgenetic gonad. The patients usually have intersexuality and primary amenorrhea. A pelvic roentgenogram characteristically demonstrates calcification.

Metastatic Tumors

Undifferentiated malignant lymphoma, or Burkitt's lymphoma, symmetrically involves the ovaries, enlarging them to as much as 10–15 cm.

Acute lymphoblastic leukemia, embryonal rhabdomyosarcoma and metastatic adenocarcinoma all can involve and result in enlargement of the ovaries. Lymphomatous involvement of the testes is also observed.

Pelvic Neuroblastomas

Relatively rare tumors, pelvic neuroblastomas are solid and, if large enough, nonspecifically displace the rectum and bladder anteriorly. Ultrasound would show a solid echogenic posterior pelvic mass.

Hydrometrocolpos

Hydrometrocolpos is an accumulation of secretions in the vagina and uterus caused by excessive intrauterine stimulation of the neonatal cervical mucous glands by maternal estrogen associated with obstruction of the genital tract by an intact hymen, a vaginal membrane or vaginal atresia. Hydrocolpos defines only fluid in the vagina. Occurring in the newborn period, an abdominal and bulging cystic introital mass results in rapid clinical diagnosis. When the cause is vaginal atresia, an introital mass is not present and diagnosis is usually delayed. In this latter group, other congenital anomalies such as polydactyly, urogenital sinus and imperforate anus occur with an increased incidence.

This condition is called hematocolpos when the above-mentioned is associated with an accumulation of menstrual flow. The menstrual discharge accumulates in the vagina with partial water absorption and becomes inspissated. If not treated, it can result in increased pressure with hematocervix, hematometra, hematosalpinx.

The ultrasound diagnosis is characterized by a lack of visualization of a normal uterus and vagina, a large cystic mass that may contain some dependent internal echoes that represent debris, made up of epithelial cells and mucoid material, and clots.

This collection of fluid, if large enough, appears lucent at the time of total-body opacification during excretory urography.

EXTRAGONADAL PELVIC MASSES

Sacrococcygeal Teratomas

Sacrococcygeal teratomas, although rare, may appear in the newborn period with a clinical picture of bladder neck obstruction, abdominal obstruction, edema of the lower extremities and venous engorgement. Even though rare, they are the most frequent tumors of the caudal region in childhood. Composed of mixed tissues, they generally involve mesodermal tissue and arise from the primitive streak and Hensen's node.

Four types are known, and include the gamut of those completely external (posterior) to those with only internal components. The tumor is midline, and can be cystic, solid or mixed. Less than 40% are malignant. No cystic lesions have been malignant, whereas all malignant lesions have been solid. A plain film of the sacrum may demonstrate congenital malformation and irregular calcification or ossification, or pressure erosion of the coccyx or sacrum.

If bowel obscures the more superior tumor extent during the ultrasound examination, consideration should be given to evaluation by computerized scanning. Usually a very vascular tumor, it can become quite large, and although the large tumor is not necessarily malignant, it makes surgical removal difficult. Depending on the acoustical pattern and clinical presentation, rectal duplication, anterior meningocele, chordoma and neuroblastoma would be in the differential diagnosis.

Anterior Sacral Meningocele

Anterior sacral meningocele is a herniation of the caudal meninges and contents through an anterior defect in the sacrum. The mass is cystic, and lies between the rectum and sacrum. Clinically, constipation may result from encroachment of the mass on the rectum, and sacral rami may be involved or compressed by the tumor, causing numbness, tingling and pain. A characteristic deformity of the sacrum is usually present. This sacral deformity consists of an oval defect on one side in the distal third, with bony deviation to the opposite side and, at the lower margin of the defect, the tip of the sacrum and coccyx hook under the mass. Although clinically lipomas, hygromas, chordomas, gliomas and teratomas can occur in the sacral hollow, the characteristic sacral deformity is pathognomonic. On occasion, ultrasound may precede the plain roentgenogram, but the cystic nature of this lesion and its position demands a subsequent roentgenogram.

Sacrococcygeal Chordomas

A rare tumor, especially in the pediatric patient, the sacrococcygeal chordoma is midline, arises from notochordal remnants, usually involves 2 adjacent vertebral bodies and can extend intraspinally and extraspinally. A partially cystic retrorectal pelvic mass may be appreciated at ultrasound, but the diagnosis is usually suggested by plain films. Roentgenographically, there is midline bone destruction with an expanded sacral anteroposterior diameter reflecting its slow growth. An extraspinal soft tissue mass may be apparent on plain film with calcification or bony fragments noted in the periphery in about 30% of patients. Usually anterior in location, the mass may have a posterior component in one third of cases. The lateral view of the rectum on plain film or during a barium enema can confirm the presence of an anterior sacral mass.

The most difficult tumor to differentiate from a chordoma is a centrally arising sacral chondrosarcoma, which can be expansile and contain calcification.

Rhabdomyosarcomas

Rhabdomyosarcomas are the most common childhood soft tissue sarcomas, and 15% arise from the prostate or bladder. This embryonic sarcoma of the bladder and urogenital sinus represents almost 10% of the malignant childhood tumors. Although the survival rate of patients with prostate rhabdomyosarcoma is low, it is excellent when the sarcoma arises from the bladder.

Pelvic Lymphadenopathy

Pelvic lymph nodes are distributed along the iliac vessels and anterior to the iliopsoas muscles. At ultrasound, enlarged nodes are rounded and usually sonolucent. Minimally enlarged nodes may not be detected, but as they increase in size they impinge on the lateral bladder walls.

Ectopic Pregnancy

The ectopic implanted gestation may be on the ovary, in the fallopian tube or in the abdominal cavity. A teenage patient who has abdominal pain, bleeding, adnexal mass with a positive pregnancy test, or amenorrhea should be studied by ultrasound to exclude an ectopic pregnancy, as an untreated ruptured ectopic pregnancy can result in hemorrhage and death.

A ruptured ectopic pregnancy may have free cul-de-sac fluid and an enlarged uterus with a decidual reaction. The uterus may be displaced by a complex adnexal mass. The mass, the residual of the gestational sac admixed with blood, has strongly reflective dense echoes, representing either some fetal echoes or blood clots. Adherent fluid-filled bowel loops, endometriosis or acute pelvic inflammatory disease may at times be difficult to differentiate by ultrasound.

With an intact gestational sac, the diagnosis is somewhat easier. As a ringlike structure, the gestational sac may be visualized in the adnexa. If implantation occurs in the fallopian tube, the sac will be surrounded by fluid. Uterine enlargement and a general increased echogenicity may be present, correlating with a general increase in uterine vascularity.

Trophoblastic Disease

Lack of expected fetal heart tones should initiate a diagnostic evaluation to exclude molar pregnancy, fetal death or a uterine mass. Ultrasound most common-ly demonstrates a uterine mass composed of a homo-geneous vesicular texture, created by hydropic villi. If degeneration and hemorrhage occur, relatively sono-lucent areas are observable.

Two percent of molar pregnancies have concomitant fetal development. There is usually little uncertainty in the diagnosis by ultrasound, but occasionally differ-entiation between degenerating leiomyomas and ne-crotic ovarian tumors is difficult. Bilateral theca-lutein cysts, usually large and multiloculated, are also identi-fiable.

The diagnosis of invasive trophoblastic disease can-not be established by ultrasound alone but requires laboratory and clinical correlation.

ENDOMETRIOSIS

Endometriosis occurs in the pediatric age group, and is characterized by dysmenorrhea, abdominal pain and a pelvic mass. In one series, 40% of patients had developmental anomalies involving the genital organs.

Endometrial implants can occur on the perito-neum, uterosacral ligaments and ovary.

Adenomyosis, so-called internal endometriosis, usually is not diagnosed sonographically although the appearance of sinuous sonolucent areas in the endo-metrium has been described and represents blood lakes.

Endometriomas can be diagnosed by ultrasound and have variable internal echogenicity. The cystic pattern is an anechoic cystic mass with irregular walls and at times septa. Some cystic endometriomas have strong, rounded, highly echogenic areas in the depen-dent portions of the cyst, indicative of blood clots. The mixed pattern of endometrioma is indistinguishable from a pelvic inflammatory or other mixed ovarian mass. Solid endometriomas have a fine uniform gray-tone texture and can be mistaken for a solid ovarian tumor.

ACUTE PELVIC PAIN

Acute pelvic pain is well suited to examination by ultrasound, particularly if the patient is too tender to examine clinically. Torsion of ovarian cysts, in-cluding benign cystic teratomas, leakage or rupture of simple ovarian cysts or hemorrhage into a cyst, causes acute pelvic pain. Rupturing or leaking ectopic pregnancies, acute tubo-ovarian abscesses and ap-pendicitis can also have overlapping clinical symp-toms. The ultrasonic findings of all of these entities also can be similar, but a decreased uterine echogeni-city and poor separation of the mass from the pelvic side walls are important findings in pelvic inflamma-tory disease.

A twisted benign cystic teratoma and leaking ectop-ic pregnancy both have dark echogenic components and may not always be distinguishable, especially if the leak is not sufficient to identify fluid in the cul-de-sac. Fluid and mucus in adherent bowel loops can appear similar to a ruptured ectopic pregnancy. The β-subunit human chorionic gonadotropin laboratory test result, when greater than 5 units, confirms the pres-ence of early pregnancy, even at 10 days after concep-tion. A normal pregnancy with a large corpus lutein cyst can have clinical findings similar to an ectopic pregnancy, but they are separable by ultrasound, especially if the fetal age is at least 5 weeks.

Between 3 and 4 weeks, pregnancy is seen by ultra-sound as an excess of dark central echoes within the uterine cavity, which are nonspecific and ap-pear similar to menstrual blood or endometrial hy-perplasia.

PELVIC INFLAMMATORY DISEASE

Gonorrhea, the most common cause of pelvic in-flammatory disease, results in a severe mucosal reac-tion with the fallopian tubes as the target organ. If prompt, adequate treatment is not instituted, adhe-sions result that can occlude the tubes and result in a pyosalpinx or hydrosalpinx. These have a known association with subsequent loss of fertility.

Staphylococci and streptococci are the agents associated most often with pyogenic pelvic disease and can occur post partum or post abortion. Spread of infection is by lymph vessels and veins creating cellulitis and phlebitis. The salpingitis is interstitial, and so adhesions and their sequelae are less frequent. The endometrium can become chronically infected following an infected incomplete abortion.

In severe, acute pelvic inflammatory disease, the uterine echogenicity is diminished as a result of the edema. Separation of the adnexa, muscle planes and bowel is difficult. With time, tubo-ovarian or pelvic abscesses develop. The abscesses are sonolucent and thick-walled, with irregular borders, and can contain debris. With incompletely treated pyogenic and gonococcal infection, the uterine texture returns to normal, but the thickened adnexa persists for a more prolonged period. A hydrosalpinx develops from a pyosalpinx following disappearance of the infecting organism and replacement by clear fluid. With time, the pelvic side walls become distinguishable, the muscle planes distinct and the adnexa thicken.

In summary, ultrasound should be the first modality used in evaluation of the pediatric pelvis, and the result can direct the proper sequence of subsequent diagnostic examination. In those special situations where the relationship to osseous structures is important, or where bowel gas significantly obscures the region of interest or surgery has distorted the normal anatomy, computerized tomography can best display the anatomy.

REFERENCES

Aarskog, D.: Maternal progestins as a possible cause of hypospadias, N. Engl. J. Med. 300:75, 1979.

Anderson, F. M., et al.: Anterior sacral meningocele: A presentation of 3 cases, J.A.M.A. 237:39, 1977.

Anikwue, C., et al.: Granulosa and theca cell tumors, Obstet. Gynecol. 51:214, 1978.

Bennett, M. J.: Puerperal ultrasonic hysterography in the diagnosis of congenital uterine malformations, Br. J. Obstet. Gynecol. 83:389, 1976.

Blumel, J., et al.: Congenital skeletal anomalies of the spine: An analysis of the charts and roentgenograms of 264 patients, Ann. Surg. 28:501, 1962.

Breen, J. L., et al.: Ovarian tumors in children and adolescents, Clin. Obstet. Gynecol. 20:607, 1977.

Burkons, D. M., et al.: Ovarian germinomas (dysgerminomas), Obstet. Gynecol. 51:221, 1978.

Carter, B. L., et al.: Unusual pelvic masses: A comparison of computed tomographic scanning and ultrasonography, Radiology 121:383, 1976.

Danforth, D. N., et al.: Endodermal sinus tumor of the ovary, Obstet. Gynecol. 51:233, 1978.

Firooznia, H., et al.: Chordoma: Radiologic evaluation of 20 cases, A.J.R. 127:797, 1976.

Fleischer, A. C., et al.: Differential diagnosis of pelvic masses by gray-scale sonography, A.J.R. 131:469, 1978.

Fleischer, A. C., et al.: Sonographic patterns in trophoblastic diseases, Radiology 126:215, 1978.

Fore, S. R., et al.: Urologic and genital anomalies in patients with congenital absence of the vagina, Obstet. Gynecol. 46:410, 1975.

Fried, A. M., et al.: Uterine anomalies associated with renal agenesis: Role of gray-scale ultrasonography, A.J.R. 131:973, 1978.

Govan, A. D. T.: Ovarian tumors: Clinical and pathological features, Clin. Obstet. Gynecol. 3:89, 1976.

Griffin, J. E., et al.: Congenital absence of the vagina: The Mayer-Rokitansky-Kuster-Hauser syndrome, Ann. Intern. Med. 85:224, 1976.

Griscom, N. T.: Total body opacification, A.J.R. 131:919, 1978.

Haller, J. O., et al.: Ultrasonography in pediatric gynecology and obstetrics, A.J.R. 128:423, 1977.

Harcke, H. T, Jr., et al.: Bladder diverticula and Menkes' syndrome, Radiology 124:459, 1977.

Jereb, B., et al.: Ovarian cancer in children and adolescents: A review of 15 cases, Med. Pediatr. Oncol. 3:339, 1977.

Korobkin, M., et al.: Computed tomography in the diagnosis of adrenal disease, A.J.R. 132:231, 1979.

Lester, P. D., et al.: Pneumopelvigraphy in childhood, A.J.R. 131:607, 1978.

Lippe, B. M., et al.: Pelvic ultrasonography in pediatric and adolescent endocrine disorders, J. Pediatr. 92:897, 1978.

Little, H. K., et al.: Hematocolpos: Diagnosis made by ultrasound, J. Clin. Ultrasound 6:341, 1978.

Maklad, N. F., et al.: Gray-scale ultrasonography in the diagnosis of ectopic pregnancy, Radiology 126:221, 1978.

Mittelstaedt, C. A., et al.: Gray-scale patterns of pelvic disease in the male, Radiology 123:727, 1977.

Novak, E. R., and Woodruff, J. D.: *Novak's Gynecologic and Obstetric Pathology: With Clinical and Endocrine Relations* (7th ed.; Philadelphia: W. B. Saunders Co., 1974).

Pritchard, J. A.: *Williams Obstetrics* (15th ed.; New York: Appleton-Century-Crofts, 1976).

Ryo, U. Y., et al.: Adrenal scanning and uptake with[131] 1-6β-iodomethyl-nor-cholesterol, Radiology 128:157, 1978.

Sample, W. F., et al.: Gray-scale ultrasonography of the normal female pelvis, Radiology 125:229, 1978.

Sandler, M. A., et al.: The spectrum of ultrasonic findings in endometriosis, Radiology 127:229, 1978.

Sandler, M. A., et al.: Gray-scale ultrasonic features of ovarian teratomas, Radiology 131:705, 1979.

Scheible, F. W.: Ultrasonic features of Gartner's duct cyst, J. Clin. Ultrasound 6:438, 1978.

Schey, W. L., et al.: Clinical and radiographic considerations of sacrococcygeal teratomas: An analysis of 26 new cases and review of the literature, Radiology 125:189, 1977.

Seymour, E. Q., et al.: Gonadoblastoma: An ovarian tumor with characteristic pelvic calcifications, A.J.R. 127:1001, 1976.

Sherman, R. M., et al.: Anterior sacral meningocele, Am. J. Surg. 79:743, 1950.

Siegel, M. J., et al.: Radiographic findings in ovarian teratomas in children, A.J.R. 131:613, 1978.

Towne, B. H., et al.: Ovarian cysts and tumors in infancy and childhood, J. Pediatr. Surg. 10:311, 1975.

Utne, J. R., et al.: The roentgenologic aspects of chordoma, A.J.R. 74:593, 1955.

Walsh, J. W., et al.: Gray-scale ultrasound in the diagnosis of endometriosis and adenomyosis, A.J.R. 132:87, 1979.

Walsh, J. W., et al.: Gray-scale ultrasound in 204 proved gynecologic masses: Accuracy and specific diagnostic criteria, Radiology 130:391, 1979.

Wepfer, J. F., et al.: Mesonephric duct remnants (Gartner's duct), A.J.R. 131:499, 1978.

Werner, J. L., et al.: Presacral masses in childhood, A.J.R. 109:403, 1970.

Wilson, D. A., et al.: Ultrasound diagnosis of hydrocolpos and hydrometrocolpos, Radiology 128:451, 1978.

Wood, E. H., et al.: Chordomas: A roentgenologic study of 16 cases previously unreported, Radiology 54:706, 1960.

Woodruff, J. D., et al.: Mucinous cystadenocarcinoma of the ovary, Obstet. Gynecol. 51:483, 1978.

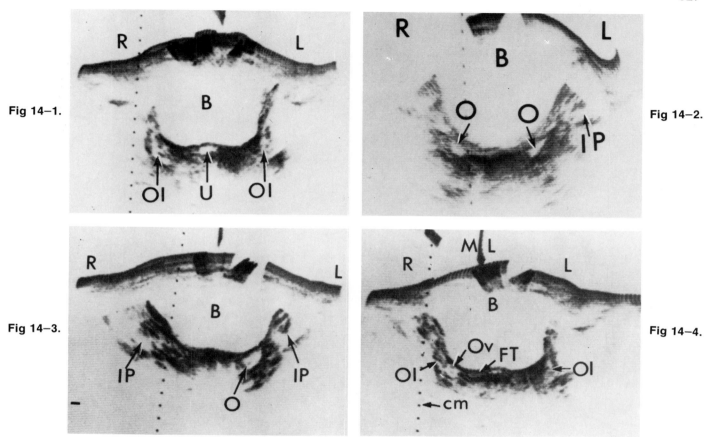

Figs 14–1 to 14–4.—Normal prepubertal pelvis. During prepubertal period, ultrasound of the pelvis involves transverse (Figs 14–1 to 14–4) and longitudinal scans with patient in supine position and full-bladder technique. Prior to patient's ability to control his or her bladder (approximately 2 years of age), sonographer has limited time to scan pelvis. In addition, pelvis is small, limiting scanning angles and making thorough examination difficult. As a result, although uterus can usually be identified in both transverse and longitudinal scans, and some of pelvic side wall muscles can be identified, it is not always possible to identify the ovaries. After 2 years of age, not only can uterus be identified but all of pelvic side wall muscles necessary for proper identification of ovaries can be seen. In addition, pelvis is of a size that allows multiple scanning angles.

In proper identification of ovaries, it is necessary to visualize obturator internus muscles as well as iliopsoas muscles. In addition, it is important to determine in which side of pelvis rectosigmoid descends. After identification of all these structures, ovary will be seen as an oval structure adjacent to obturator internus muscle. R = right; L = left; B = bladder; OI = obturator internus muscle; U = uterus; IP = iliopsoas muscle; O and Ov = ovary; cm = centimeter marker; ML = midline; FT = fallopian tube.

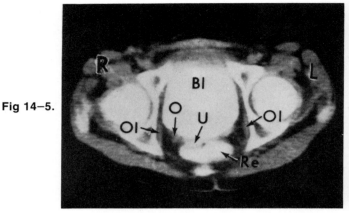

Fig 14–5.

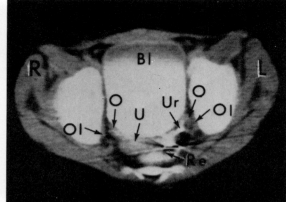

Fig 14–6.

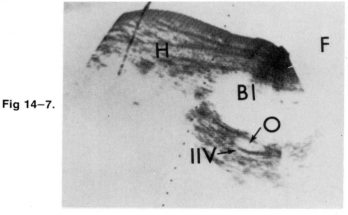

Fig 14–7.

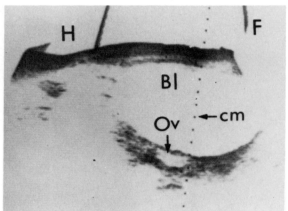

Fig 14–8.

Figs 14–5 to 14–8.—Normal prepubertal pelvis. Computed tomographic scans can also be utilized to identify uterus and ovaries of prepubertal child over 2 years of age (Figs 14–5 and 14–6). Identification is aided by rectal and urinary iodinated contrast material. Many deeper muscles of pelvis are readily identified and rectum is more thoroughly visualized than on ultrasound. Nevertheless, ovaries are small at this age and partial volume phenomena make measurement difficult. In addition, reconstructive techniques have to be performed to obtain all dimensions of ovary, which require thinner sections and therefore additional radiation.

Longitudinal scans of ovaries, however, can be obtained readily on ultrasonograms (Figs 14–7 and 14–8). These scans are frequently best obtained with scanning plane angled outward. Frequently tubular structure can be seen beneath ovary, which represents either ureter or one of internal iliac vessels. With this measurement of the ovary, in addition to those obtained for thickness and width on transverse scans, ovarian volume can be calculated based on modified prolate ellipsoid formula: Ovarian volume

$$\text{Volume} = \frac{\overset{(X)}{\text{length}} \times \overset{(Y)}{\text{width}} \times \overset{(Z)}{\text{height}}}{2}$$

In prepubertal age group, this volume should not exceed 1 cu cm. R = right; L = left; OI = obturator internus muscle; O and Ov = ovary; Bl = bladder; U = uterus; Re = rectum; Ur = ureter; IIV = internal iliac vessel; cm = centimeter marker; H = head; F = feet.

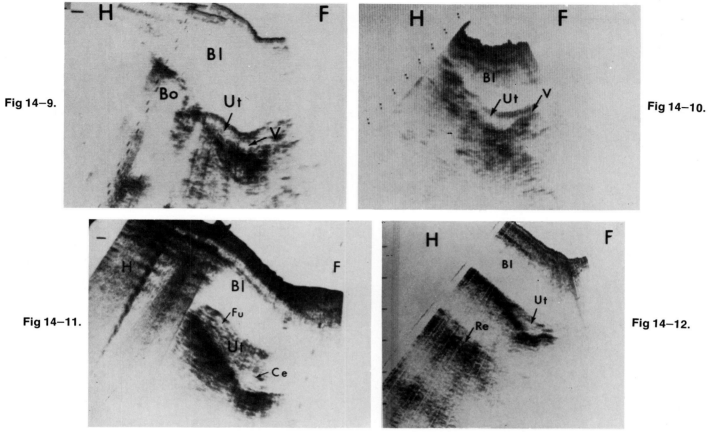

Figs 14–9 to 14–12.—Normal prepubertal uterus. After determining axis of uterus, longitudinal scans along long axis of uterus can be obtained. During immediate neonatal period, fundus of uterus may be equal to or even slightly thicker than cervix due to hormonal stimulation (Fig 14–9). However, after 4 to 6 weeks, maternal hormone stimulation is absent and uterus takes on shape it will maintain until puberty, with fundus thinner than cervix region (Figs 14–10 to 14–12). H = head; F = feet; Bl = bladder; Bo = bowel; Ut = uterus; V = vagina; Ce = cervix; Fu = fundus; Re = rectum.

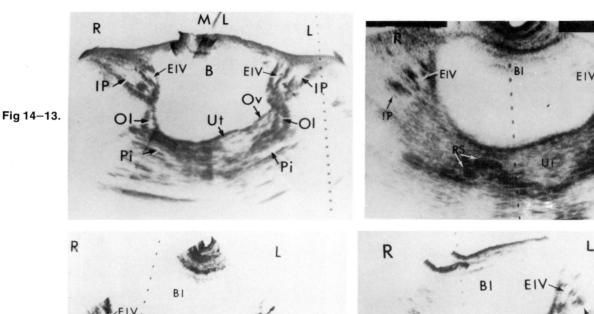

Figs 14–13 to 14–16. — Normal postpubertal pelvis. Postpubertal pelvis is also studied in transverse and longitudinal scans performed with patient in supine position with full-bladder technique. Proper muscle identification is again necessary in order to properly localize ovaries (Figs 14–13 to 14–16). Iliopsoas, obturator internus and piriformis muscles representing pelvic side walls should be specifically identified. In addition, the echogenic mucus pattern or shadowing gas pattern of rectosigmoid region should be visualized for it can mimic a mass (Fig 14–14). Ovaries usually will be found between uterus and pelvic muscle side walls, unless uterus is severely tipped to one side. In this situation, ovary on ipsilateral side may be found posterior or superior to uterus. In addition, external iliac and internal iliac vessels may be seen immediately medial to pelvic side wall muscles. Ovary may lie very close to iliopsoas muscle; however, end of this muscle is predicted by the echogenic region representing fibrofatty section of tissue around main nerves (Figs 14–13 and 14–14). Muscle usually ends approximately 1 cm medial and inferior to this landmark. R = right; L = left; ML = midline; IP = iliopsoas muscle; EIV = external iliac vessels; B and Bl = bladder; O and Ov = ovary; Ut = uterus; OI = obturator internus muscle; Pi = piriformis muscle; RS = rectosigmoid; Bo = bowel gas; Re = rectum.

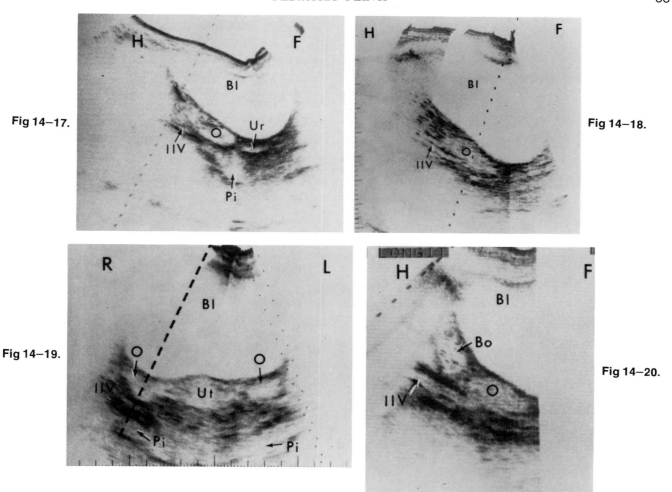

Fig 14–17.

Fig 14–18.

Fig 14–19.

Fig 14–20.

Figs 14–17 to 14–20.—Normal postpubertal ovaries. Longitudinal scans are necessary to obtain 3d dimension necessary for calculating ovarian volume. Scans performed parasagittally are inclined outward (Fig 14–20). Parasagittal scans performed in this fashion should demonstrate ovary immediately underneath bladder and either internal iliac vessel or ureter passing deep to ovary between ovary and piriformis muscle (Figs 14–17 to 14–19). It is not always possible to differentiate the blood vessel from the ureter unless one can see the blood vessel branch or the ureter continue down to base of bladder. Utilizing transverse and longitudinal scans and modified ellipsoid formula based on height, width and thickness measurements, ovarian volume can be obtained. Upper limits of normal for postpubertal primipara patient is 6 cu cm. Ovaries greater than 1 cu cm in volume are considered a manifestation of puberty. H = head; F = feet; R = right; L = left; Bl = bladder; Ur = ureter; O = ovary; Pi = piriformis muscle; IIV = internal iliac vessel; Bo = bowel; Ut = uterus.

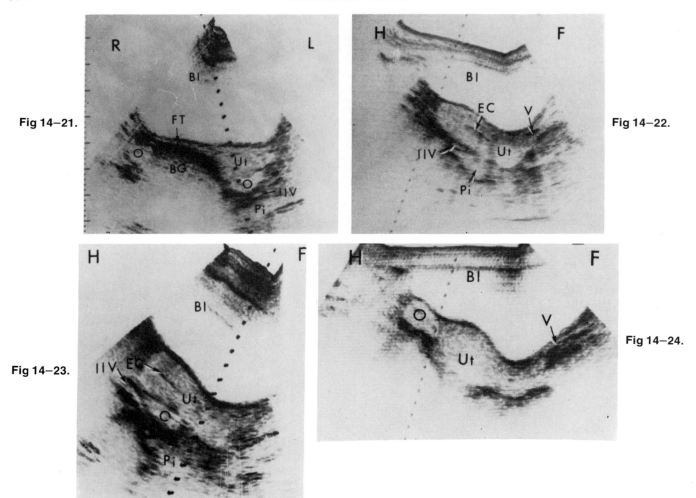

Figs 14–21 to 14–24.—Normal variations in postpubertal ovary. When uterus is tipped to one side, ovary may be located immediately posterior (Fig 14–21) to uterus. In this location, it is particularly critical that scan be performed through long axis of uterus and that piriformis muscle be specifically identified (Fig 14–22). Furthermore, identification of internal iliac vessel or ureter is mandatory, for both will course posterior to ovary and anterior to piriformis muscle (Figs 14–22 and 14–23). Alternatively, the ipsilateral ovary may be found superior to uterus (Fig 14–24) and should not be mistaken for uterine or adnexal abnormality. Furthermore, it may require a greatly distended bladder to push bowel high enough to visualize this ovary. This may be somewhat uncomfortable for patients. R = right; L = left; H = head; F = feet; Bl = bladder; FT = fallopian tube; O = ovary; BG = bowel gas; Ut = uterus; IIV = internal iliac vessel; Pi = piriformis muscle; V = vagina; EC = endometrial canal.

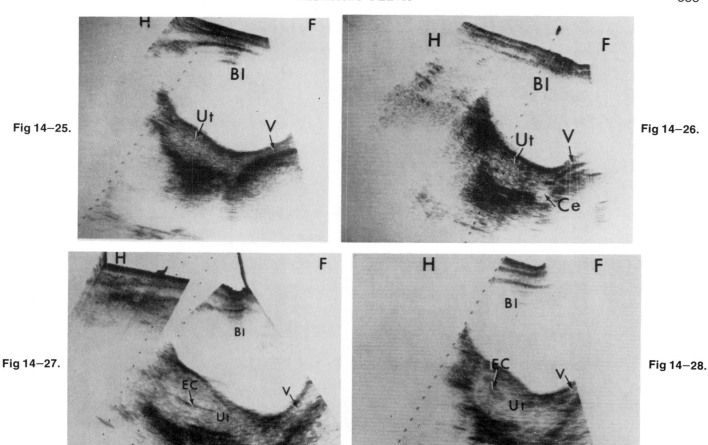

Fig 14–25.

Fig 14–26.

Fig 14–27.

Fig 14–28.

Figs 14–25 to 14–28.—Normal variations in postpubertal uterus. Normal postpubertal uterus may have a variety of texture patterns depending on stage of menstrual cycle. In general, uterine myometrial tissue has a coarse medium-level echogenic pattern. There may be no delineation of endocervical, endometrial or vaginal canals (Fig 14–25). This most likely occurs during 1st half of menstrual cycle. Alternatively, vaginal mucus and mucosa can be delineated as echogenic line separating the 2 vaginal walls (Fig 14–26). This may extend into endocervical canal, which remains secretory throughout menstrual cycle. Following ovulation, endometrial canal echo is visible (Fig 14–27). This may increase in prominence, being maximal just prior to menstruation. Prominent endocervical canal echo around the time of menstruation can be mistaken for early intrauterine pregnancy and sometimes only by serial examination can this differential be ascertained (Fig 14–28). Similarly, this echo complex may mimic the decidual cast of ectopic pregnancy. H = head; F = feet; Bl = bladder; Ut = uterus; V = vagina; Ce = cervix; EC = endocervical canal.

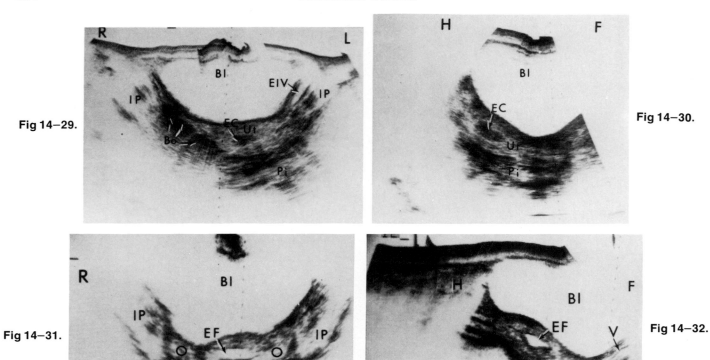

Figs 14–29 to 14–32. — Normal variations in uterus during menstruation. During actual menstruation a variety of endometrial canal echoes can be visualized. Prominent echogenic region centrally surrounded by slight halo probably reflects blood clot and edematous sloughing endometrium (Figs 14–29 and 14–30). Alternatively, one may simply see endometrial fluid representing fresh bleeding (Figs 14–31 and 14–32). Finally, pattern of endometrial fluid with deeper echogenic region may represent combination of fresh and old blood clot or fresh bleeding and sloughing endometrium. R = right; L = left; H = head; F = feet; Bl = bladder; IP = iliopsoas muscle; EIV = external iliac vein; EC = endometrial cavity; Ut = uterus; Bo = bowel; Pi = piriformis muscle; O = ovary; EF = endometrial fluid; V = vagina.

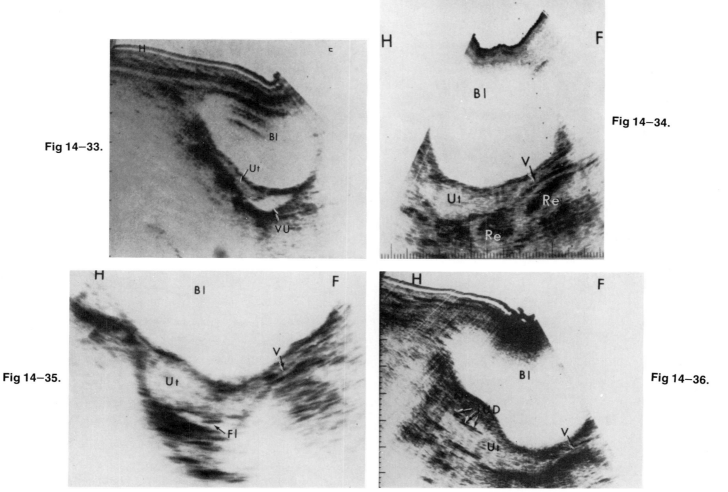

Fig 14–33.

Fig 14–34.

Fig 14–35.

Fig 14–36.

Figs 14–33 to 14–36.—Normal variations in pediatric pelvis. A variety of normal variations will be seen in pelvis in pediatric age group. One common finding in young girls is effects of physiological incontinence. Small amount of urine may accumulate in posterior fornix of vagina (Fig 14–33) and mimic fluid in cul-de-sac. However, this fluid does not usually extend more cephalad than posterior lip of cervix in contrast to cul-de-sac fluid, which may extend up posterior aspect of body of uterus. Another normal variant is prominent rectosigmoid, acoustical texture of which may mimic dermoid or even ectopic pregnancy (Fig 14–34). If confusion exists, fluid can be instilled per rectum to better define rectosigmoid region.

If patient is examined at the time of ovulation, a small amount of fluid may be observed in cul-de-sac (Fig 14–35).

Since such a finding may also be secondary sign of pelvic inflammatory disease, ectopic pregnancy or free peritoneal fluid, it is important to correlate this observation clinically with ovulation. Serial examinations could be performed for differentiation.

In postpubertal age group, it is not uncommon to find intrauterine devices that patient may be too embarrassed to mention. Intrauterine devices commonly generate very strong reflections, frequently in pattern that can identify type of intrauterine device and, with higher-frequency transducers, usually cast acoustical shadows (Fig 14–36). H = head; F = feet; Bl = bladder; Ut = uterus; VU = vaginal urine; V = vagina; Re = rectum; Fl = fluid; IUD = intra-uterine device.

335

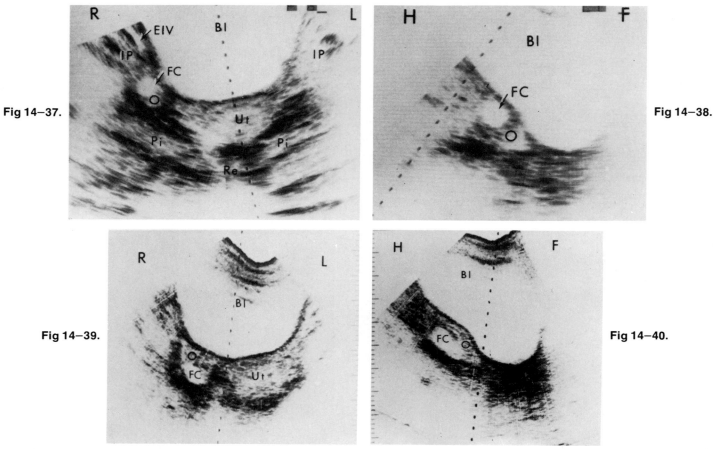

Fig 14-37.

Fig 14-38.

Fig 14-39.

Fig 14-40.

Figs 14–37 to 14–40.—Functional ovarian cysts. Functional ovarian cysts may develop during preovulatory and postovulatory portions of menstrual cycle. These are commonly seen on ultrasonograms as 1- to 2-cm fluid collections within ovary (Figs 14–37 to 14–40). This will increase ovarian volume, sometimes to 6 cu cm or greater. If any question exists regarding possibility of fluid collection representing pathologic process, serial examination through 1 menstrual cycle is appropriate. R = right; L = left; H = head; F = feet; Bl = bladder; EIV = external iliac vessel; IP = iliopsoas muscle; FC = functional cyst; O = ovary; Ut = uterus; Re = rectum; Pi = piriformis muscle.

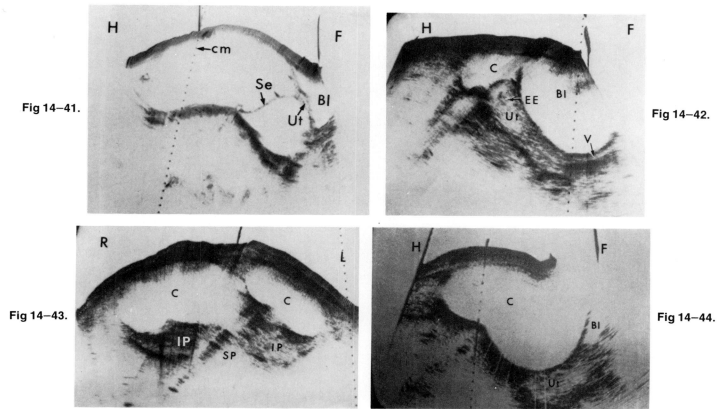

Figs 14–41 to 14–44.—Benign ovarian cysts. A variety of benign ovarian cysts appear in young girls, including serous cystadenoma, mucinous cystadenoma and follicular cyst. These generally appear as large circumscribed fluid collections that may have completely smooth walls or various degrees of septation and undulation (Figs 14–41 to 14–43). When septations or irregularities of the wall exist, then differential diagnosis from malignant process may not be possible. If these cysts are very large and reside in supravesicular region anterior to uterus, they may simulate the bladder (Fig 14–44). A scan following evacuation of bladder will allow differentiation. Benign ovarian cysts may develop bilaterally and therefore both ovaries should always be identified when possible. H = head; F = feet; R = right; L = left; C = cyst; Bl = bladder; Ut = uterus; Se = septum; cm = centimeter marker; EE = endometrial echo; V = vagina; IP = iliopsoas muscle; SP = spine.

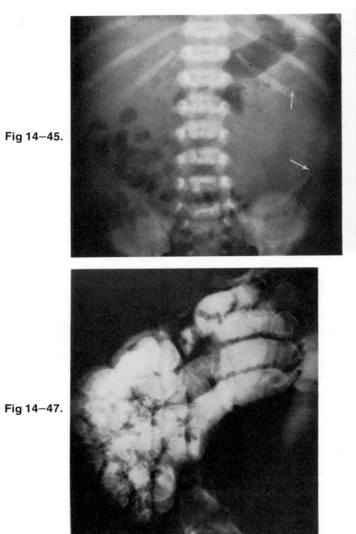

Fig 14—45.

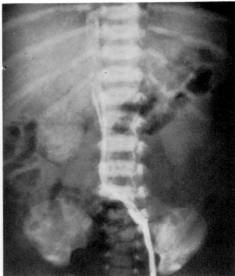

Fig 14—46.

Fig 14—47.

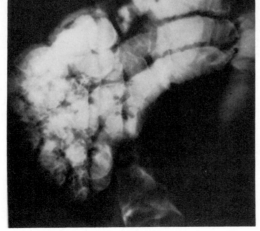

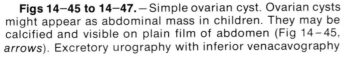

Figs 14—45 to 14—47.—Simple ovarian cyst. Ovarian cysts might appear as abdominal mass in children. They may be calcified and visible on plain film of abdomen (Fig 14—45, *arrows*). Excretory urography with inferior venacavography (Fig 14—46), will clearly demonstrate an extrarenal origin. Contrast studies of gastrointestinal tract (Fig 14—47) will demonstrate displacement of loops of bowel.

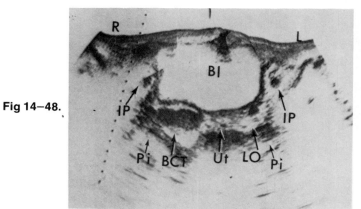

Fig 14−48.

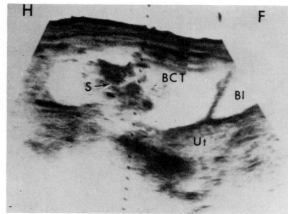

Fig 14−49.

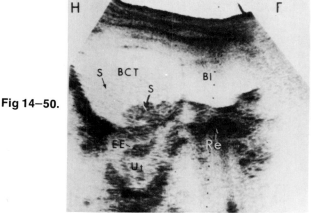

Fig 14−50.

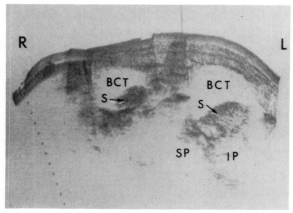

Fig 14−51.

Figs 14−48 to 14−51. − Benign cystic teratoma. Benign cystic teratomas are common tumors in young adults. One ultrasonic hallmark is presence of high-level echoes within these tumors, usually secondary to fat, dermal elements or skeletal elements (Fig 14−48). There may be variable degrees of solid and cystic components. The tumors frequently lie in supravesicular location (Figs 14−49 and 14−50). Since in 10% of patients benign cystic teratomas may be bilateral (Fig 14−51), it is important to try to identify other ovary. Completely solid benign teratomas may be difficult to identify in pelvis as they merge with other strong echoes from fibrofatty tissue. Nonetheless, if close attention is paid to bladder contours, which will be deformed by solid benign teratoma and not deformed by normal retroperitoneal tissues, such a tumor usually will not be overlooked. Another feature of solid benign teratomas is frequent high attenuation of sound. Therefore, close attention should be paid to degree of acoustical penetration on both sides of pelvis. R = right; L = left; H = head; F = feet; IP = iliopsoas muscle; BI = bladder; Pi = piriformis muscle; BCT = benign cystic teratoma; Ut = uterus; LO = left ovary; S = solid elements; EE = endometrial echo; Re = rectum; SP = spine.

Fig 14–52.

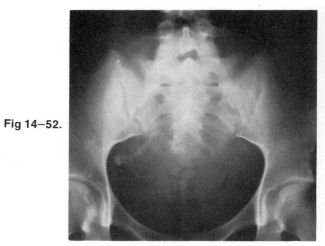

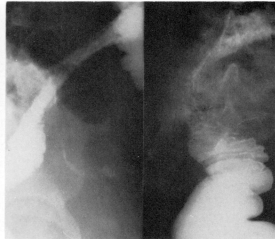

Fig 14–53.

Fig 14–54.

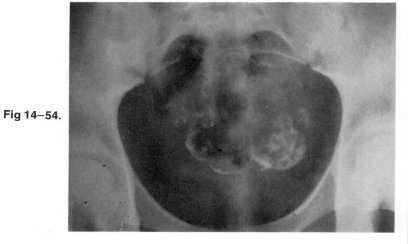

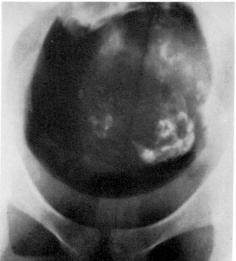

Fig 14–55.

Figs 14–52 to 14–55.—Ovarian dermoid. If ovarian dermoid is calcified, it will be visible on plain film of the pelvis. Sometimes calcification has typical appearance (Fig 14–52) similar to extremity, or tooth, etc., and no further diagnostic study is necessary. These lesions might cause extrinsic compression of gastrointestinal tract (Fig 14–53) or ureters. Pelvic pneumography, which was used with more frequency in the past, can localize the lesion to ovary (Figs 14–54 and 14–55). However, use of ultrasonography has tremendously diminished use of pelvic pneumography in pediatric pelvic lesions.

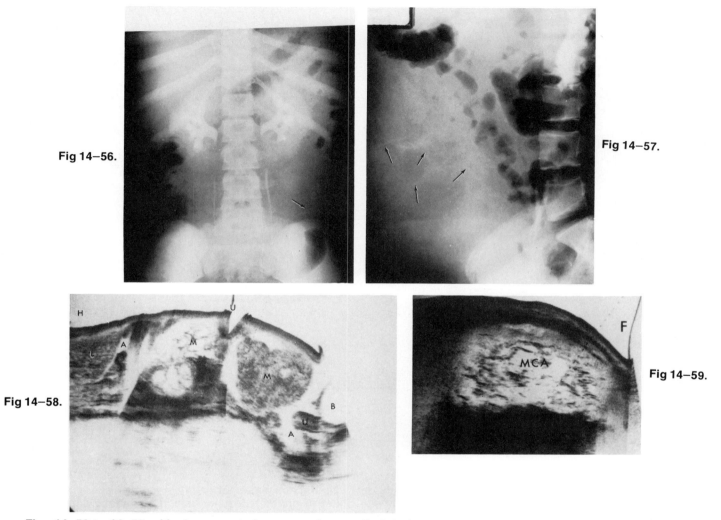

Figs 14–56 to 14–59.—Mucinous cystadenoma and mucinous cystadenocarcinoma. On excretory urography, these lesions would appear as anterior mass with areas of septations (Figs 14–56 and 14–57, *arrows*). It is not possible, ultrasonographically, to differentiate between cystadenocarcinoma (Fig 14–58) and cystadenomas (Fig 14–59). Both lesions appear as mixed lesions with septations. They may also be associated with ascites (see Fig 14–58). H = head; F = feet; L = liver; A = ascites; M = mucinous cystadenocarcinoma; U = uterus; B = bladder; MCA = mucinous cystadenoma.

Fig 14–60.

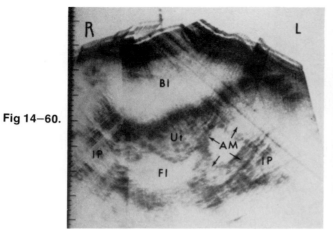

Fig 14–61.

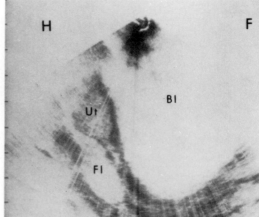

Fig 14–62.

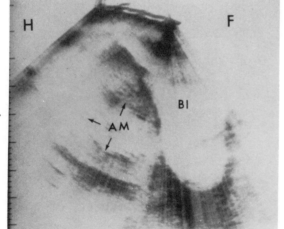

Figs 14–60 to 14–62.—Ovarian carcinoma. Although ovarian carcinoma is rare in pediatric and young adult age group, it may occur. The same findings associated with adenocarcinoma in adults are observed, with mixed (cystic and solid) adnexal masses frequently associated with ascites (Figs 14–60 to 14–62) demonstrated as free fluid in cul-de-sac or upper abdomen. Unfortunately, there is nothing specific about acoustical texture to distinguish these masses from either pelvic inflammatory disease or such entities as endometriosis or benign complex ovarian cysts. In fact, present case in 17-year-old girl correlated with clinical findings of pelvic inflammatory disease. However, serial examination demonstrated continued growth, particularly of solid elements. R = right; L = left; H = head; F = feet; Bl = bladder; Ut = uterus; IP = iliopsoas muscle; FL = fluid in cul-de-sac; AM = adnexal mass.

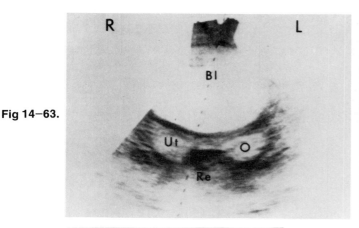

Fig 14-63.

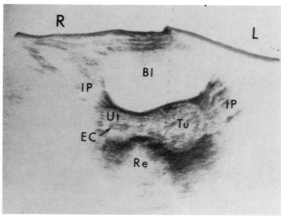

Fig 14-64.

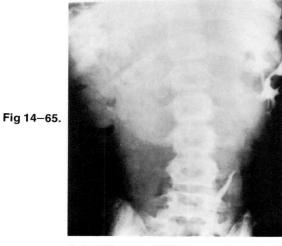

Fig 14-65.

Figs 14-63 to 14-67. — Dysgerminoma. Dysgerminoma is a more commonly occurring tumor in pediatric age group and is highly malignant. Rapid course of this malignancy is well illustrated in present case. This 14-year-old girl demonstrated normal left ovary on initial examination (Fig 14-63). Six weeks later, reexamination demonstrated tumor mass in left ovary with solid but clearly abnormal acoustical texture (Fig 14-64). Six months later, in spite of therapy, massive metastasis to retroperitoneum had occurred, as evidenced by marked displacement of left kidney and ureter laterally and nonfunctioning right kidney on excretory urogram (Fig 14-65) and obvious solid mass on ultrasonograms (Figs 14-66 and 14-67). R = right; L = left; BI = bladder; Ut = uterus; Re = rectum; O = ovary; IP = iliopsoas muscle; EC = endometrial canal; Tu = tumor; M = mass; Sp = spine.

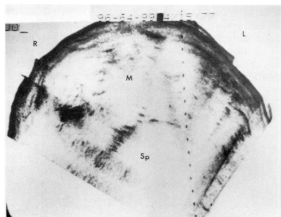

Fig 14-66.

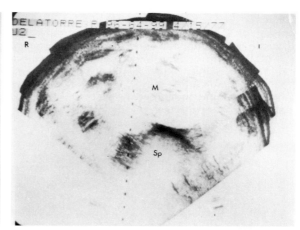

Fig 14-67.

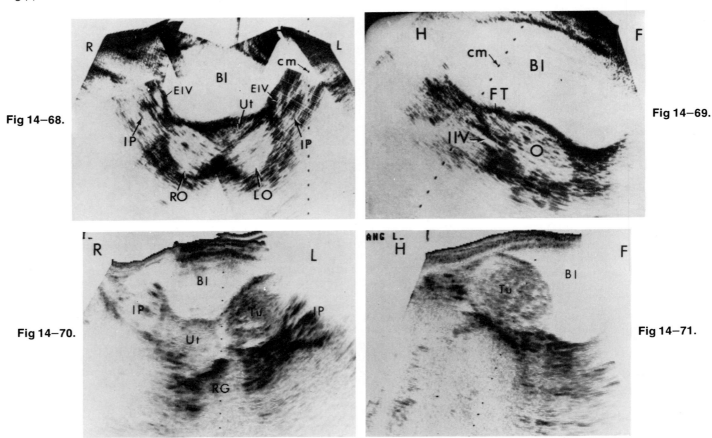

Fig 14–68.

Fig 14–69.

Fig 14–70.

Fig 14–71.

Figs 14–68 to 14–71. — Hirsutism. Hirsutism in pediatric age group may be secondary to polycystic ovaries in post-pubertal patient or functional ovarian tumor in any age group. Polycystic ovaries appear as enlargements of ovary greater than 6 cu cm in volume and frequently reaching 10–15 cu cm. Texture pattern within ovaries frequently contains multiple sharp lines indicating incompletely resolved tiny cysts (Figs 14–68 and 14–69).

Functional tumors of ovary have no distinguishing char-acteristics, usually having a solid acoustical texture with medium- to low-level reflections (Figs 14–70 and 14–71). Occasionally, fluid areas will develop, presumably secondary to necrosis. R = right; L = left; H = head; F = feet; IP = iliopsoas muscle; Bl = bladder; EIV = external iliac vessel; Ut = uterus; cm = centimeter marker; LO = left ovary; RO = right ovary; FT = fallopian tube; IIV = internal iliac vessel; O = ovary; Tu = tumor; RG = rectal gas.

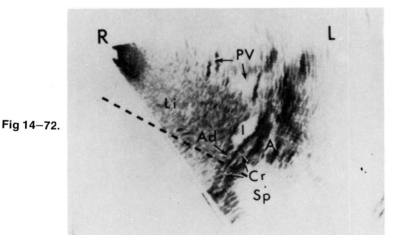

Fig 14–72.

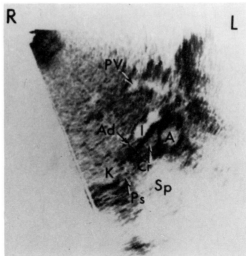

Fig 14–73.

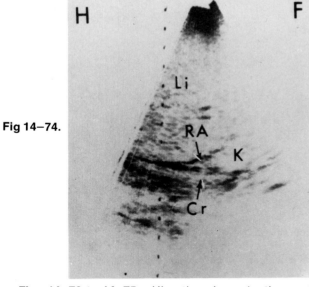

Fig 14–74.

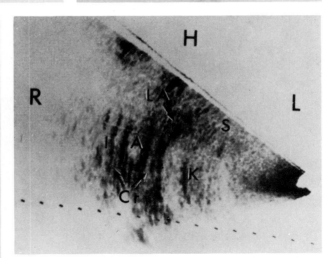

Fig 14–75.

Figs 14–72 to 14–75.—Hirsutism. In evaluating pediatric patient for hirsutism, adrenal glands should also be examined (Figs 14–72 to 14–75). A variety of clinical syndromes are associated with adrenal hyperfunction that may mimic those of ovarian cause. Adrenal glands are examined as described in Chapter 7. In various forms of adrenal hyperplasia, children may have ambiguous genitalia or, later on, various masculinizing syndromes. Adrenal glands may or may not be enlarged. As a result, ultrasonograms are most effective in showing functional benign tumor rather than establishing diagnosis of hyperplasia. R = right; L = left; PV = portal vein; Li = liver; Ad = adrenal gland; I = inferior vena cava; Cr = crus; A = aorta; Sp = spine; Ps = psoas muscle; K = kidney; RA = right adrenal gland; H = head; F = feet; LA = left adrenal gland; S = spleen.

Fig 14–76.

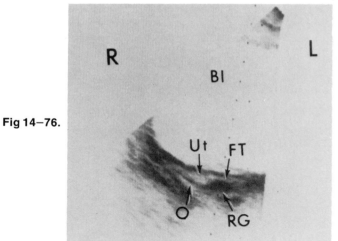

Fig 14–77.

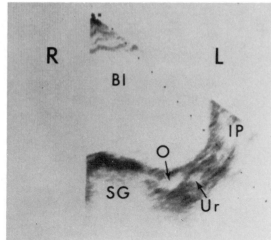

Fig 14–78.

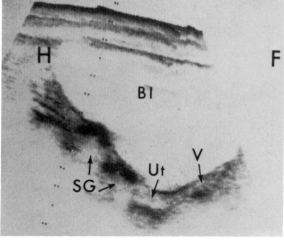

Fig 14–79.

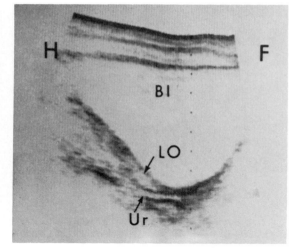

Figs 14–76 to 14–79.—Amenorrhea. Many children may have a delayed menarche. Most of the time this is related to biological amenorrhea. However, occasionally there is indeed primary ovarian failure, which can be demonstrated on serial ultrasonograms. Uterus remains prepubertal in shape and size and ovaries never attain a size greater than 1 cu cm (Figs 14–76 to 14–79). R = right; L = left; Bl = bladder; Ut = uterus; FT = fallopian tube; O = ovary; RG = rectal gas; IP = iliopsoas muscle; Ur = ureter; SG = sigmoid gas; V = vagina; LO = left ovary; H = head; F = feet.

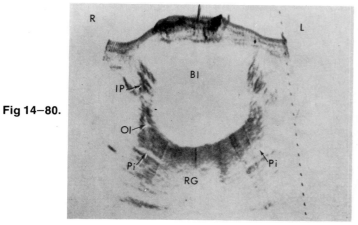

Fig 14–80.

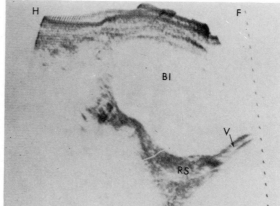

Fig 14–81.

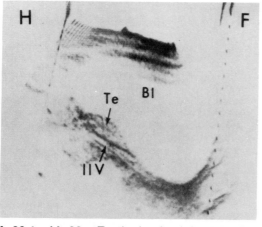

Fig 14–82.

Figs 14–80 to 14–82.—Testicular feminization. Another cause of apparent amenorrhea and delayed menarche is testicular feminization. Individuals with testicular feminization go on to develop secondary sex characteristics and appear as normal, often attractive, females. Nevertheless, uterus and ovaries are absent in these patients (Figs 14–80 and 14–81) and, therefore, they cannot menstruate. In fact, they generally have intra-abdominal or high pelvic testicular tissue. Ultrasonograms will demonstrate absence of uterus.

Ovaries cannot be identified; however, there may be tissue in high adnexal region that in fact represents testicular tissue (Fig 14–82). This may be mistaken for an ovary; however, texture is more homogeneous and medium-gray in tone. R = right; L = left; H = head; F = feet; BI = bladder; IP = iliopsoas muscle; OI = obturator internus muscle; Pi = piriformis muscle; RG = rectal gas; V = vagina; RS = rectosigmoid; IIV = internal iliac vessel; Te = testis.

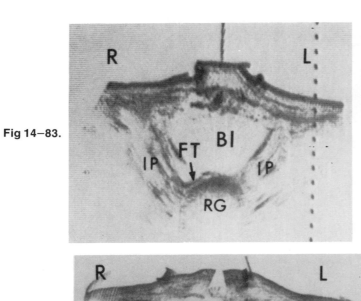

Fig 14–83.

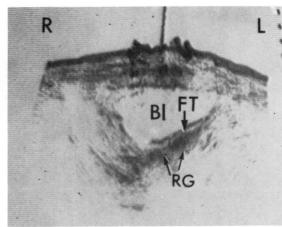

Fig 14–84.

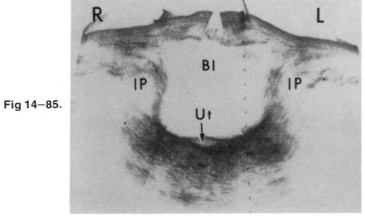

Fig 14–85.

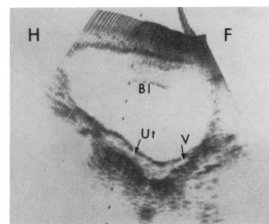

Fig 14–86.

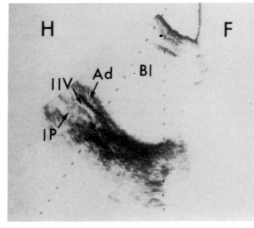

Fig 14–87.

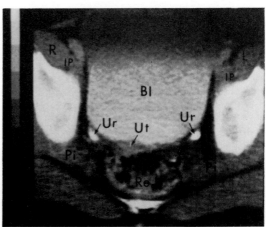

Fig 14–88.

Figs 14–83 to 14–88.—Gonadal dysgenesis. A variety of chromosomal abnormalities will lead to syndromes associated with amenorrhea. Perhaps the most common is Turner's syndrome or a Turner's variant (mixed gonadal dysgenesis). In these patients, uterus will be prepubertal in size, unless they are taking exogenous estrogen to attempt to stimulate their menstrual cycle. Although adnexal structures, including fallopian tubes, can be visualized on ultrasonograms (Figs 14–83 and 14–84), an adnexal enlargement representing an ovary cannot be visualized (Figs 14–85 to 14–87). If problem with bowel exists in these patients, computed tomograms (Fig 14–88) can be used to try to locate a high ovary. R = right; L = left; H = head; F = feet; Bl = bladder; IP = iliopsoas muscle; FT = fallopian tube; RG = rectal gas; Ut = uterus; V = vagina; IIV = internal iliac vessel; Ad = adnexa; Ur = ureter; Pi = piriformis muscle; Re = rectum.

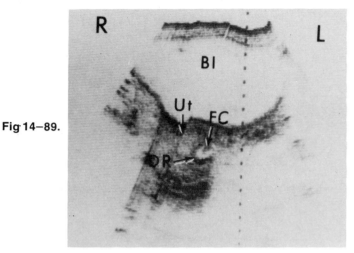

Fig 14–89.

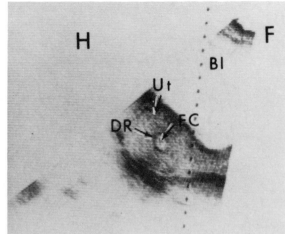

Fig 14–90.

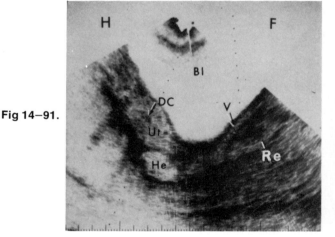

Fig 14–91.

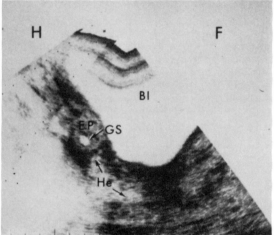

Fig 14–92.

Figs 14–89 to 14–92. — Ectopic pregnancy. In postpubertal pediatric age group, ultrasonograms are frequently performed to rule out intrauterine or ectopic pregnancy. Ultrasonography is most effective when reliable pregnancy test, such as the β-subunit immunoradioassay, is available. If this test is positive, then ultrasonographer's main job is to determine whether there is an intrauterine gestational sac. In order to avoid confusion with decidual casts within uterus which frequently accompany ectopic pregnancy, it is necessary to demonstrate both ringlike decidual reaction plus fetal complex (Figs 14–89 and 14–90). In cases of ectopic pregnancy, one may also demonstrate associated findings, such as fluid collection within cul-de-sac and an adnexal mass frequently containing highly reflective gestational components (Figs 14–91 and 14–92). R = right; L = left; Bl = bladder; Ut = uterus; FC = fetal complex; DR = decidual reaction; DC = decidual cast; V = vagina; He = hematoma; EP = ectopic pregnancy; GS = gestational sac; H = head; F = feet; Re = rectum.

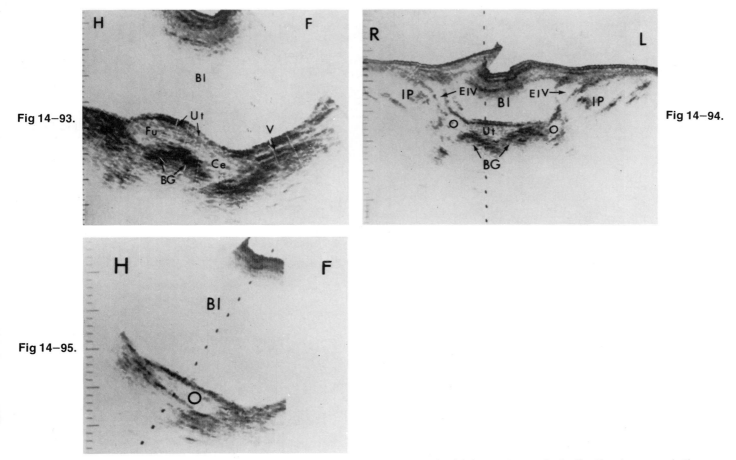

Fig 14–93.

Fig 14–94.

Fig 14–95.

Figs 14–93 to 14–95.—Precocious puberty. Many female children go through transient period of breast enlargement that is of no clinical significance. However, the question of true precocious puberty may be raised, and ultrasound is an excellent way to exclude or confirm this diagnosis (Figs 14–93 to 14–95). In true precocious puberty, ovarian volume will be greater than 1 cu cm. In addition, although uterus may not be grossly enlarged, fundus is frequently equal to cervix, indicating hormonal stimulation. In cases of exogenous hormonal intake, mimicking precocious puberty, uterus may be enlarged and menses may have occurred. However, in these children, ovaries will be normal prepubertal size under 1 cu cm. H = head; F = feet; R = right; L = left; Bl = bladder; Ut = uterus; Fu = fundus; Ce = cervix; BG = bowel gas; V = vagina; IP = iliopsoas muscle; EIV = external iliac vessel; O = ovary.

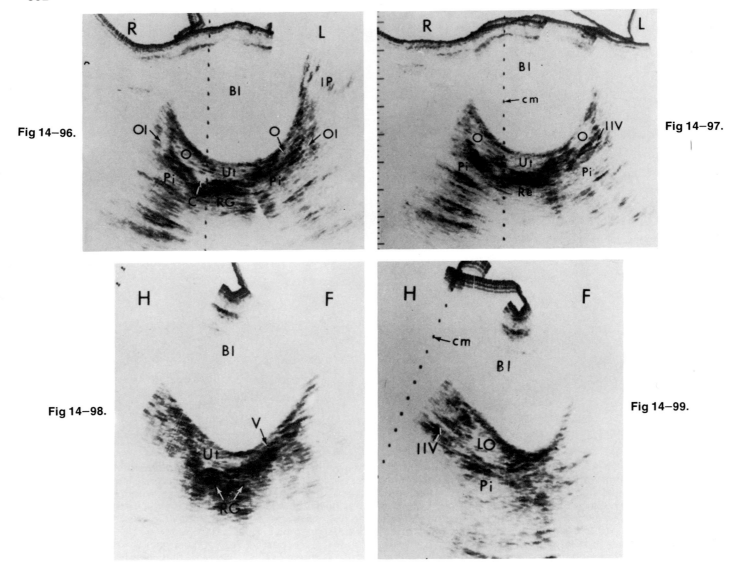

Fig 14—96.

Fig 14—97.

Fig 14—98.

Fig 14—99.

Figs 14–96 to 14–99. — Precocious puberty. In some cases of true precocious puberty, not only will ovaries be enlarged but functional cysts can be identified within the ovary indicating ovulatory process (Figs 14 – 96 to 14 – 99). Not in all cases of true precocious puberty will the uterus be enlarged or the fundus thickened. Uterine changes may lag substantially behind those of ovary. R = right; L = left; H = head; F = feet; Bl = bladder; OI = obturator internus muscle; O = ovary; Pi = piriformis muscle; C = cyst; RG = rectal gas; cm = centimeter marker; Re = rectum; IIV = internal iliac vessel; V = vagina; LO = left ovary; IP = iliopsoas; Ut = uterus.

Fig 14–100.

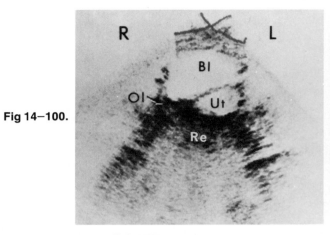

Fig 14–101.

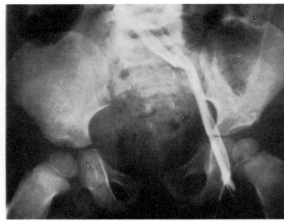

Fig 14–102.

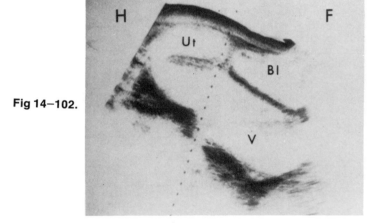

Fig 14–103.

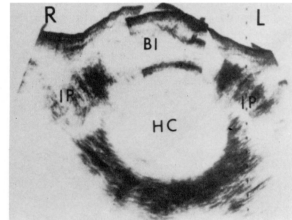

Fig 14—105.

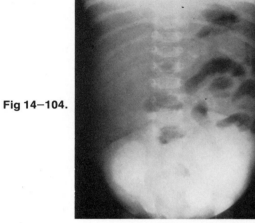
Fig 14—104.

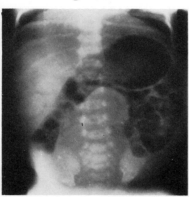

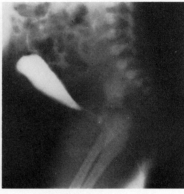
Fig 14—106.

Figs 14—100 to 14—106.—Other causes of uterine enlargement. In young children, uterus may be enlarged secondary to rhabdomyosarcoma. On ultrasonograms, this represents nonspecific increase in size of uterus (Fig 14–100). The nonspecificity of sonographic findings and clinical presentation may delay diagnosis, and patient may return with larger pelvic mass (Fig 14–101) with displacement of iliac vessels and ureters. Another cause of uterine enlargement, usually associated with apparent delay of menarche, is hematocolpos. Hydrocolpos, as well, is manifested by enlargement of uterus (abdominal mass). In these situations, blood or secretions fill vaginal and uterine cavities and distend size of uterus such that it would be palpable on physical examination. These lesions might be associated with renal anomalies (see Chapter 3). History, in conjunction with ultrasonography (Figs 14–102 and 14–103) or roentgenograms (Figs 14–104 to 14–106), will aid in making accurate diagnosis. R = right; L = left; H = head; F = feet; Bl = bladder; OI = obturator internus muscle; Ut = uterus; Re = rectum; V = vagina; IP = iliopsoas muscle; HC = hematocolpos.

Fig 14–107.

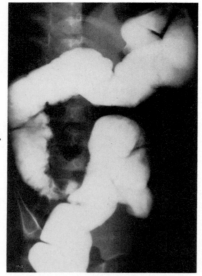

Fig 14–108.

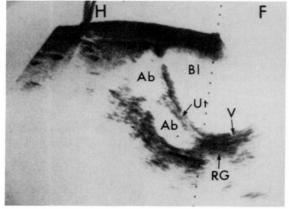

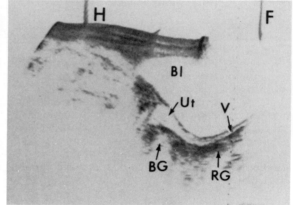

Fig 14–109.

Figs 14–107 to 14–109.—Pelvic inflammatory disease. Pelvic abscesses may be secondary to other intra-abdominal disease as well as venereal disease. In the case of appendicitis, roentgenographic studies such as the barium enema may suggest the diagnosis (Fig 14–107). Ultrasonogram in this case documents irregular fluid area around uterus extending into cul-de-sac consistent with abscess (Fig 14–108). Patient had an appendectomy and was treated with antibiotics. Follow-up scan two weeks later (Fig 14–109) demonstrated dissolution of abscess and normal appearance of pelvis. H = head; F = feet; Bl = bladder; Ut = uterus; V = vagina; Ab = abscess; RG = rectal gas; BG = bowel gas.

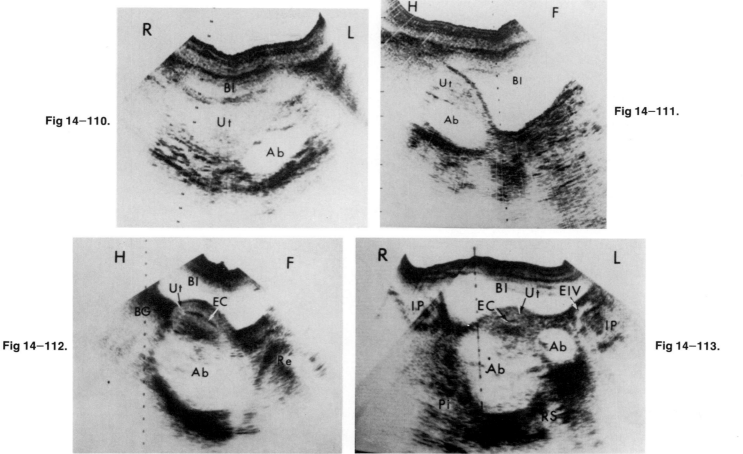

Fig 14–110.

Fig 14–111.

Fig 14–112.

Fig 14–113.

Figs 14–110 to 14–113.—Pelvic inflammatory disease. The most common cause of pelvic inflammatory disease in postpubertal pediatric age group still remains venereal disease. On ultrasonograms, in acute phase, uterus may be slightly enlarged and decreased in its acoustical texture. Irregular fluid areas may be demonstrated in adnexa or culde-sac, representing developing abscesses (Figs 14–110 and 14–111). Alternatively, adnexa may be just slightly thickened, particularly very early in the disease. Additional findings may be generalized difficulty in discerning various muscle planes as well as thickening of bladder wall.

Uterine changes will frequently return to normal very quickly following antibiotic therapy. On the other hand, adnexal changes may respond much slower (Figs 14–112 and 14–113). Ultrasound is an excellent way to serially observe patients who continue to have pelvic pain to see if abscesses are recurring or responding to therapy. R = right; L = left; Bl = bladder; Ut = uterus; Ab = abscess; H = head; F = feet; BG = bowel gas; EC = endometrial canal; Re = rectum; IP = iliopsoas muscle; EIV = external iliac vessel; Pi = piriformis muscle; RS = rectosigmoid.

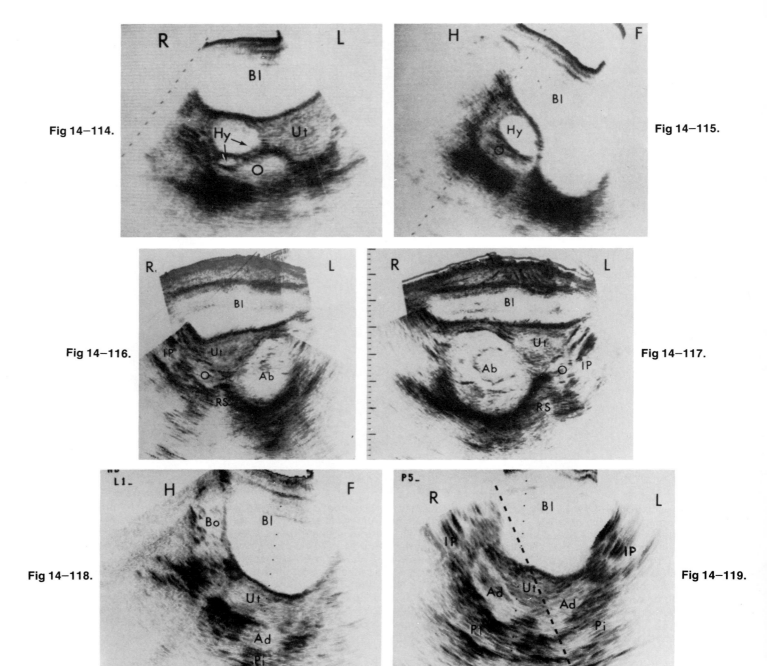

Fig 14—114.

Fig 14—115.

Fig 14—116.

Fig 14—117.

Fig 14—118.

Fig 14—119.

Figs 14–114 to 14–119. — Pelvic inflammatory disease. A number of sequelae can follow an episode or recurring episodes of acute pelvic inflammatory disease. Hydrosalpinx may develop within fallopian tube secondary to adhesions, and on ultrasonograms thick-walled, sometimes multiloculated, mass can be delineated, sometimes separable from ovary (Figs 14–114 and 14–115). Alternatively, abscesses may shift from one adnexa to the other, particularly when antibiotic therapy is not given for a long enough period (Figs 14–116 and 14–117). Or patient may have chronically thickened adnexa. On ultrasonograms, adnexae are found to be adherent to uterus and frequently muscle planes are difficult to clearly separate from pelvic organs (Figs 14–118 and 14–119). R = right; L = left; H = head; F = feet; Bl = bladder; Ut = uterus; O = ovary; Hy = hydrosalpinx; IP = iliopsoas muscle; RS = rectosigmoid; Ab = abscess; Bo = bowel; Ad = adnexa; Pi = piriformis muscle.

Fig 14–120.

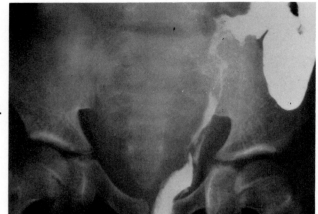

Fig 14–121.

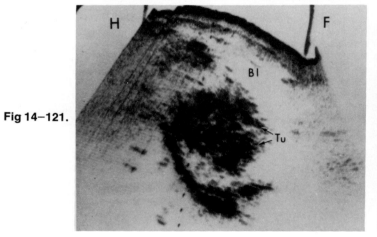

Fig 14–122.

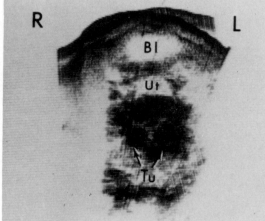

Figs 14–120 to 14–122.—Neuroblastoma. Although presence of pelvic mass may be identified with other roentgenographic procedures, such as barium enema (Fig 14–120), ultrasound has advantage of delineating size of the mass as well as providing some acoustical texture differential diagnostic information. In present case, pelvic mass is large and has very dense echo pattern (Figs 14–121 and 14–122). One process that can give this type of pattern is microscopic calcification, which was present in this patient with pelvic neuroblastoma. H = head; F = feet; R = right; L = left; Bl = bladder; Tu = tumor; Ut = uterus.

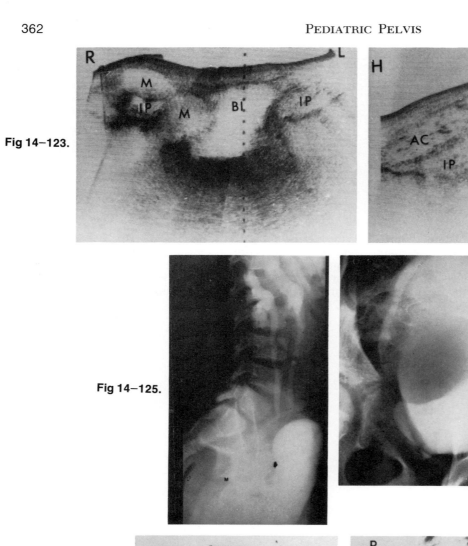

Fig 14–123.

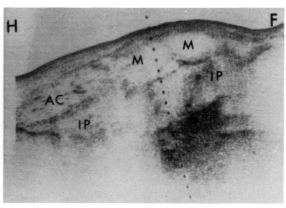

Fig 14–124.

Fig 14–125.

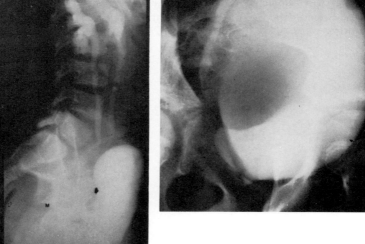

Fig 14–126.

Fig 14–127.

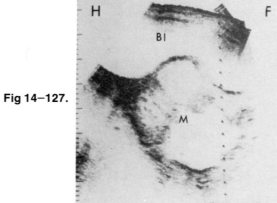

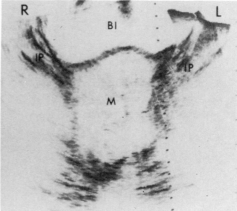

Fig 14–128.

Figs 14–123 to 14–128.—Pelvic lymphoma. Lymphoma most frequently manifests itself in pelvis by enlargement of internal or external pelvic side wall lymph nodes. These will appear as homogeneous solid masses indenting bladder and obscuring muscle planes of pelvic side wall (Figs 14–123 and 14–124).

Lymphoma may also appear as presacral mass displacing other pelvic structures anteriorly (Fig 14–125, *arrow*). This is identified on other imaging modalities, such as excretory urography (Figs 14–125 and 14–126). However, extent of the process can frequently be better evaluated on ultrasonograms (Figs 14–127 and 14–128). R = right; L = left; M = mass; IP = iliopsoas muscle; Bl = bladder; AC = ascending colon; H = head; F = feet.

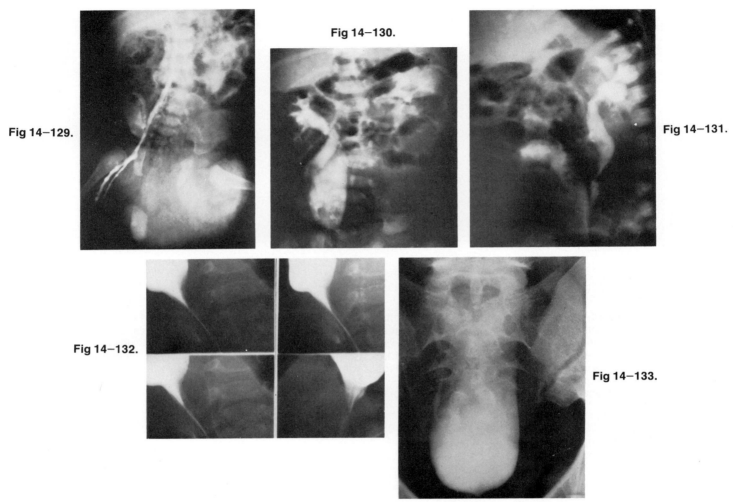

Figs 14–129 to 14–133.—Pelvic masses. Figures 14–129 to 14–132 demonstrate a pelvic hemangioma in a patient with Klippel-Trenaunay syndrome that shows characteristic early pooling of contrast material in the hemangioma (see Fig 14–129) during excretory urography, with posterolateral displacement of the bladder and bilateral hydronephrosis (see Figs 14–130 and 14–131). The mass has wrapped around the rectum, causing almost complete obstruction (see Fig 14–132). Figure 14–133 illustrates the typical appearance of pelvic lipomatosis with elevation of the bladder base and lateral compression of the bladder by a relative radiolucency.

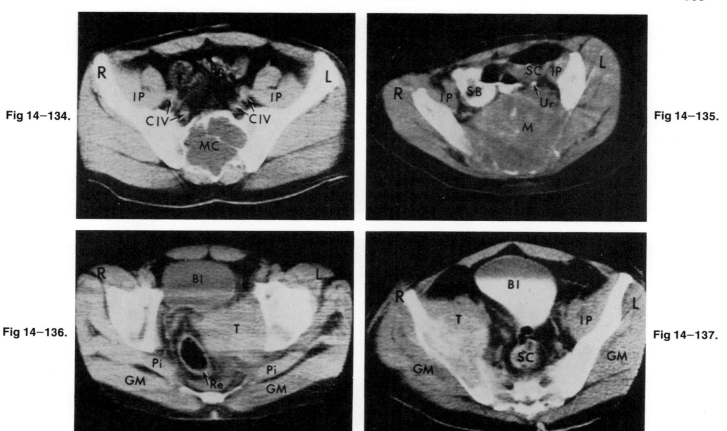

Fig 14–134.

Fig 14–135.

Fig 14–136.

Fig 14–137.

Figs 14–134 to 14–137. — Computed tomography of pelvis. The greatest role for computed tomography of pelvis involves diseases affecting bony and muscular elements. In cases of presacral or sacral abnormality, destruction or erosion of bone as well as solid or cystic nature of process can be determined by computed tomography. In this way such entities as meningocele (Fig 14–134) can be distinguished from other more solid masses, such as chordoma (Fig 14–135) or giant cell tumors. In cases of malignant tumors, such as sarcoma of mesenchymal tissues (Fig 14–136), or malignant tumors of bony elements, such as Ewing's sarcoma (Fig 14–137), computed tomography is an excellent means of determining degree of bony destruction as well as size of soft tissue mass. R = right; L = left; Bo = bowel; IP = iliopsoas muscle; CIV = common iliac vessels; MC = meningocele; SB = small bowel; SC = sigmoid colon; Ur = ureter; M = mass; T = tumor; Re = rectum; Pi = piriformis muscle; GM = gluteus maximus; Bl = bladder.

Index